Occupying Disability: Critical Approaches to Community, Justice, and Decolonizing Disability

Pamela Block • Devva Kasnitz
Akemi Nishida • Nick Pollard
Editors

Occupying Disability: Critical Approaches to Community, Justice, and Decolonizing Disability

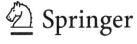

Springer

Editors
Pamela Block
Disability Studies, Health
and Rehabilitation Sciences
School of Health Technology
and Management
Stony Brook University
Stony Brook, NY, USA

Akemi Nishida
Disability and Human Development
Gender and Women's Studies
University of Illinois at Chicago
Chicago, IL, USA

Devva Kasnitz
Disability Studies
School of Professional Studies
The City University of New York
New York, NY, USA

Nick Pollard
Occupational Therapy
Faculty of Health and Wellbeing
Sheffield Hallam University
Sheffield, UK

ISBN 978-94-017-7746-9 (PB)
ISBN 978-94-017-9983-6 (HB)   ISBN 978-94-017-9984-3 (eBook)
DOI 10.1007/978-94-017-9984-3

Library of Congress Control Number: 2015943316

Springer Dordrecht Heidelberg New York London

Cover credit:
© Neil Marcus
Tent City 2011, Oakland, California City Center. Image Description: Somewhat battered protest posters, "Occupy Colonize" and "Everything Oakland," line a subway stairwell behind a metal hand rail. A bike wheel protrudes from the right, seeming to climb the stairs. The space is not accessible, yet it is claimed.

Printed on acid-free paper

Springer Science+Business Media B.V. Dordrecht is part of Springer Science+Business Media (www.springer.com)

Foreword

The editors of *Occupying Disability* have given us a book that is bold, critical, and radical. Its core project consists in "decolonizing disability." Toward this end, the editors offer a synthesis of three disparate kinds of sources:

- Occupational therapy, **a health profession** concerned with prevention and remediation of barriers to function and social participation of people with disabilities
- Anthropology, **an academic discipline** concerned with understanding the global and local forces—the discourses and practices—that reproduce cultures but also produce cultural transformations
- Disability studies, the intellectual side of **a social movement** that demands full citizenship and personhood for people with embodied differences

These disparate sources—their languages, perspectives on the human condition, conventional modes of action, and practical concerns—can overlap only partly, not fully. They also collide, threatening to career an unwary visitor into the "discomfort zone," a term the editors use to describe the bumpy, multiuse terrain of this book. What is so potentially uncomfortable or discomforting about this place? Why should anyone—anthropologist, disabled activist, occupational therapist—choose to go there?

The answer has to do with the idea of **occupation**. To be colonized is to have control taken away, to have the cultural and material foundations of our homeland seized by an occupying power. But the politics of liberation—with pain and joy—encourages us to do what is necessary so that we ourselves and everyone else can meet our human potential for individual growth and social participation. We insist on occupying the places where we belong.

Among the editors, contributors, and readers of *Occupying Disability* can be found anthropologists who are disabled and produce research on disability; critical occupational therapists who endorse disability rights over medicalization; and disabled artists and activists who aim to unsettle and transform exclusionary cultures. None are waiting around for others to agree with them or to give them permission to act. We are at a point of passage beyond stigma and inclusion. We are engaged and occupied.

Tensions do exist, however, among these multiple positions, standpoints, and intersections. For some of us to experience colonization, others of us must be colonizers, at least in some times and in some places, as situations shift. So the discomfort zone comes with a certain amount of risk. Identifying or being identified strongly with a profession, discipline, or disabled viewpoint may easily put one at odds with others in the collective project. In fact, it may put us maddeningly at odds with ourselves.

Welcome, then, to the discomfort zone. Prepare to read a post-disciplinary manual about occupation. You will find yourself in a place where a certain intellectual anarchy—the refusal to fit into set boundaries—restores a missing wholeness. What a challenging and liberating place to be.

Gelya Frank
Author of *Venus on Wheels: Two Decades of Dialogue on Disability, Biography, and Being Female in America* (Berkeley and Los Angeles: University of California Press, 2000)

Division of Occupational Science and Occupational Therapy,   Gelya Frank
Ostrow School of Dentistry and Department of Anthropology,
Dana and David Dornsife College of Letters, Arts, and Sciences,
University of Southern California, Los Angeles, CA, USA
9/14/16

Acknowledgments of Partnerships

There are many intersecting networks here that describe our collective and individual pathways: our literal and intellectual geologies. Editors Pamela, Devva, Akemi, and Nick would like to thank Maria Milazzo for her assistance in copy-editing chapter drafts. We must thank our contributing authors, too many to list here. And then there are the people who influenced all of us—albeit differently considering our varied ages and life histories—some as mentors, some as colleagues, some as friends, and some as partners in struggle. The lists are long. We thank Neil Marcus for setting the most productive and welcoming tone to the project and providing us with our cover image, and Leroy Moore and our many activists and artists collaborators for their knowledge, perception, wit, and juice. Then we would like to thank the people who straddle anthropology and occupational therapy: Anne Blakeney, Gelya Frank, Amy Paul Ward, and Sherri Briller. We all are also profoundly in debt to the following progressive occupational therapists: Lilian Magalhães, Frank Kronenberg, Dikaios Sakellariou, Mansha Mirza, Sue Magasi, and Sandra Galheigo. We are all influenced and supported by anthropologists of disability including Russell Shuttleworth, Lakshmi Fjord, Sumi Colligan, Gerald Gold, Nora Groce, Elaine Gerber, Michele Friedner, Pamela Cushing, Patrick Devlieger, Karen Davis, Rayna Rapp and Faye Ginsberg. And then there are the founders and definers of disability studies and the Society for Disability Studies (an organization of which both Devva and Pamela are past presidents), many with a foot/wheel in anthropology or a related social science or even occupational therapy: Kate Seelman, Richard Scotch, Mariette Bates, Helen Meekosha, Joan Ostrove, Joy Hammel, Nirmala Erevelles, Alison Carey, Noam Ostrander, Alberto Guzman, Petra Kuppers, Marjorie McGee, and Tammy Berberi.

Pamela: In addition to those mentioned above, Pamela would like to thank her mentors in disability studies (Christopher Keys and James Rimmer), in occupational therapy (Vera Jean Clark Brown in memoriam), and anthropology (Richard G. Fox) who influenced her emerging scholarship and helped her along this journey. She would also like to thank Dean Craig Lehman of the School of Health Technology and Management at Stony Brook University as well as Sue Ann Sisto, Deborah Zelizer, Eva Rodriguez, and Richard Johnson for supporting her scholarship and initiatives to build disability studies programs in our school and across campus. A special thanks to the growing list of disability studies colleagues at Stony Brook, especially Eva Kittay, Lisa Diedrich, Michele Friedner, Patricia Dunn, Michael Dorn, Carla Keirns, Kathleen McGoldrick, Stephanie Patterson, Sharon Cuff, and Lori Scarlatos. Finally, she thanks the Society for Disability Studies and all its leaders and members throughout the years that have sustained this vital community. Pamela is grateful for the love and support of her husband Matthew Lebo, children Shoshana, Isaac, and Harrison, sisters Hope and Karen, and honors the memory of our mother Barbara Kilcup and father Harvey Block, who left us too soon.

Devva: Along with those we all thank, I would like to highlight Russell Shuttelworth, my longtime anthropology/disability studies collaborator and revoicer, now MIA somewhere in Australia. I thank my fellow SDSers for 32 years of brilliance, in particular Elaine Makas, Susan Fitzmaurice, and Tammy Berberi. I thank the family who helped me keep house and home and chicks and child together while working on this and my past projects: My husband Earl Wyland, son AJ, and the whole mishpocheh: Saul, Mira, Berel, Doro, Estella, Dre, and Deborah and Lauren, you have my heart. I must mention Stephan Smith and Jean Ashmore of AHEAD; Mariette Bates of CUNY; Tom Seekins of RRTC-Rural; Joan Leon, Judy Heumann and Marsha Saxton of WID; Susan Schweik, Katherine Sherwood, Fred Collignon, and all our wonderful postdocs at UCB; Cyndi Jones and other activists in APRIL and NCIL; and so many others so important to my 64 years of growth. And then there are my mentors living and dead but remembered from Clark, Michigan, Northwestern, and UCSF: Jim Blaut, David Stea, Bill Lockwood, Arthur Vander, Skip Rappaport, Ronald Cohen, Margaret Clark, and Joan Ablon. I honor those with whom I had the privilege of working who are no longer here but help me daily nonetheless including Irv Zola, Ed Roberts, Harlan Hahn, Linda Gonzales, Daryl Evans, David Pfeiffer, Judy Ross, and Sam, Dorothy, Reva and Harold Kasnitz, and June and Bill Stone. And I cherish all my students and my fellow anthropologists with special personal hugs to those working on disability: Pamela Block, Lakshmi Fjord, Carol Goldin, Joe Kaufert, Lenore Manderson, Louise Duval, Steven Kurzman, Zev Kalifon, Mathew Kohrman, Linda Mitteness, Susan Gabel, Margaret Perkinson, and the list goes on (I'm sure I'll miss someone important) who helped me to establish the mutual listening skills of anthropologists and disability studies thinkers. Thanks to my sister Rabbi Naomi Steinberg for being.

Akemi: I would like to thank my fellow editors—Pamela, Devva, and Nick—for their patience and rigorous guidance as I learn how an edited book is collaboratively created. My gratitude also goes to Park McArthur and Joe Martello for their physical and intellectual labor of editing my writings. Acknowledgments are needed for my academic mentors, Michelle Fine, Dan Goodley, Wendy Luttrell, and Nirmala Erevelles, as well as activist mentors Leroy Moore, Patricia Berne and Sebastian Margaret for their constant nurturing and educating of me (and the world) and for reminding me to keep myself accountable to my academic work and standpoint.

Nick: I would like to thank my wife, Linda, and Molly, Joshua, and Daisy for putting up with me working at home (again), and Sally, Ben, and Crystal for tolerating me working at their house too. Thanks to my colleagues and students in the Faculty of Health and Wellbeing at Sheffield Hallam University for their support and interest during this project and especially those who share my office. Thanks to Dikaios Sakellariou for his patience as sometimes this took precedence in our projects and he has carried the load. Thanks to Mark Doel, Sarah Cook, and Gordon Grant for keeping me on track while finishing the PhD that ran alongside this editing. Thanks to everyone at Pecket Learning Community and the Writing Occupation group from whom I've had a lot of useful mentoring. Thanks to my fellow editors and all the contributing authors for making this such an enjoyable and stimulating time.

Contents

Part I

Decolonizing Disability

Editors' Note: For an introduction to Part I see Sect. 25.1

Occupying Disability: An Introduction

Pamela Block, Devva Kasnitz, Akemi Nishida, and Nick Pollard

Abstract

Inspired by disability justice and the fall 2011 "Disability Occupy Wall Street/Decolonize Disability" movements in the US and related activism elsewhere, we are interested in politically engaged critical approaches to disability that intersect academic fields—principally occupational therapy, disability studies and anthropology—as well as community organizing and the arts. The "occupy" international movements claim collective identities as does *Occupying Disability: Critical Approaches to Community, Justice, and Decolonizing Disability*. International disability movements claim disability as a collective identity rather than a medical category and recognize the political and economic dimensions of disability inequity as it intersects with other sources of inequality. Different political positions have evolved within different disability perspectives, all of which demand audience. Working with them and understanding them

P. Block (✉)
Disability Studies, Health and Rehabilitation Sciences, School of Health Technology and Management, Stony Brook University, Stony Brook, NY, USA
e-mail: pamela.block@stonybrook.edu

D. Kasnitz
Disability Studies, School of Professional Studies, The City University of New York, New York, NY, USA
e-mail: devva@earthlink.net

A. Nishida
Disability and Human Development, Gender and Women's Studies, University of Illinois at Chicago, Chicago, IL, USA
e-mail: anishida922@gmail.com

N. Pollard
Occupational Therapy, Faculty of Health and Wellbeing, Sheffield Hallam University, Sheffield, UK
e-mail: N.Pollard@shu.ac.uk

© Springer Science+Business Media Dordrecht 2016
P. Block et al. (eds.), *Occupying Disability: Critical Approaches to Community, Justice, and Decolonizing Disability*, DOI 10.1007/978-94-017-9984-3_1

3

requires broader social critiques not usually part of most clinical educations. Some activists would not, as a matter of principle, engage clinicians because of their unfettered access to agency and operations of power. Negotiation of separatist consciousness is a stage to forming identities in many political movements. Yet we, as editors and authors strive to move beyond simple binaries: the goal is true participation, meaningful occupation, and disability justice.

Keywords
Occupation • Occupational • Occupying • Occupational therapy • Occupational science • Disability • Disability studies • Anthropology • Theory • Practice • Activism • Justice • Decolonize • Community • Movements

1.1   Anthropology, Disability Studies, and Occupational Therapy

This book provides a discursive space where the concepts of disability, culture, and occupation meet critical theory, activism, and the creative arts. There are books that challenge occupational therapists to engage in innovative, community-based and politically relevant practice, however, there are no books that draw from anthropology and disability studies together to push the boundaries of how occupational therapy/science approaches disability. Similarly, the "Occupational Therapy without Borders" literature has great relevance to anthropology and disability studies— offering (as Gelya Frank has been telling us for many years) innovative ideas about what to *do* with all this theoretical training—but this literature is regrettably not known to most anthropologists and disability studies scholars (Frank et al. 2008). Even the use of "occupational science" and "applied anthropology" nomenclature has not served to bridge contested and negatively value-loaded academic and professional boundaries that variously characterize occupational therapy as clinical and atheoretical, anthropology as an esoteric soft science, and disability studies as an interesting self-indulgence for the disabled.

Our contributing authors come from a variety of professional, academic, and activist backgrounds in order to include perspectives from theory, practice, and experiences of disability. The authors are premiere scholars and practitioners, as well as emerging theorists and activists drawn from all three fields of study and from around the globe. Our principal themes include: all the permutations of the concept of "occupy;" disability activism and decolonization work; marginalization and minoritization; technology; and struggle, creativity, and change. Moving well beyond traditional clinical formulations of disability, this book will engage clinicians, social scientists, activists and artists in dialogues about disability as a theoretical construct and as lived experience. In other words, the goal of this volume is to consider disability, not in terms of pathology or impairment, but as a range of unique social identities and experiences that are shaped by a full spectrum of always visible—sometimes perceivable—usually invisible— diagnoses/impairments/embodied differences, connected to socio-cultural values, assumptions, and environmental barriers. We try to look at disability analytically but without confining it to any particular definition. We allow authors to define their own terms appropriate to their purpose. Terminological definitions should be tied to theoretical positions, and these in turn should be chosen not only by what intellectually satisfies, but by what supports action toward human flourishing. We probe deeper and broader than usual visible/invisible, physical/psychiatric, acute/chronic binaries.

Negotiation of separatist consciousness is a stage to forming identities in many political movements. In this evolving dialogue there may be some issues of coherence, it is not an arena where everyone speaks in the same academic language, because it is a space shaped by inequality—in access to places and platforms, in opportunities for education and expression, and in struggles for resourcing and a right to daily existence. The languages used are themselves determined by these experiences and at times there will be no consensus about appropriate terms, no clear agreement. An emergent discourse is not an easy one to follow. We have had to step back from taking the traditional academic editorial role, which in this project would have stifled the authors. It is not appropriate here to correct the way people have written in their own words what they have wanted to say, except perhaps to make some adjustments for clarity. Instead, we hope we have tried to let the conversation flow. We're excited about working with the authors to present these discussions in the same volume, and look forward to the arguments and debates that we hope it may stimulate the reader to take up. In the course of editing this book, we have had some of those debates ourselves and so feel at first hand that it is an emergent discourse. As editors and authors we strive to move beyond simple binaries: the goals are true participation, meaningful occupation, and justice for disabled people.

The concept of "occupation" is also intentionally a moving target in this book. Some authors will discuss occupying spaces as a form of protest or, alternatively, protesting against territorial occupations. Others will discuss occupations as framed or problematized within the fields of occupational therapy and occupational science and anthropology as engagement in meaningful activities. Others will frame it, as Friedner (Chap. 14) does explicitly, in terms of occupying time and space in or out of the workplace.

There are marked tensions about just who occupies disability in the sense that countless professional jobs have been created to "support" disabled people across the life course in educational, rehabilitation, and service fields, while disabled people themselves struggle for employment. There are disabled occupational therapists and anthropologists, but they are pretty rare and barriers are legion: from licensing specifications or expectations of exotic fieldwork that can be used to exclude students from these fields, to the inaccessibility of national conferences that deter the participation of all disabled professionals—a new and particularly disturbing experience for those with late onset disability (Murphy 1987). "Independence/interdependence" and "meaningful occupations" remain real unmet goals in which occupational therapy has an important but too often unrecognized or unrealized role. We seek to explore critical reassignment of those terms. At present the occupational therapy profession seems to consider "occupation" in ways that underpin the professional relationship to medicine and other health roles. It has yet to demonstrate—even in its foundation theoretical field of occupational science—how occupation is experienced as a human quality encompassing all behaviors in all varied cultural contexts. In terms like productivity (Wilcock 2006) there is a tendency for the meaningfulness of occupation to be separated from the positive meanings that many people experience in occupations that lead, for example, to sexual intimacy, fun, taking action, or, negatively, to exploitation or drudgery. As a "service" field, occupational therapy tends to be focused on individual experiences of meaning rather than supporting collaborative growth through interdependence, or being facilitative such as in the generation of spaces where people can experience each other and joint occupations. This latter approach is explicit in the application of disability studies and anthropology.

Our specific aims are to:

- Give occupational therapy scholars, students, and practitioners more complex theoretical approaches to disability using anthropology and disability studies,
- Give disability studies and anthropology scholars, students and practitioners examples of occupation-based practices of direct relevance to disability studies and anthropology,
- Engage students, professionals and academics with disability activist concepts as articulated directly by the activists themselves, with the goal of preserving the power and authority of activist voices.

Too often scholars of disability studies and anthropology are content to observe, document and theorize. Examples of this include the *Disability Studies Reader* (Davis, 3rd edition 2010) and *Disability in Local and Global Worlds* (Ingstad and Whyte 2007). Meanwhile, occupation-based practices focus on active engagement but are often under-theorized. Disability studies has emerged as the multi/inter-disciplinary home to incubate theoretical and methodological perspectives toward disability in society, not just any disability content. Anthropology and disability studies can inform and enhance critical reflections on the nature of occupation-based engagement with disabled people and disability communities. Occupational therapy can focus theory on the content of human occupation. Our goal is a dialogue that is balanced among the people who study, practice, and work for justice: some of us utilize these "occupations" of occupational therapy, anthropology, and disability studies, while some contest these occupations with our lived experiences as disabled people. In documenting various means of translation from theory to practice we span the spectrum from clinical practice to activism and performance.

This dialogue has taken place over the past decade in spaces like the Society for Applied Anthropology, the Society for Medical Anthropology, the Society for Disability Studies, and the Society for the Study of Occupation, and in the 2008 special issue of the Journal *Practicing Anthropology* (edited by Block, Frank, and Zemke). There are books that challenge occupational therapists to engage in innovative, community-based and politically relevant practice. Examples include *Occupational Therapy without Borders* (Kronenberg et al. 2005, 2010), with a planned second edition to these first volumes, *A Political Practice of Occupational Therapy* (Pollard et al. 2008), and *Politics of Occupation-Centered Practice* (Pollard and Sakellariou 2012). However, there is no book that specifically discusses how occupational therapy engages with disability studies *and* anthropology. It is time to move the conversation forward through a book project allowing for a deeper and more richly comprehensive exchange of ideas.

1.2   The Discomfort Zone

We are aware of our responsibilities in creating a collection that includes critical scholarship, research reports, and activist narratives. We must remain accountable to all the participating communities both in terms of regional power dynamics and tensions between therapeutic, scholarly, and activist modes of representation and practice. For example, Petra Kuppers (Chap. 5) cautions that anthropologists and occupational therapists would do well to join "[w]estern disability researchers [who] need to take better heed of the concept of sovereignty and culturally specific knowledge, and allow these understandings to complicate universal human rights frames and ways of conceiving of aid," (p. 70). Activists also confront western scholars about elitism and the lack of accessibility in academic formulations of disability. For example, activists heatedly protested the original framing of a call for proposals (CFP) for a forum on gender and disability issues for the online publication called *The Feminist Wire* (TFW). After receiving numerous complaints about the inaccessibility of the CFP, the program committee responded with the following statement:

> Given the sustained exclusion and economic vulnerability of those with disabilities, the academic language of our call was pointed to as yet another method of exclusion. Reduced access to formal higher education works to perpetuate a cycle of ableism. The unfortunate reality is that there's a disjuncture between disability studies (and academia at large) and disability justice organizing. We honor that many communities on the frontlines of oppression regard the academy itself as a major site of violence, trauma, and ableism. While TFW seeks to blur the demarcation between activism and scholarship, it is also an "academic-ish" publication. We are committed to making our forum widely accessible, and we also want to acknowledge and politicize the location from which we ourselves are located and form critical analysis.
> (The Feminist Wire Call for Submissions 2013, http://thefeministwire.com/2013/08/call-for-submissions-tfw-forum-on-disabilities-ableism-and-disability-studies/, retrieved 7/20/2014)

The TFW forum organizers were in a fertile but disquieting space that we term "the discomfort zone," (Block et al. 2011). Unrelated to Jonathan Franzen's (2006) book of the same name, our concept of "the discomfort zone" was first introduced in a panel *The Discomfort Zone: Exploring juxtapositions of Applied and Theoretical DS in Research and Practice*, organized by Pamela Block and moderated by Pamela Cushing, at the Society for Disability Studies in 2009, Tucson Arizona (Block 2009) which included the following presentations: "The Discomfort Zone: Collaborative

Disability Studies Research with Clinicians, Activists, and Youth with Multiple Sclerosis" (Block et al. 2009), "Using the Discomfort Zone to Create a Disability Studies Informed Rehabilitation Practice" (Magasi and Kramer 2009), as well as presentations by Kasnitz (2009) and Cushing (2009).

This *discomfort zone* is where we acknowledge and respect boundaries while at the same time pushing them. This is an ongoing struggle when moving between activist versus scholarly, clinical, and professional formulations. And from the other end, in some contexts, scholars fear the appropriation of disability studies for partisan political purposes, as Mello and Block discuss (Chap. 20), as well as the appropriation of disability activism by academia as just described above. Similarly, the discomfort zone emerges when engaging topics that highlight the intersectionality of race, sexuality, nationality, and disability as it has been articulated in Bell (2012), Erevelles (2011), and by many others. Such a discomfort zone actually prepares and continues to nurture the ground for critical theories, activist practices, and art to sprout. This is where this book idea first emerged; readers will witness the ongoing struggle when moving between and interweaving activism, artistic, scholarly, clinical, and professional spheres.

Language differences exist across cultural and regional boundaries but also across disciplinary, professional and activist ones. In June 2013, Block gave a presentation in Brazil about neurodiversity and her family experience growing up as the concept of autism changed dramatically over a 45 year period from the late 1960s to the second decade of the twenty-first century. She used autistic-first language as is preferred in autistic self-advocacy contexts in the United States and many northern countries. However, Brazilian activists and scholars embrace the people-first language of the Convention on the Rights of People with Disability (CRPD), long-ratified in Brazil. Even though Block was careful to explain in detail why she made her language choices, she could see the audience cringing every time she used disability-first language. Though jarring to readers used to other formulations based in other political realities, the respectful language choices in individual chapters, such as Aoyama (Chap. 3) who refers to Minamata Disease survivors as "victims," accurately represent the sometimes politically-charged language choices made by specific disability groups from around the world. In addition, the academy often specifies how knowledge should be expressed and privileges certain writing styles. This constriction of diverse and creative expression narrows our understanding of people's experiences. Instead, this book embraces various writing styles that are authentic to the authors and topics and we also include a few images to expand how the authors' wisdom is communicated. We have tried to edit the chapters in this book in ways that are sensitive to how different experiences are described by different people and that allows the authors' perspectives to be shared unobscured.

We are indeed in *the discomfort zone*, and this is where we want to be. Not all contributors are in agreement on how the concept of occupation should be used and how occupation works in practice. Not all contributors agree with how disability should be defined and spoken about, what language to use, and even who is allowed to join the discussion. Some use "people first" language and some do not. Because our chapter authors represent UK, US, and Australian English speakers, as well as many for who English is a second or third language, we preserve local vocabulary and syntax while trying to communicate intent. Retaining the creativity of the discomfort zone is work in need of doing and one of our occupations for this book.

1.3 Decolonizing Disability, Disability and Community, and Struggle, Creativity and Change

These are the three *Parts* of this volume. Any and all of the chapters can stand alone and be understood separately. In fact, in our new era of publishing flexibility, the chapters may be purchased separately. The *Parts*, while not specifically chronological, do have a mood of temporality about them—past, present, future.

Part I: Decolonizing Disability, does take as its focus disability in the context of oppressive social structures of power that create and recreate disability out of difference in part as a system of control—methods of settler colonialism of the past or that which we hope is past. It is not pessimism, just that to come to a point of proactively decolonizing, we must first recognize the state of being colonized or how the settler colonialism deeply intersects with the mechanism of ableism. This section title as well as the book title is a direct reflection of the second half of the "Occupy Wall Street" movement: "Decolonize Wall Street." We strongly agree with indigenous scholars' statements that "Decolonization is not a metaphor" (Tuck and Yang 2012). While not all chapters directly engage with the work of decolonization, our intention for the use of this word is in order not to stop our conversations at Occupy disability and in order to acknowledge and join the work to decolonize and occupy wall street, the ableist medical industry, and many other spaces." This *Part* spans from the personal to the statistical—from Taylor et al. (Chap. 2) life change narrative from sites of US activism against class injustice, to Geddes (Chap. 9), a formal analysis of post-colonial inequality in the Caribbean. As in Geddes, decolonization is directly relevant to Kuppers' view of disability in Aboriginal Australia (Chap. 5), while Aoyama's (Chap. 3) story of Minamata Disease in Japan, and Yergeau's (Chap. 6) of autism are examples of decolonization reinterpreted intraculturally. Ames (Chap. 7) and Perez et al. (Chap. 8) are both about art funded as therapy for colonized cultures—Wales and Brazil respectively. Without denigrating art as therapy, and good therapy as art, both of these chapters ask "who benefits?" Perhaps the essence of understanding disability in colonialism is to ask that question.

Part II: Disability and Community, takes as its starting point that disability can be a basis for community. This is the present in our quasi-temporal order. Community is a deceptively simple word and concept. We think we know what it is, particularly if it is intentional. We speak of multiple kinds of intentionality. There is the extreme intentionality of planned or "Intentional Communities" such as utopian experiments that have and will seduce those with a touch of escapism (Zola 1982). Disabled people could be ripe for this kind of future if we were not so diverse. However, current trends in intentional communities that involve disability are either still nursing-home-esque, single-impairment, defined by others, and often involuntary; or, they are loosely structured and fluid and based on the collective experience of disability, not on the individual experience of impairment. The *community* we explore here can be based on social identities or occupational activities. Whether the community we discuss is "real" or "imagined" or "wishful," whether it is defined from within or without or both, whether it is physical or "virtual," it is contemplated, from a structuralist point of view, because someone found the idea "good to think."

Clearly community can be geographic and permanent, but its physicality can also be temporary and episodic. A community can be communicative or linguistic, a type, a style, a mode of intersecting networks of information and feelings. Many combine both aspects: geography and communication, such as the Welsh case, but this is changing. Nepveux (Chap. 12) and Friedner (Chap. 14) are the most geographically bounded discussions of community. They both talk of the unrecognized importance of a place to be that is fluid in how people can use it as a site for interconnection and communication. Both are examples of geographic communities that continue to exist, at least partially, due to service providers' all-too-precarious support. "Naturally" occurring US Deaf communities using American Sign Language (ASL) are clearly communicative, but usually share proximity only episodically and with sustained effort.

Some chapters, like Nishida (Chap. 10) and Mirza et al. (Chap. 11) speak to a clash, or potential clash, of communities, in these cases communities directly related to occupation in its most formal sense—what you do for a living. Nishida introduces the idea of occupational "hyper-productivity" and applies it to academia. Hyper-productive occupational expectations can in themselves exclude many groups of people and are inherently ableist and saneist everywhere and in any field. Nishida demonstrates that in academia, where knowledge is supposedly created and shared, the disability community, in particular as it intersects with other minoritized communities, conflicts with the academic. Mirza et al. look at the occupation of being an occupational therapist and of how this occupational community can conflict with that of "their" not always so "patient" customer (although we can argue that insurance providers are the actual customer). They suggest a more open and interdisciplinary approach to *training for collaboration*, a recurrent theme, as one corrective for the narrowness of monocular clinical occupations. This myopia is a direct foil for the creation of the community described in de la Haye (Chap. 16): the service users' movement. She wants to see this community visible in a policy world and active in research. Will reaching out to the professionals be accepted as true participation?

Three of the chapters in this *Part II: Disability and Community*, tell a story of how an individual negotiates communities. Stoddart and Turnbull (Chap. 13) relate Stoddart's journey as someone denied a professional occupation by a speech impairment who tries to create an occupation as a trainer in how to communicate with people with speech impairments. With Turnbull as his university-based partner, he succeeds conceptually, but not yet fiscally. However, while Stoddart does not embrace disability as a collective identity, Dupree (Chap. 15) most explicitly does. Is this related to their different experience of satisfaction? Dupree seeks out community in one of the most densely populated places on earth, Manhattan, NY. As a ventilator user he demonstrates true physical risk as part of the business of building community. He is an example of how luck and life can meet disability and create activist communities in the process. This is not to idealize Dupree's lived experience, which includes life-threatening struggles, discomfort, pain, and weariness. Accompanying the triumphs come roller-coaster rides of hope and disappointment. Perhaps the most optimistic picture of emerging disability community is that of Eva Rodriguez (Chap. 17). She relates how simple but profound changes in how an educational planning meeting is structured, centering the priorities of family and disabled child, may make a huge difference in the child's future. We want to educate for choice and collaborative communities that enshrine the needs, hopes and opportunities of all children.

Part III: Struggle, Creativity and Change is the future in this quasi-temporal schema and our many paths to a cautious optimism. This endeavor is not academic, it is not a sequestered case study, nor is it a random sample. It is the best of what we know that drives us to know more. It is the best of what we have seen that works and satisfies. *Part III* also resides in the discomfort zone as reader and writer both struggle in ways that bring the kind of creativity that sparks substantive change. All are underrated. Some of these chapters capture us in their unusual formats: with a poem, a dialogue, an image, we promise creativity. We close the effort on the upbeat with Marcus et al. (Chap. 24) which uses all of these creative formats. However, even here the pain to arrive at such a hopeful place is just below the surface. Hecht (Chap. 19), among other dark chapters, is perhaps the darkest foil to Marcus et al.'s optimism. It is a discomforting but riveting short story by Hecht upon which Mello et al. (Chap. 20) reflect, as they do a groundbreaking job of discomforting English language disability studies specialists with a surprising sibling, Brazilian disability studies. Our message is simple: change and grow—collectively, it is both possible and necessary.

Struggle is such a recurrent theme. Even Seelman (Chap. 18), as she embraces technology, worries not only about the politics of economic access, and of the unhappy consequences of surveillance potential, but about what creates daily meaningful occupation with low or high tech help. Chaplin (Chap. 22), a Deaf/blind author, welcomes us into his everyday world. Occupational therapists will appreciate how he analyzes his own experience of participation. His greatest instrumental need is for people to relax their hyper-productive drive for constant simultaneity. The use of focus in time recurs as a theme in all discussions of communication impairment. Kasnitz has noted conflicts of reality in this area. She describes to us all how blind interlocutors who have not touched her, held her hand, or stroked her cheek as she speaks, often don't realize the effort her speech entails nor body language cues of conversational turn taking. A chapter such as Chaplin's fills some of the "Now I got it!" gaps in our experience of each other's struggle and how creative we need to be to have voice.

The poems and text of the Stevenage Survivors (Chap. 23) do this explicitly. There should be no real surprise that art, particularly preformed or written word art, is a powerful vehicle for psychiatric survivors. As Moore, Garcia, and Thrower (Chap. 21) demonstrate, the written word also reveals often overlooked violence—police brutality against disabled people of color or political gentrification by mainstream activism—as well as challenges it and sheds a light on the path to justice. Ben-Moshe's (Chap. 4) perspective as a disabled Israeli illustrates how violence manifests at the intersections of ableism and other social injustices when living with a legacy of military occupation. In other parts of the world, we are not so close to death, but neither is it as far away as we would like. The Stevenage group call themselves "Survivors" appropriately, and the term could just as well be applied in Dupree (Chap. 15) or Peres et al. (Chap. 11) or withheld in Moore et al. (Chap. 21) or Hecht (Chap. 19). Many disabled people experience a lack of *voice*. Whether autistic (Chap. 6), a psychiatric survivor (Chaps. 11, 16 and 23), learning disabled (Chaps. 7 and 17) or speech impaired (Chaps. 13 and 24), we are haunted by a sense that no one is listening, we are silenced, misrepresented, or erased. Is it any wonder that we hone our performance skills to hold an audience's attention, once we have won the battle to get them to still their inner chatter and really listen—a reborn art we demand of our environment?

1.4 Recurrent Themes and Open Futures

This book is not a random collection but it is very diverse. Two of us, Block and Kasnitz, are American Jews who sit here in solidarity with Liat Ben-Moshe (Chap. 4), safe, and feel horrified but powerless to stop the death and disability-making going on at this moment (August 2014) in Israel/Palestine except in our voices of protest recorded here. This war time disability-making is of course not new. In *Moving Violations* (1995), Hockenberry describes it in haunting accounts of his experiences as a wheel-chair using journalist in the Middle East between 1988 and 1992. He describes dark times, and these tales seem prescient to our post 9/11 era and the current war in Gaza. Moore et al. (Chap. 21) describe the disability-making of police violence. Minamata Disease (Chap. 3) is the disability-making of corporate greed. The colonization of Australia created disability from difference as seen by Kuppers (Chap. 5). And being people of color in white supremacist societies, brings disability closer to them, whether it is through racial violence or over- and under-diagnosis.

Once made, disability is best lived in community. Any struggle for community is worthwhile. A creative struggle is the most satisfying. This volume is rife with contributions by people who consciously engage in word art as an act of resistance. We really want to see these and the other innumerable skills of disability recognized and taught. However satisfying these occupations may be to spirit, we also want to break through the barriers to formal *occupations*, what we are remunerated for, how we support our families. Everyone needs to be paid for what they can do, not warehoused for what they can't. We have not yet scratched the surface of disability as an ingenious way to live.

We close this introduction with a note about our style. As this book developed, and with such dramatic changes in publishing, many of you may never hold this volume in your hands. You won't feel its weight or flip its pages. You may not even have the whole thing. You may have just purchased chapters. Well, if you are reading this, we invite you to also read Chaps. 25 and 26, the last two. Like this chapter they are also written by the four of us and in serving as introduction, development, and conclusion are the three legged stool on which we sit thinking about the problems and delights of the ramifications of "occupying" and "decolonizing" disability.

Disability is not a 'brave struggle' or 'courage in the face of adversity'

DISABILITY IS AN ART

It's an Ingenious way to live

© 2002 graphics & graphic by Neil Marcus
Used with permission of the author & DisAbility Media Agency
All rights reserved
© 2012 layout by Marina Jubran/Butterfly Wheel Designs

Disability is an Art: This is an example of poster art by Neil Marcus. It is a self-portrait, a loopy rope-like ink drawing of a figure in a wheelchair accompanied by the text: "Disability is not a 'brave struggle' or 'courage in the face of adversity.' DISABILITY IS AN ART (this last phrase in large bolded, ink-stroked text in all capital letters). It's an ingenious way to live." (Drawing by Neil Marcus)

References

Bell C (2012) Blackness and disability: critical examinations and cultural interventions. Michigan State University Press, East Lansing

Block P (2009) Organizer, "The discomfort zone: exploring juxtapositions of applied and theoretical DS in research and practice." Session at the annual meetings, Society for Disability Studies, Tucson, Arizona

Block P, Frank G, Zemke R (2008) Anthropology, occupational therapy and disability studies: collaborations and prospects. Pract Anthropol 30(3):1–31

Block P, Milazzo M, Rodriguez E, Nishida A (2009) The discomfort zone: collaborative disability studies research with clinicians, activists, and youth with multiple sclerosis. Presentation at the annual meetings, Society for Disability Studies, Tucson, Arizona

Block P, Rodriguez E, Milazzo M, MacAllister W, Krupp L, Nishida A, Slota N, Broughton A, Keys CB (2011) Building pediatric MS community. Res Soc Sci Disabil 6:85–112

Cushing P (2009) Where is DS at today? Systematic overview and analysis of current distribution of disability studies courses and degrees. Presentation at the annual meetings, Society for Disability Studies, Tucson, Arizona

Davis L (ed) (2010) Disability studies reader, 3rd edn. Routledge, New York

Erevelles N (2011) Disability and difference in global contexts. Palgrave MacMillan, New York

Frank G, Block P, Zemke R (2008) Introduction to the special issue. Pract Anthropol 30(3):2–5

Franzen J (2006) The discomfort zone: a personal history. Farrar, Straus and Giroux, New York

Hockenberry J (1995) Moving violations. Hyperion, New York

Ingstad B, Whyte SR (eds) (2007) Disability in local and global worlds. University of California Press, Berkeley

Kasnitz D (2009) Thoughts on the application of disability studies and the maintenance of theory. Session at the annual meetings, Society for Disability Studies, Tucson, Arizona

Kronenberg F, Simo Algado S, Pollard N (eds) (2005) Occupational therapy without borders – learning from the spirit of survivors. Elsevier Science, Edinburgh

Kronenberg F, Pollard N, Sakellariou D (eds) (2010) Occupational therapies without borders, vol 2. Elsevier Science, Edinburgh

Magasi S, Kramer J (2009) Using the discomfort zone to create a disability studies informed rehabilitation practice. Presentation at the annual meetings, Society for Disability Studies, Tucson, Arizona

Murphy RF (1987) The body silent. W. W. Norton, New York

Pollard N, Sakellariou D (eds) (2012) Politics of occupation-centered practice. Wiley, Oxford

Pollard N, Sakellariou D, Kronenberg F (eds) (2008) A political practice of occupational therapy. Elsevier Science, Edinburgh

"The Feminist Wire Call for Submissions" (2013) http://thefeministwire.com/2013/08/call-for-submissions-tfw-forum-on-disabilities-ableism-and-disability-studies/

Tuck E, Yang KW (2012) Decolonization is not a metaphor. Decolonization: Indig Educ Soc 1(1):1–40

Wilcock AA (2006) An occupational perspective of health. Slack Incorporated, Thorofare

Zola I (1982) Missing pieces: a chronicle of living with a disability. Temple University Press, Philadelphia

Sunaura Taylor, Marg Hall, Jessica Lehman, Rachel Liebert, Akemi Nishida, and Jean Stewart

Abstract
This chapter includes a collage of reports from disabled (and their ally) occupiers of different cities. The collage is contextualized by Taylor's involvement in Occupy/Decolonize Oakland through journals she wrote while she stayed at the camp site. As much as this chapter acknowledges and celebrates the powerful force of Occupy Movement, it also points out the movement's challenges to make the sites accessible to all. Stewart and Hall illustrate works of CUIDO (Communities United in Defense of Olmstead) and its intersection with the Occupy movement. Nishida introduces KOWS (Krips Occupy Wall Street), the disability community representation at New York City, Occupy Wall Street (OWS), and multiple roles it plays at the site. Liebert reads OWS from radical

Originally published in Occupy! a broadsheet newspaper inspired by the Occupy movement. Edited by n + 1 with Sarah Leonard, Sarah Resnick, and Astra Taylor.

S. Taylor (✉)
American Studies, New York University, 20 Cooper Square, 4th Floor New York, NY 10003, USA
e-mail: sunaurataylor@gmail.com

M. Hall • J. Stewart
CUIDO (Communities United in Defense of Olmstead), Berkeley, CA, USA

J. Lehman
Senior and Disability Action, San Francisco, CA, USA

A. Nishida
Disability and Human Development, Gender and Women's Studies, University of Illinois at Chicago, Chicago, IL, USA
e-mail: anishida922@gmail.com

R. Liebert
Critical Social Personality Psychology, The Graduate Center, The City University of New York, Fifth Avenue 365, New York, NY 10016, USA

psych perspective, and shares ways people are working to educate OWS to ensure safety for all within the movement. Lehman points out relations between Occupy and general disability rights and suggests mutual education take place between these movements. This chapter ends as Taylor reflects on awareness she gained through her participation in the movement; where she learned the depth of structural police violence and her own privileges in intersection with her disability identity.

Keywords
Community • CUIDO (Communities United In Defense of Olmstead) • Decolonize • KOWS (Krips Occupy Wall Street) • Occupy Oakland • Occupy Wall Street (OWS) • Oscar Grant Plaza • Police brutality

2.1   Introduction

Sunaura Taylor

January, 2012

Inspired by Occupy Wall Street and the numerous other encampments that were spreading across the country, first time protestors and seasoned activists began occupying a public plaza in downtown Oakland, California on October 10, 2011. What began as a relatively small protest on a rainy evening turned into a powerful movement that has had ramifications well beyond the city of Oakland.

My partner and I were there that very first day and it didn't take long before we were hooked–spending hours at the General Assemblies, and (when we could) camping out in our sleeping bags and tent. We were there during countless inspired moments of community building and we were there during many of the (often scary) confrontations with the Oakland police.

Early on I was invited to write my experiences of Occupy for the Occupy! gazette, a project put out by n + 1. What follows are five pieces written for the gazette. They appear here in the order they were originally released. The first three are reflections and updates I wrote on my experiences as a protestor in Oakland. The next is a piece I edited that brought together the voices of other disabled protestors who were participating in the Occupy movement locally and nationally. The last returns to my voice.

Looking back on fall, 2011 I am aware that being a part of the Occupy movement has truly been one of the most remarkable experiences of my life. Of course it has sometimes been challenging, inaccessible, and deeply disappointing—it was and is not perfect. Even the name chosen for the movement, Occupy, has garnered a lot of criticism for the ways in which it uses the language of colonization, leading many to argue for a name change: Decolonize Wall Street (and similarly Decolonize Oakland). Despite its flaws however, the Occupy/Decolonize movement has been inspiring in a way I don't think I've ever felt before.

Occupy Oakland, like the Occupy movement more generally, is not over or dead as the media so often declares. However, it has transformed into something that at least for a time is a lot less visible than the unruly tent cities that were sparking our imaginations last fall. People are busy stopping foreclosures, striking debt and saving their schools. In the past year Occupy Oakland has organized many successful events, it has survived (albeit in a different form) the increasingly intimidating police presence and it has celebrated its first birthday.

My Queer (dis) Abled: Black and white drawing done in pen of a woman with glasses and long hair pulled back by a bandana. She is smiling slightly and wearing a t-shirt with an image and the word Propagandhi in capital letters. She holds up a crutch that is used as a sign post, with a sign saying: "My Queer (dis) Abled Welfare Chicana Ass Demands Structural Change." "Welfare" is in smaller letters than the rest of the words. "Change" is vertical, in parentheses on the bottom right of the sign, also in smaller letters. (Drawing by Sunaura Taylor)

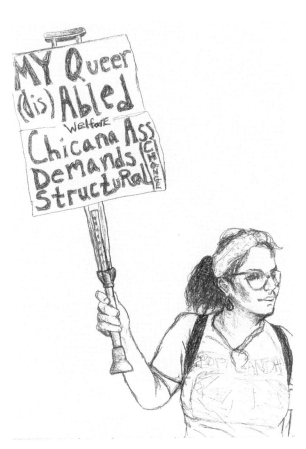

2.2   Occupy Oakland

Sunaura Taylor

October, 2011: I write this as a participant and admirer of Occupy Oakland. Not as a representative of Occupy Oakland.

I just woke up in my tent at Occupy Oakland. This is the first night my husband and I (and our dog) have camped out here, and although I can't say we slept well over the sounds of the city and people talking into the early hours of the morning, we woke up still deeply enthused and excited to be part of such an event in Oakland. We've been stopping by the encampment pretty regularly since it started last Monday. It's in downtown Oakland, in Frank Ogawa Plaza, which is right in front of the city hall. Within hours of the protest starting, there were signs renaming the location. The new name: Oscar Grant Plaza.

Frank H. Ogawa was a Japanese American who was a long time Oakland City Council Member. He served time during WWII in a concentration camp. He died while the plaza was being renovated and so it was renamed in his honor. Oscar Grant was a young African American man fatally shot by BART (Bay Area Rapid Transit) police on New Year's Day, 2009. The case, which made headlines nationwide, has become a symbol of the city's problem of police brutality and racial inequality. The movement for justice that has emerged from Oscar Grant's shooting has no doubt played a powerful role in how Occupy Oakland has been organized.

It was clear from the first signs that went up at the encampment, and the first organizers who spoke, that Oscar Grant Plaza was going to be as much about addressing and healing Oakland's wounds as it was about uniting the 99 %. This was not going to be an encampment that ignores issues of race, class, nationality and gender–and as I've found out over the past few days, in at least some ways, they've also been trying to address issues of disability.

Although I'm the only wheelchair user I've seen staying at the camp (which doesn't mean I necessarily am), the Bay Area's disability community has been coming out to support the events and participate in the protest. This weekend over 2,500 people made it to Oscar Grant Plaza for a march and rally calling for "Jobs Not Cuts." The protesters included many individuals from various unions, including Service Employees International Union SEIU. CUIDO, a radical activist group made up of disabled people and allies, was also present. CUIDO, which stands for, Communities United in Defense of Olmstead (a landmark court decision that declared that disabled people have a right to live in their own communities), is no stranger to protest encampments. In the summer of 2010, dozens of members of CUIDO camped out in tents on a traffic median in Berkeley to protest the proposed budget cuts to services poor, elderly and disabled folks rely on. Arnieville (named after our then governor Arnold Schwarzenegger) was a remarkably accessible tent city and thrived for over a month.

Although Oscar Grant Plaza has yet to be as accessible to a broad range of disabled people as Arnieville, I've been pleasantly surprised by how an awareness of disability has been at least somewhat present over the past week. Ableism was mentioned during the General Assembly meeting as an issue that the "Safe Place" committee wanted to address, and I've seen signs for "access for all," demanding people keep ramps clear.

Still, 7 days into the protest and there is no longer any room for tents on the plaza's large lawn. Tents are squeezed together so tightly that in many areas there is no room to move in between them, for me in my wheelchair or for someone who walks. There is more access to the community tents. There is a free school, an art station, a Sukkot tent, a medical tent, a children's area, a people of color tent, and a quite remarkable food station, where huge batches of soups and beans are made, and tea, coffee, and healthy snacks seem to be abundant. The various projects the camp is working on include installing solar panels, and reclaiming parts of the park as a community garden.

One of the most amazing aspects of being at Oscar Grant Plaza is witnessing how moved people are. People who may never have said a word to each other a week ago are now neighbors. The General Assembly meetings, which happen every evening, are often very beautiful. Of course people bicker, or get bored, or are sometimes disrespectful, but much of the time the meetings are thoughtful and patient.

The assembly talked very vulnerably about issues ranging from how to deal with sexism and violence at the campsite, to what role alcohol and partying should play in the encampment. We talked about the complexity of discouraging certain behaviors like drinking and partying, while also trying to respect people's individual freedoms. There was a strong sense of support for watching out for each other, and for not wanting to give the police or the city any reason to try to kick us out. The Security Committee, which enlists volunteers to take shifts watching out for the campers throughout the night, encouraged more people to sign up.

Negotiating what different people want for the atmosphere of the camp is undoubtedly a challenge. Some of the protesters seem adamant that there can't be a revolution without a party, while others repeated numerous times that although they weren't strangers to partying themselves, "this camp is not Burning Man!"

Participating in this movement is intimidating in many ways, especially for people who are shy, or those who feel that there is no one "like them" at the protests. I'm certainly intimidated by camping with strangers, by being one of the only visibly disabled people present, and by the lack of access and simple comforts. However, I want to be out there, because I realize this sort of opportunity to come together doesn't happen every day. But also, I want to be there because I am hella proud of Oakland for creating this sort of encampment—an encampment that often fails in its desire to be a safe and accessible place for all people, but that is nonetheless trying.

2.3   Oakland Raid

Sunaura Taylor

October 27, 2011

Early Tuesday morning, Occupy Oakland encampments at Oscar Grant Plaza and Snow Park were raided and destroyed by police. There were numerous reports of excessive use of force and violence. Nearly 100 people were arrested and held on $10,000 bail. The emergency text alert system, which apparently had over 1,000 people signed on, failed to go off for many people, and so occupiers were left alone to defend the camps in the early hours of the morning. The police blocked off streets, rerouted buses, and shut down the closest BART stop. Because of the police blockade, it was reportedly next to impossible for media or legal observers to see the raid. Photos from the raided Oscar Grant Plaza show an utterly destroyed encampment, with tents cut up and intentionally destroyed.

At 4 pm that day, people who had not been arrested, as well as supporters of Occupy Oakland, rallied at the Oakland public library to show support of those arrested and outrage over the destruction of the camps. What began as a rally and march of about 500 people turned into a march of thousands. We marched through Oakland reclaiming our streets and demanding our parks be returned to us. Over and over again, we were met with tear gas and extreme police force. Many people were injured, including Scott Olsen, a 24-year-old veteran who survived two deployments to Iraq. He was hit in the head with a police projectile (either a tear gas canister or a flash bang grenade) and was in critical condition up until last night when he was downgraded to serious but stable condition. Videos show that as protesters rushed in to help the man, police threw another teargas canister or flash bang grenade at them. One photo shows a woman in a wheelchair, a member of CUIDO, in a cloud of tear gas. The energy, although often very scary, was amazing—passionate and brave and dedicated. The protesters vowed to be out there every evening at 6 pm until our parks were reclaimed.

As the world turned its attention to Oakland, my partner and I had to leave, taking the red eye out that night to NY for a family engagement. We are both glued to the reports that have been flooding in of the amazing rally that took place last night. 3,000 people reclaimed Oscar Grant Plaza, tearing down (and neatly stacking) the fence the police had encircled the plaza with. There seems to have been very little police presence. The gathering held a general assembly where nearly 1,600 people voted on proposals of what to do next. The general assembly passed a decision to have a general strike and mass day of action next Wednesday, November 2nd.

As the website for Occupy Oakland says, "The whole world is watching Oakland. Let's show them what's possible."

2.4   Oakland Rises! Oakland Strikes!

Sunaura Taylor

November, 2011

In the past 2 weeks Occupy Oakland has undergone massive change. On October 25th, Oscar Grant Plaza was raided and destroyed by riot cops. Only a week and a half later, you never would have known it had gone. The tent city was resurrected only 1 day after being brutally torn down. That same night Occupy Oakland held a General Assembly of 3,000 people.

I had no idea a movement could grow so quickly. Occupy Oakland is not even a month old and yet it has become an incredible force in this city. It held the nation's first General Strike in over 65 years (the last general strike was also held in Oakland in 1946). Thousands of people came. The exact numbers are unclear, but it seems likely it was between 5,000–10,000 people, although some estimates put it anywhere from 20,000–40,000. The day was glorious and peaceful (even the mayor and the city council members had to admit it was remarkable). Unfortunately, it ended in the yellow fog of nighttime tear gas and police violence.

The strike was a huge success, with a sustained energy from the early morning hours until the late hours of the night. Multiple banks were forced to close throughout the day and a massive march and sit-in during the evening hours shut down the Port of Oakland. For the whole day and into the night, protesters occupied 14th and Broadway, the main intersection beside the encampment. Huge hand-made banners hung across roads and in front of banks declaring things like, for example, "Death to Capitalism." The intersection and the camp itself was the central hub of the protest, but throughout the day groups of hundreds or thousands would leave, march across Oakland to a bank or to participate in an action or event, while thousands of others stayed at Oscar Grant Plaza, to dance, make political signs, and celebrate. Hot food was provided and cooked by local businesses, union representatives, firefighters, Occupy campers, and countless others. The atmosphere was festival-like, but only better, as everyone seemed to be talking about changing the world—and actually believing in it. Even by night, after sitting at the port in the cold for many hours, people still seemed overjoyed. One person told me it was the best day of his life.

People had been urged throughout the days leading up to the event to organize their own actions, and that's clearly what happened. Everywhere you went you'd find different pockets of people self-organizing. From the Children's Brigade to the Disability Action Brigade, to a flash mob singing "I will Survive (Capitalism)," to a 99 % storytelling tent, countless groups of people made their own creative and powerful moments of resistance.

At the port we split up into groups, each blocking a separate entrance. It is hard to say how many people were there, but some estimate that at its peak there were 20,000 people marching to the port. At 7 pm a new work shift was going to begin and we were to block the workers from entering by creating massive community picket lines. This action had largely been developed to show solidarity with the Longshore Workers in Longview, WA who have been battling EGT (Export Grain Terminal) for months over anti-union practices. The port closure was also a way of directly stopping Capitalist trade. Many Longshore Workers announced solidarity with the strike, even as the International Longshore and Warehouse Union was unable to officially authorize it. Although, there were reports of some frustrated truckers (and two marchers were injured by an angry driver), the vast majority honked their horns enthusiastically in support of us and some even let protesters climb atop their containers for a better view of the seemingly endless parade of people. Spontaneous General Assemblies were held at each gate using the human microphone, where a lot of conversation seemed to focus on the importance of occupying foreclosed spaces, especially as winter nears. After many hours it was announced that we had successfully shutdown the Port of Oakland! My partner and I cheered and then began the long march back.

During the day the cops were absent, despite a few incidents of property damage to some banks and a Whole Foods grocery store. A small number of protesters smashed windows, broke ATMs, and spray-painted messages on the outside of banks. Youtube videos show other protesters trying to stop the vandalism, sometimes with force. People debated the vandalism throughout the day–with many staunchly opposed to it, and others arguing that property damage isn't violence (what the banks do is violence). Still others argued that, either way, these tactics are unhelpful and turn people away from the movement.

After the police violence of the week before, which drew international attention and which left people hurt, it was clear that the city of Oakland did not want any more bad press. However, as the night wore on things began to change.

When my partner and I arrived back to Oscar Grant Plaza, exhausted and ready for our second night at the new camp, we were told that a group of protesters had occupied a nearby foreclosed building and that the police were coming. It is hard to know what exactly happened before or after the police raid, but within 20 min hundreds of cops in full riot gear descended on Occupy Oakland and were blasting the crowds with tear gas. I felt confused by what was going on, as I had left the port with no knowledge that a building occupation had been planned. Later large fires were lit by some of the protesters (supposedly to combat tear gas), and some bottles were hurled at the cops.

I have been preoccupied since that night with the debate that has ensued over the use of "violent" tactics by some of the protesters. I myself had certainly felt frustrated by the atmosphere of that night. Besides being disheartened once again by the brutality of the cops (who, along with tear gas, shot rubber bullets at people, one of which hit a homeless man), I also personally felt dismayed by some of the protest activity itself. As I watched from a distance it seemed to me that the crowd was largely very young and very able-bodied. It is easy for me to assume they were also predominantly white and male–but as I was not on the frontlines, I'm not sure. I do know though, that as a disabled woman and wheelchair user, I felt little of the diversity of people that makes this movement so beautiful and so revolutionary to me–and that makes it a safe place for me.

As I've watched the debate unfold it seems that one of the main points of contention is over whether or not destruction of property is violence. In my opinion destruction of property has had its place even within nonviolent movements, but it is a tactic that needs to be used carefully. After all, the 1 % were not the ones out in the streets of Oakland the next morning cleaning up the shattered glass, or picking up the burned debris. I do think there can be a kind of violence in the way property destruction affects others without their consent. A small group of people making decisions that affect the safety and reputation of the whole movement is not what democracy looks like. That is what violence looks like.

However, the violence perpetrated by the protestors was minimal compared to the violence perpetrated by the police in response. Yet another person was seriously injured, and bizarrely, it was another young Iraq war veteran. According to an interview he gave to The Guardian, Kayvan Sabehgi was walking alone when he was stopped by a group of cops who proceeded to beat him with batons. Kayvan was in jail for 18 h calling for help and in excruciating pain. When he finally got to the hospital it was found his spleen had been ruptured.

I awoke at my home on November 3 and was incredibly relieved to hear that the camp had not been destroyed; I was also relieved to see that the media coverage of the violence had not completely overshadowed all the spectacular moments of the day.

What has ensued since November 2nd is an important debate among protesters and community members over nonviolent versus violent tactics. The day of the General Strike proved that there are thousands, if not tens of thousands, of people who support Occupy Oakland. To me, the only thing the broken windows, spray paint, and fires have done thus far is make some groups, small businesses, and unions more hesitant to support us, and it has made many individuals feel less safe.

The evening after the strike, Occupy Oakland held a forum on violence and nonviolence. Occupy Oakland supports a diversity of tactics, but as one woman said at the forum, respecting a diversity of tactics must go both ways. When a few people choose violence, they need to be aware of how their tactics can trump the tactics of those who choose nonviolence. I would hate to see this movement slowed down or destroyed by infighting. I'd also hate to see it fall apart because of violence. To me, it's essential that we really think complexly about what respecting a diversity of tactics—and a diversity of people—really means. Our future depends on it.

2.5   Disabled People Occupy America!

Sunaura Taylor

November, 2011

Disabled people are most commonly viewed as people who "suffer" from medical problems, versus as members of a disenfranchised community whose suffering largely stems from inequality, prejudice, stereotypes, and limited access to basic necessities like housing, health care, education, and jobs. Because of this, disabled people are far too often left out of political movements. Although this is often still the case within the Occupy Wall Street movement, disabled people have taken the matter into our own hands and are loudly declaring "We are here!"

We have been really excited by the ways in which disabled people have been participating in the OWS movement, coming together to build community, raise awareness, and make the movement accessible. From the Occupy at Home movement, which gives a space to those who can't be physically present at protests, to the disabled individuals who put themselves on the frontlines risking arrest, disabled people are showing that they are an important force in this movement. What follows are the voices of just a few of the disabled people occupying America.

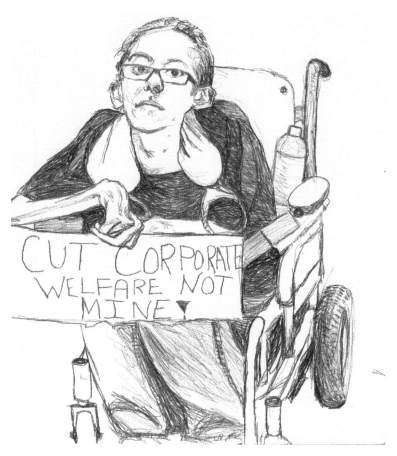

Cut Corporate Welfare: A black and white drawing done in pen of a young man in a power wheelchair. The man has short hair and he is wearing glasses. A pillow hangs around the back of his neck to support his head. A water bottle sits behind him in the right side of his chair. He looks determined. One thin arm is holding a sign that says in all capital letters: "Cut Corporate Welfare Not Mine!" (Drawing by Sunaura Taylor)

2.6   Other Voices: OWS and CUIDO

Jean Stewart

Marg Hall

We were born in an occupation. Communities United in Defense of Olmstead (CUIDO) grew out of a 2010 month-long disability protest encampment in Berkeley, California. We oppose budget cuts to programs serving people with disabilities, elders, and poor people. These brutal austerity measures threaten the right of people with disabilities to live in our homes and communities—a right affirmed by the Supreme Court's Olmstead decision of 1999.

We think and act outside the box. CUIDO engages in nonviolent direct action to affect both immediate and systemic change. Through sit-ins, occupations, street theatre, propaganda, and letter-writing, we demand our human rights, in alliance with the 99 %, especially poor people. Disability usually ushers in poverty, which in turn can lead to homelessness, hunger, pain, illness, institutionalization in nursing homes and jails, and death.

Like the Occupy movement, CUIDO boasts fabulous diversity, though of a different sort; we encompass a rainbow of disabilities. We ride wheelchairs, we're deaf, we're blind, we have learning disabilities, psychiatric disabilities, chemical sensitivities, and a host of other hidden whatnot.

Why does the Occupy movement thrill us? Because, like CUIDO, it acts outside the box, challenging legitimacy and encouraging resistance. The corporate stranglehold on government threatens our very lives. (Headline of yesterday's flyer, which we handed out as we marched with tens of thousands toward the Port of Oakland, successfully shutting it down: MEMO TO GOVERNMENT: GET YER FILTHY MITTS OFF OUR SAFETY NET!)

We who resist, who civilly disobey, are our only hope.

www.cuido.org www.facebook.com (CUIDO)

2.7 Other Voices: Krips* Occupy Wall Street (KOWS) or Disabled (Un)Occupy Wall Street

Akemi Nishida

KOWS started with a growing desire of disabled people to have collective and supportive presence at Occupy Wall Street. With DIA (Disabled in Action), disabled people and allies of multiple generations gather at OWS every Sunday at noon. KOWS' presence there has been powerful and ever growing.

We go to OWS to represent our community, especially those who cannot be there physically for various reasons; to show diversity within the 99 %; to inform and educate people about ableism; to welcome disabled people who do not know about the community; and to be with each other.

Even though OWS has a wheelchair accessible entrance, this does not mean that it is an accessible and safe space for all. The OWS is often too crowded to maneuver and overwhelming. Its lack of disability politics makes some feel unsafe. Also its fast-pace organizing is inaccessible and unsustainable to many. Therefore, the next agenda of KOWS is to develop a web space where those who do/cannot join KOWS physically can still participate.

KOWS is in the middle of learning and practicing more collective, interdependent, accessible, safe, and sustainable organizing and protesting.

Come join us at OWS every Sunday at noon or through web-based space.
*Krips = Crips = Cripples = Insider word for disabled people.
www.facebook.com (Krips Occupy Wall Street!!!!! Every Sunday at NOON)

2.8   Other Voices: Doing Radical Psych at Occupy

Rachel Liebert

Occupy weaves together communities refusing to go on carrying the burdens of an unjust economic-structure; burdens that land especially in communities who are poor, of color, queer, trans, and/or disabled.

And burdens that can manifest as madness.

Yet, backed by a medico-industrial complex that profits from turning madness into sickness, these issues are by-and-large framed as an individual's "mental illness;" diverting critical attention from our crazy-making world. These mainstream approaches are therefore both a product and tool of imperialism, capitalism, neoliberalism, and securitization; those very systems that Occupy is striving to undo.

It follows that madness connects deeply with Occupy. Yet, conflated with aggression and disturbance, mental illness is instead increasingly seen as a threat that needs to be screened out or eliminated. (While conveniently used to depict the movement as unstable to "the outside," and distract from the ever-present state-sanctioned threat of police violence.)

Alternatively, using a lens of diversity, protest, and community, radical psych sees madness as containing seeds of expertise and revolution, one that offers learning and growth to the movement, and that deserves to be included (not just tolerated) in "the 99 percent." We have been organizing for mad justice, and offering social and emotional support on-site to all protestors—no matter what form their protest takes—through written materials, teach-ins, counseling, peer-support, and community-building.

We are working hard to create a space within Occupy for diverse connections, particularly as mad voices disproportionately represent bodies already marginalized and policed by society.

In solidarity.

2.9   Other Voices: Thoughts On Occupy From A Disabled Community Organizer

Jessica Lehman

Disability activists have been participating in Occupy protests all over the country. While the Occupy movement appeals to many white, non-disabled people who have lost their jobs and homes and are feeling oppression for the first time, people with disabilities were already in the middle of a horrendous years-long fight to protect and maintain basic survival services like personal attendant services and health care. As one disability activist said recently, "We have been working hard and doing a great job, but we just don't have enough people." Maybe the Occupy movement provides a chance to fight with a large enough group that we can win.

Access has been a problem in every city. Camping out is challenging for many people with disabilities (as well as seniors, families with children, women and queer people who question safety). Occupy sites need ASL interpreters, captioning, accessible porta-potties, ramps not blocked by bikes, and air not contaminated with smoke. Ensuring access is challenging given the nature of a "leaderless" movement. It has been pointed out, however, that rather than saying that none of us are leaders, we must say that all of us are leaders. Rather than fighting for someone in power to provide access, as we are used to, people with and without disabilities are taking it upon themselves to provide access and to educate each other. It is a transformative experience for our movement for us to have the opportunity and the responsibility of creating the access we wish to see in our community.

Some disability groups have pointed out that the Occupy movement gives the disability community a chance to educate other activists about the threats facing people with disabilities, a chance to bring others into our fight. For others, the Occupy movement is an opportunity to transform our own movement, a chance to connect the fight for health care and access with a broader fight for social and economic justice. We have an opportunity to educate our own community about how our fight is linked to the fight of all oppressed people, all people who are fighting to have power in their own lives and communities. This recognition can make space for people of color with disabilities, queer people with disabilities, immigrants with disabilities, and people with non-apparent disabilities to have power in the disability community.

As a community organizer, I'm always looking for ways to bring more people into the disability rights movement and ways to broaden and grow our movement. I see and hear from people with disabilities around the country – on Facebook, email, and phone – who are drawing new energy from the Occupy movement. After years of cuts and defeats, this movement is creating sparks in individuals, groups, and in the disability community as a whole – sparks that can lead us to action, transformation, and justice.

2.10   Sunday, November 13th

Sunaura Taylor

December, 2011

On November 10th, as Oscar Grant Plaza prepared to celebrate its 1-month anniversary, a young man was shot and killed a few yards from the plaza. The tragic event has engendered many responses—from those who have used it as a justification to evict the campers, to others who say that this sort of tragedy is nothing new to Oakland—it is in fact deeply related to the systemic issues that Occupy Oakland is protesting. The Occupy Oakland medics were the first to respond on the scene. As one of the medics, a young black man, said later, "I have been to 79 funerals in my 22 years of life. This is what happens in Oakland." Later other people made the point that if a young black man is shot in Oakland it usually never makes the news.

I am young, female, a wheelchair user and I am white. I have had an intense education in the past month, on what my city is really like for much of its population—and it is devastating. The very first day Oscar Grant Plaza was erected people yelled, "fuck the cops!" and it was made clear this was not a space that would welcome or negotiate with police. I remember thinking, "This is too bad. We should give the cops a chance." I have learned over the past few weeks just how privileged that sentiment was.

I have been arrested twice in my life, both times with a relatively small group of disabled people. Both times the police for the most part were careful and polite, albeit clearly patronizing (this is not always the case, as police violence against disabled people is common). What I have seen the cops do to Occupy Oakland, Occupy Cal and countless other occupations across the country, is nothing short of criminal. The cops are not polite and careful if you are homeless, if you are poor, if you are a person of color and if you are part of a movement that they understand as actually threatening to change things.

I have seen video of cops brutally beating students at UC Berkeley with batons, pulling their hair and jabbing them forcefully in the stomach. I've been a short distance away from cops who shot tear gas into spaces they knew included children, disabled people, homeless people, and animals. I've seen footage and read stories of cops shamelessly shooting rubber bullets at people, including those with cameras. Across the country in dozens of locations the cops are surrounding, destroying, and brutalizing protesters. From Occupy Atlanta to Occupy Salt Lake City to Occupy Denver, police are attacking our cities. It is hard to believe these are just isolated instances–it seems much more like a national organized attack on the movement.

The police brutality is new to many of us. Like me, many people were surprised by the level of violence the cops have used. But to many communities in Oakland this is simply more of the same—there is nothing surprising about it. I am ashamed I was so naïve about the cops in Oakland, but even more than this I am furious. I am furious that the police are allowed to brutalize people.

I am also furious that the cop violence makes these protests so unsafe that many of us who are more vulnerable for whatever reason (age, immigration status, disability, and so forth) cannot even risk exercising our right to be out there and protest. Every time I go down to Oscar Grant Plaza now I weigh the risks I take on as a disabled person who can't run away, a person who can't cover my mouth or my eyes if they tear gas me. And this makes me furious, because I have just as much right to voice my dissent as anyone else.

How is it, that as a supposedly just and democratic nation, we find it justifiable for police to use violence? Even if a handful of protesters are throwing rocks or breaking things, how could this possibly justify the sorts of violent tactics the police routinely use? The cops have proven themselves again and again over the past few weeks (and really throughout history) to not be working for the people; they are the thugs and bullies sent out to protect the rich, the powerful and the status quo. All people, whether part of the Occupy movement or not, should be horrified by what the police have been doing.

The day after the shooting there was a Veterans Against Police Brutality march. A few hundred veterans and allies marched down to the police station, where the Veterans told the cops they should be ashamed. They told the cops they should be protecting the people. They should not follow orders if they are unethical orders.

As Occupy Oakland undergoes a barrage of criticism (some valid, but much not) over some violent tactics a few protestors have used, the police force that has hurt, maimed and nearly killed numerous protestors, has slipped by with little more damage than a bit of bad press.

Occupy Oakland currently braces for another raid. I will now have much more understanding for those who yell, "fuck the cops!" even if I choose not to yell this myself. Privilege is a complicated thing. Where my wheelchair often makes me more at risk of violence, it has also, in conjunction with my whiteness and my gender, most likely shielded me from police violence in the past. However, this situation, this movement, is different than protests I have been involved in previously. It has woken me up—the cops in Oakland and at UC Berkeley have been brutal to everyone and anyone. They are not working to protect the people; in fact they are more than willing to harm us.

The police need to be held accountable for their actions. Even more than this, police violence needs to be publically disgraced as the unlawful, unjust and corrupt tactic that it is.

Editors' Postscript If you enjoyed reading Chap. 2 by Taylor, Hall, Lehman, Liebert, Nishida, and Stewart and are interested in reading more on disability communities' responses to the Occupy Wall Street, we recommend Chap. 15 "My World, My Experiences with Occupy Wall Street and How We can go Further" by Nick Dupree and Chap. 21 "Black & Blue: Policing Disability & Poverty Beyond Occupy" by Leroy Franklin Moore Jr., Lisa 'Tiny' Garcia, and Emmitt Thrower.

Mami Aoyama

Abstract

Minamata disease is a type of poisoning caused when mercury from a chemical factory in southwest Japan polluted the sea, accumulating in fish and shellfish, and affecting people who consumed contaminated seafood. This chapter reviews the historical background of Minamata disease and analyzes the suffering experienced by the victims of the Minamata disease incident, showing how damage to the environment caused multiple disabilities including health and livelihood impairments, poverty and discrimination, and loss of occupational meanings and identities.

Keywords

Disability • Environmental pollution • Minamata disease • Japan post-1945

3.1 Introduction

Modernity has brought material affluence and convenience to people's lives, but has also brought health impairments, poverty and inequality, and has damaged the natural environment on a global scale. Environmental problems such as global warming and the decline in biodiversity have become serious problems that threaten human health, welfare and sustainability (Millennium Ecosystem Assessment 2005). To build resilience in the face of such crises, we have to understand both the "light" and the "dark" sides of modernity.

M. Aoyama (✉)
Department of Occupational Therapy, Faculty of Health Sciences, University of Ljubljana,
Zdravstvena pot 5, Ljubljana 1000, Slovenia
e-mail: AoyamaLjubljana@yahoo.co.jp

© Springer Science+Business Media Dordrecht 2016
P. Block et al. (eds.), *Occupying Disability: Critical Approaches to Community,
Justice, and Decolonizing Disability*, DOI 10.1007/978-94-017-9984-3_3

31

Minamata disease is a type of poisoning caused when mercury from factory wastes polluted the sea and accumulated in fish and shellfish; people who then ate contaminated seafood became ill. Humans have used mercury since antiquity and there have been numerous cases of mercury poisoning, especially from industrial uses of mercury in silver production (UNESCO 2012). In contrast to these incidents, Minamata was the first known case of mercury poisoning through the food chain and Minamata became widely known as one of the most serious examples of postwar industrial pollution (Harada 2004). Other examples of mercury poisoning through the food chain have occurred in Niigata, Japan and in rural Ontario (George 2001; Erikson 1994) and the name "Minamata disease" is widely applied to such cases.

As well as a disease, the Minamata disease incident is a microcosm of modernity, a concrete example of the history experienced by Japan from modernization in the Meiji period (1868–1912) until the era of high growth after World War II (Gotō 1995). The Chisso chemical factory in Minamata City brought jobs and happiness to many people, but also brought unimaginable sorrow to others. The Minamata disease incident clearly shows the light and the dark sides of modernity.

Research on the Minamata disease incident has been conducted in many fields such as medicine, environmental science, sociology, and law. Minamata also has many lessons for disability studies and occupational therapy. The basic cause of Minamata disease was pollution of the ocean. The Minamata disease incident allows us to examine the links between environmental destruction and disability, to understand the social structures that produced those disabilities, to learn from this "negative heritage" and think about ways to use the lessons of Minamata. This chapter will concentrate on the links between environmental destruction and disability; the role of Minamata as "negative heritage" is discussed in Aoyama and Hudson (2013). After briefly reviewing the historical background of Minamata disease, this chapter summarizes the disabilities experienced by victims of Minamata disease, showing how damage to the environment caused multiple disabilities including health and livelihood impairments, poverty and discrimination, and loss of meanings.

Unlike many of the other examples discussed in this book, the disabilities resulting from the Minamata disease incident were a type of social trauma affecting a whole group of people in what was perceived to be an assault on their whole way of life. This trauma has many similarities with the historic trauma experienced by Indigenous peoples around the world. At the same time, it is a type of trauma that is being repeated in Japan as a result of the nuclear meltdown at Fukushima. The author hopes that the analysis in this chapter will deepen understandings of the complex relationships between disability and environmental damage. In this context, the Minamata disease incident can teach us about the way various types of disability (not just physical but social and psychological) result from environmental damage, about how to assign responsibility for such an incident, and about how the incident has impacted society over the last 60 years. Due to limits of space, however, this chapter will focus on the first of these issues. The terminology used in this chapter does not come from a disability empowerment stance but rather reflects the standard usage in Japanese wherein Minamata disease is seen as a criminal "incident" and those people affected by Minamata disease have "suffered" as "victims" of a conscious crime from which they deserve relief— a victim empowerment approach to their various experiences of suffering and disability.

3.2 Minamata Disease and the History of the Minamata Incident

3.2.1 What Is Minamata Disease?

Minamata disease is methylmercury (organic mercury) poisoning caused by pollution from the Chisso chemical factory in Minamata City, Kumamoto Prefecture.

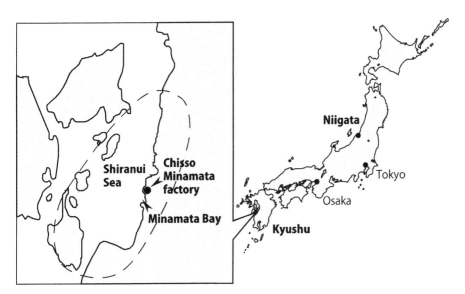

Map of Japan: On a map of the islands of Japan major cities and islands, Niigata city (which is another area with Minamata Disease outbreak as described in the chapter) is shown at the northern part of the main island, and Kyushu island at the south bottom. The coastal cities of Tokyo and Osaka are marked on the main island of Japan: Tokyo south of Niigata and Osaka south of Tokyo and north of Kyushu. In the Shiranui sea, a western inlet of the island of Kyushu, there is a dot showing the location of Minamata Bay. In a square balloon to the left of this image, growing out of the dot, there is a blown-up inset map showing the Shiranui Sea, Minamata Bay and the Chisso Minamata factory

The mercury moved up the food chain to fish and shellfish and then to people who consumed seafood. Methylmercury taken into the body is carried to the internal organs where it accumulates and damages all bodily functions beginning with the brain and nerves. The major symptoms include peripheral neuropathy (sensory impairment of upper and lower limbs), ataxia, tunnel vision, hearing impairment, loss of balance, muscle weakness, speech disorders, convulsions, and eye movement disorders. Severe cases were accompanied by extreme pain and many such people seemed to become deranged and lost consciousness before death.[1]

Many people who developed Minamata disease in the 1950s–1960s died within 3 months and in 1965 the mortality rate was 44.3 %. Later, people were found with only partial or light symptoms (Minamata City 2008). By 2012, a total of 2,273 certified patients was known[2]; 620 of these were still living in 2008 (Minamata City 2008). However, around 11,000 people accepted payments in the 1995 reconciliation and more than 65,000 applied under the Minamata Disease Special Measures Law that was passed in September 2009 and held open for applications until July 2012.[3] Despite these numbers, it is thought that further hidden victims still remain uncounted.

3.2.2   The History of the Minamata Incident

Before the Chisso factory opened in 1908, Minamata was a small town with surrounding fishing villages along the Shiranui Sea.

> The Shiranui Sea was called "the sea where fish gushed out." The fisher folk of Minamata built their houses on hills by the sea, caught fish, planted vegetables in their gardens and traded fish for rice . . . If a visitor came, they would put the kettle on the fire, then go down to the sea, catch a fish or an octopus and be back just as the kettle started boiling. As long as they had this rich and beautiful sea, they enjoyed a life nestling close to nature. (Kurihara 2000)

This quiet, humble life in Minamata was massively transformed by the Chisso chemical factory. In the following I summarize the history of the Minamata incident in three stages.

3.2.3   Minamata Becomes a Chisso "Castle Town"

In 1908, Nihon Chisso Hiryō K.K. (Japan Nitrogenous Fertilizers, Inc.) was established in Minamata. The name of the company was later changed to Shin Nihon Chisso Hiryō (abbreviated to "Chisso") and it grew as a semi-governmental corporation. Many people from neighboring areas moved to work at the Chisso Minamata factory. In 1932, wastewater containing methylmercury—the cause of Minamata disease—began to be discharged from a plant producing acetaldehyde. After World War II, the Minamata factory was quickly reopened and became a

---

[1] A recording of such a patient can be seen at www.youtube.com/watch?v=oxB_SXbxY28.

[2] Up-to-date data on the number of certified patients can be found at www.soshisha.org/kanja/toukei.htm.

[3] Mainichi Shinbun newspaper, 30 August, 2012.

symbol of hope for the reconstruction of Japan. With its population surpassing 40,000, Minamata was designated as a city in 1949 and a former Chisso factory manager became mayor. More than half of the inhabitants of Minamata worked at Chisso, or in Chisso related companies, and Minamata became a so-called "castle town" dominated by Chisso, just as feudal lords had ruled towns in Japan's earlier history (Minamata City 2008; Harada 2008).

3.2.4 The Outbreak of Minamata Disease and the Search for Its Causes

From around 1954, cats in local fishing villages began to "go mad" and die and almost all cats disappeared. In 1955 there was an outbreak of congenital Minamata disease and May 1956 saw the official discovery of the disease when it was reported to the local health center. At first, it was handled as a "strange disease" without a known cause and, fearing that it was infectious, patients were hospitalized in an isolation ward. Rumors of a strange epidemic quickly led to discrimination against victims of Minamata disease.

In November 1956, Kumamoto University Faculty of Medicine reported that poisoning from fish and shellfish caught in Minamata Bay was a possible source of the disease. As a result, Minamata City passed a voluntary directive against fishing and shellfish collecting and it became impossible to sell seafood from Minamata Bay. In that year, 54 people developed symptoms of Minamata disease and 17 died. Kumamoto University made public its methylmercury theory in July 1959. In the same month, the Chisso company hospital began an experiment wherein wastewater from acetaldehyde production was put on food given to cats. By October, one cat had developed symptoms of Minamata disease. This clearly demonstrated that the effluent was the cause of Minamata disease, but Chisso hid these results and continued producing acetaldehyde until 1968 (Minamata City 2008; Harada 2008).

3.2.5 The Search for Responsibility

The directives against fishing and retail boycotts of seafood took away the livelihoods of the Minamata fishers, who were already burdened by having to care for family members sickened by Minamata disease. In November 1959, fishermen forced their way into the Chisso factory, demanding a stop to operations and over 100 people were injured. In the following month, the Minamata Disease Patients' Families Mutual Aid Society agreed to Chisso's so-called "solatium agreement." ¥300,000 was paid to families of people who had died and patients who were still alive were given an annual payment of ¥100,000 (¥30,000 for children).[4] This agreement included a clause stipulating that, "even if Minamata disease should be

---

[4]Until 1971, the US dollar exchange rate was fixed at ¥360. These payments were thus equivalent to $833 for deceased family members and $277 for adults still living ($83 for children).

found to be derived from the [Chisso] factory in the future, the plaintiffs shall make no further claims for compensation" (Minamata City 2008).

For almost 9 years after this contract there was a blank period in which no one was held responsible for the suffering of Minamata disease. In May 1968, after Chisso stopped production of acetaldehyde, the Japanese government concluded that Minamata disease was caused by methylmercury in the waste discharge from Chisso's Minamata factory. Lawsuits began between 1969 and 1973 ruled that Chisso had corporate responsibility and compensation was paid to certified patients. In 2004, the responsibility of the national and prefectural governments was also recognized. Due to Chisso's financial difficulties, however, certification as a Minamata patient became very hard after 1977 and the number of people whose applications were rejected increased.

3.3   The Historical Background to Minamata Disease

In Japan at the end of World War II, it was not unusual for people to starve to death and, for people who experienced this period of hardship, the sight of smoke spouting from chimneys was not a sign of pollution but a symbol of salvation from starvation and the promise of a bright future (Toranomon K.H.J. 2010). Using the Korean War as a springboard toward reconstruction, Japan entered the "era of high growth." From the mid-1950s until the early 1970s, the Japanese economy experienced unprecedented average growth of 10 % and in 1968 Japan's GNP reached second place after the United States. By the mid-1960s, 80 % of households in Japan had the so-called "three treasures" of television, refrigerator and washing machine. Electric rice-cookers, cameras, lipsticks and a range of other goods became widely available and were followed by the "3C" consumables: cars, color TVs and "coolers" (air conditioners/heaters) (Yoshikawa 1997). Japan became economically and materially affluent. The 1964 Tokyo Olympics held a symbolic meaning for a Japan that had accomplished reconstruction after World War II and had been re-admitted into international society.

As in other nations, plastics were essential to economic growth in postwar Japan. Plastics were cheap, hygienic and open to countless uses: "Plastics promised a material utopia, available to all" (Freinkel 2011). Acetaldehyde was necessary to make many plastics and Chisso had two-thirds of the market in this substance. As part of the production process of acetaldehyde, waste containing methylmercury was discharged into the sea.

3.4   The Disabilities and Suffering of the Minamata Disease Victims

The main disabilities and loss of meanings experienced as a result of the environmental damage at Minamata can be summarized as follows.

3.4.1 Pollution of the Sea: The Loss of Occupational Places That Formed Spiritual Cornerstones

For the fisher folk of Minamata, fish were *norisa* or gifts from the ocean. The fishing people prayed to the sea god Ebisu, giving thanks for the rich blessings from the sea. Into that sea flowed "large, oily-looking patches of an unknown stuff, shining black, red and blue" (Ishimure 2003). Polluted with mercury, large numbers of fish with "their fins twitching" (Araki 2000) floated on the surface and there was a terrible stench from rotting shellfish. The fisher folk had not only lost their fishing grounds, which were the source of all life and provided their livelihoods, but they had also lost the place that connected space with spirits. Ogata (2001) remembered that, "Being out on the Shiranui Sea was like rocking in life's cradle" and "my soul felt like it was dancing," but he was shocked that "poison was fed" into that same sea. In Michiko Ishimure's famous book on Minamata, the Shiranui Sea became the "sea of sorrow" (Ishimure 2003).

3.4.2 Sickness and Death of Families: The Loss of Peaceful Households

In 1970, the character 怨 *urami* (meaning "bitterness" or "anger") was displayed at the Chisso shareholders' meeting to represent the feelings of those who had been deprived of family members. One after another, parents, brothers, sisters and children all became sick with Minamata disease. Masato Ogata's father died 2 months after becoming sick without knowing the name or cause of his illness (Oiwa 2001). Ogata (2008) recalls that, "the most important and irreplaceable person in my life was killed by poison from a company that I had never seen. This was the motive for my deep resentment and hatred over the following years." The unnatural death of the great father that he respected and trusted had a big effect on Ogata.

Mothers passed the methylmercury in fish they had eaten to their placentas and their fetuses developed Minamata disease in utero. One mother cried that, "When my baby was in my belly, I ate a lot of fish to give it plenty of nourishment. But then the baby was born with Minamata disease. The baby was a Minamata disease patient from the moment it was born, but there was nothing at all wrong with me" (Higashijima 2010). A father lamented for his child who was born with Minamata disease and only lived a short life: "She was born into this world and a life without light ... A child without sin received a punishment. I don't know how many times I watched her face and thought if only I could exchange myself with this child. (...) But as a parent I couldn't do anything for [my child] who wanted to live" (Kamimura 2005). A patient interviewed by Ishimure at the Minamata City Hospital in 1959 was pregnant when hospitalized, but "The doctors said that my life was more important than the baby's. When they pulled it out with their horrible instruments, my baby writhed in pain, and kicked with its tiny arms and legs. I don't know how

I managed to survive the operation, and the shame and grief afterwards" (Ishimure 2003). This testimony by Yuki Sakagami clearly shows the great sorrow of victims who were unable to protect their loved ones. Irreplaceable parents, siblings and children died one after another or lived with profound disability from the terrible chronic disease; watching this was like being sick oneself—or sometimes an even worse mental strain—and the households that were places of calm and repose began to break down.

Ogata remembers that he was so angry, he "once thought of planting a bomb at Chisso" (Oiwa 2001). But the "reverence for life" held by the Minamata fishers "was the major reason that the victims of Minamata disease did not kill anyone responsible for their condition" (Oiwa 2001). They are disabled but seek justice, not revenge for their *urami*.

3.4.3 Damaged Bodies: Impairments of Function and Capability, Loss of Feelings of Self-Control, and Fear of Sickness and Death

As seen from the following examples, the suffering of people affected by Minamata disease included aspects that cannot be fully described in medical terms like "sensory impairment."

> I was taking a nap beside my father. There was a strange smell so I got up and looked at him. His right hand was moving a little and was scratching his left shoulder. When I looked at that shoulder I was horrified: it was bright red with blood. The skin and flesh had been scratched off and you could see the bone below. But still the hand moved. (. . .) [But] my father did not feel any pain himself (Sasaki 2000).

> Minamata Disease is hell. . . . I have no grip. I cannot hold my husband's hand in mine. My arms shake so hard I cannot even draw my own son close to me. I might even bear this if I could go on living somehow, but I can't eat. I can't bring the rice bowl to my mouth. I can't hold my chopsticks. When I walk, it's not like putting one leg in front of another on the ground, but like floating on air (Ishimure 2003).

Many victims could not understand or accept their illness. At the Minamata City Hospital, Ishimure saw several Minamata patients who were unconscious; others still had some "ill-fitting scraps of consciousness." The latter "emaciated, ghostly-transparent people clearly knew that they were going to die, but the puzzled expressions, the unnatural, contorted postures in which they were lying, the silent accusation in their eyes showed that they were not prepared to die" (Ishimure 2003). A man called Old Sensuke asked, "'How could I come down with Minamata disease, that ugly, shameful illness?' . . . He argued that this monstrous man-made illness ought not to, could not possibly exist" (Ishimure 2003). People who developed Minamata disease were hospitalized but impairments of function and capability progressed rapidly and they lost control of their own bodies. Unwillingly, they faced sickness and death; amidst the bitterness of being unable to accept that they had fallen into this state, they could not face their own deaths.

3.4.4 Can't Fish and Can't Sell the Fish: Loss of Income, Identity and Reasons to Live

Fisher folk who had great pride in their work and who lived modestly became sick one after another. Their actions became jerky and they were unable to conduct tasks such as mending nets and landing fish. Furthermore, the advisory against fishing in Minamata Bay meant that people stopped buying seafood. The fishing harbor at Minamata became a "boat cemetery" full of "empty, half-rotten boats" (Ishimure 2003).

Shunji Araki recalled that, "As a fisherman, not being able to fish at Minamata was the saddest thing. (. . .) If I could recover from Minamata disease, I would go back to get my boat and go out fishing" (Kurihara 2000, p. 70). The spread of Minamata disease ruptured the traditional occupation of fishing in the area: "Deserting the village in ever increasing numbers . . . the young people settled elsewhere. They never came back. In spite of their efforts, the old fishermen could no longer initiate the succeeding generations into the secrets of their profession" (Ishimure 2003). The fisher folk began to go out to sea when they were young, developing their skills, catching fish and supporting themselves. They would work hard to get their own boats. For the fishers, fishing was the occupation through which they realized their full abilities facing the sea and the fish. Engaging in this occupation brought them happiness, healing and pride in addition to their "daily bread." With the outbreak of Minamata disease, however, their health was damaged and they could no longer sell their fish; even by going fishing every day they could no longer support their families. Thus, the loss of the occupation of fishing was the loss of regular work, the loss of an occupation that challenged a lifetime of knowledge and technique, the loss of the role of supporting one's family, and the loss of the occupation of teaching the next generation. In short, it was the loss of occupations that faced the soul with nature. With the loss of these occupations that brought both income and something to live for, the Minamata disease disabled also lost their identity as fisher folk, their dreams in which they entrusted the future, and the hope to live.

3.4.5 Poverty: Impairments to Daily Activity

Despite their own symptoms, people affected by Minamata disease had to look after their own families even though they could not sell their fish. Harada, a doctor from Kumamoto University, described the poverty in Minamata: "The houses where the patients lived were in disrepair and tilting to one side. They would close the storm screens and hide inside, never coming out. (. . .) The tatami mats . . . were old and in disrepair and there was nothing to eat. If you went to the kitchen, there was one pot and if you lifted the lid you saw that it contained only boiled fish. This was a time when everyone was too frightened to eat fish. But they had to eat fish or else would hardly have been able to make ends meet" (Harada 2004).

When 16 members of the Diet, the Japanese parliament, visited Minamata in 1959, a housewife named Satsuki Nakaoka read out a petition:

Our children are dying of Minamata Disease. . . . Our husbands are suffering from the same terrible illness and so are no longer able to sail out to catch fish. Those who can still handle their nets face poverty and hardship because no one will buy their catches. Restrained by conscience, we cannot make a living by stealing. We tried to put up with our suffering by convincing ourselves that it was our fate, and that we couldn't change it, but now we have reached the limit of our endurance. (Ishimure 2003)

The sad plight of the Minamata disease disabled had already reached such a state where they were no longer able even to protect the barest minimum of their lives and yet there was no one who admitted responsibility or tried to save them.

3.4.6 Discrimination: Alienation from the Community

People who had done nothing wrong bore the brunt of the disease amidst poverty and discrimination. At the beginning, when people became ill they were forcibly hospitalized in isolation wards. When a family member got sick, officials would come from the city office and "would disinfect the whole house. We were ostracized and when we went shopping, shopkeepers would not take the money in their bare hands but would use chopsticks or bowls. When people walked in front of the house they would hold their noses" (Shimoda 2000). At primary school, when it was time to clean the classroom, "we were told not to touch desks or chairs because the strange disease was catching" (Shimoda 2000). Sugimoto (2000) recalls that when her mother walked outside, a neighbor pushed her down a bluff saying, "You lot stay indoors!"

In 1969, discrimination was escalated by a lawsuit seeking responsibility from Chisso. Bringing litigation against Chisso in Minamata meant making enemies of almost all inhabitants of the city, who worked in industries connected to Chisso (Higashijima 2010). Fumi Hiyoshi remembers that, "Windows were broken, people urinated against the house, the phone would ring after 12 o'clock at night . . . and men who looked like [gangsters] came to pressure us" (Higashijima 2010). In 1971, a handbill in newspapers delivered to all households in Minamata City included comments such as, "That lot ate rotten fish and got a strange disease;" "Please be aware that if you don't choose the right way, you will make enemies of the citizens of Minamata as well as the company;" "You give the impression both inside and outside the town that you bear a grudge not only against the company but also against the town. Please be more aware that the citizens of Minamata are angry that you have brought the image of the town to the lowest level"; and "How dare you lay it on like this? ¥30 million is too much for neuralgia or alcoholism" (Higashijima 2010). In this way, "citizens" and "patients" became opposed to each other and there was widespread discrimination against "fake patients with dirty money" and "Fishermen from other places who ruined Minamata."

That this discrimination continued for a long time is clear from the following story by national broadcast network NHK reporter Higashijima. At a year-end party held by a certain company in 1992, one employee raised his hand and said, "'I'm gonna do an impression of a patient!' He began to stagger slowly around. He stuck out his hands in front of him and continued with exaggerated tremors. With a sloppy open mouth he implored, 'Give me money! Give me moneeey!' and wandered around the tatami room like an old goat. The room exploded with laughter [and] he returned to his seat amidst a huge round of applause" (Higashijima 2010). Higashijima noted there were several company employees present who were children of Minamata victims, but they also felt compelled to clap and smile.

The misconception that Minamata disease is catching can still be found today. Examples of continuing discrimination include cases where children from Minamata are refused accommodation on school trips, people who refuse to take part in swimming competitions with participants from Minamata, and instances where people from Minamata have been prevented from getting jobs or even getting married when their hometown becomes known. As the very name "Minamata disease" has been the cause of discrimination against Minamata City residents, there have been calls to change the name of the illness. At the same time, there is an argument that because Minamata disease was not a one-off accident involving methylmercury, but a type of man-made environmental pollution that works up the food chain, the name should not be changed so that the existence of this incident is not forgotten.

In addition to the discrimination between "citizens" and Minamata "patients" and between "locals" and "outsiders," as the process of official certification of Minamata disease patients progressed, new splits have developed between certified and non-certified patients. Kiyoto Sasaki explained the impact of the certification process in the following example: "When I left Meshima [village] in 1960, all the houses were old and falling apart. When I came back 18 years later, the uncertified people were living even harsher lives, but the lives of the certified people had completely changed due to their compensation payments and pensions. The old atmosphere where the whole village seemed like one big family had completely broken down' (Kurihara 2000, p. 120)". Experiencing discrimination from people who had been like family and being alienated from the community added to the health and lifestyle impairments and made the sorrow of the Minamata victims even greater. Many people continued to hide the fact that they had Minamata disease in order not to impede their children's chances of employment or marriage. Moreover, not only is it very hard to dismantle feelings of discrimination once they have been constructed, but rebuilding broken communities requires a long time and great perseverance.

3.4.7 The Long Absence of Responsibility: Coerced "Self-Responsibility"

In 1973, the Kumamoto District Court ruled in favor of Chisso's responsibility, stating that, "if the factory had conducted sufficient tests of the wastewater and had responded appropriately to the environmental changes, it could have minimized the damage." The court ordered between ¥16–18,000,000 (at that time US $60,000–68,000) to be paid to the plaintiffs. Seventeen years had passed from the official recognition of Minamata disease to this ruling. It took a total of 31 years before the responsibility of the national and prefectural governments was recognized in 2004. The victims of Minamata disease had themselves done nothing wrong, but because no one accepted responsibility for a long time, they had to manage by themselves, with profound health and lifestyle impairments, poverty and discrimination, and eating polluted fish. Even today, after the responsibility of the company and government authorities has been legally recognized, there are still disputes over the criteria for patient certification. Almost 60 years after Minamata disease was recognized, the Minamata affair is still not over.

3.4.8 Summary of Disabilities

As shown above, Minamata disease is not limited to physical disabilities but also involves many other layers of turmoil including the loss of occupational places that form spiritual cornerstones, emotional distress and the breakup of families due to family sickness, the loss of bodily self-control through impairments to function and capability, functional disabilities, fear of sickness and death, employment deprivation and loss of purpose in life, the loss of occupations providing monetary income and the loss of identity and useful roles, the lifestyle impairments of poverty, alienation from the local community, and coerced self-responsibility due to the failure of the real culprits to take responsibility.

Prejudice and discrimination from the local community worsened the loss of the Minamata victims. This prejudice continued for a long time because class discrimination between metropolis and province, between different ranks in the factory, between Chisso employees and farmers, and between farmers and fishers was still deeply rooted in Japanese society. This discrimination can be said to have contained elements of self-protection whereby people attempted to maintain their own rank by keeping others in a position lower than themselves. Another factor promoting discrimination was related to the fact that Chisso supported the fluorescence and income of Minamata City: if Chisso declined people would find their incomes cut off and be unable to maintain their livelihoods. Thus for the citizens/workers of Minamata, the victims of Minamata disease were threats to their own lives. This feeling that those disabled from Minamata disease were a hindrance or obstacle led to intense prejudice and discrimination.

These social injustices resulted in the deprivation of many basic human rights, including the right to a clean environment, the right to existence, the right to health, the right to occupation, the right to happiness, and the human right of equality.

3.5   Conclusions

After the deprivations and hardships that resulted from Japan's colonial expansion into Asia and the following war, most Japanese people wished for economic growth and shouldered together the reconstruction and rapid growth of the postwar years. Japan quickly attained economic affluence. It was during this period that Minamata disease produced many victims. Minamata disease did not only involve physical impairments resulting from mercury poisoning, but also involved a range of other disabilities as summarized in Sect. 3.4.8.

As discussed in Aoyama and Hudson (2013), responsibility for the outbreak of Minamata disease and for its expansion and prolonged nature lies with the following groups:

- Chisso: responsibility for the outbreak and expansion of Minamata disease.
- Government: responsibility for not instituting measures to prevent the spread of the disease and for prolonging its effects.
- Academics: responsibility for acting in complicity with the government to expand and prolong the impacts of the disease.
- Mass media: responsibility for reporting that gave priority to economic growth.
- The mayor and inhabitants (workers) of Minamata City: responsibility for prejudice and discrimination in protecting their lifestyles.
- Companies who bought Chisso products: responsibility for supporting Chisso.
- Consumers and citizens: responsibility for ignorance and indifference in consumption and voting.

In other words, almost all of the people who made up Japanese society bore some responsibility for the Minamata disease incident and the subsequent disabilities and discriminations described in this chapter. In their inability to question the nature of their "affluence," the Japanese people lost their capability for autonomy and became caught up in the dark side of modernity and its socials powers and structures that give priority to economic growth even at the expense of victims such as those with Minamata disease. This happened even though Japan had in theory become a democracy after World War II. On March 11, 2011, Japanese society once again produced a crisis after the explosions and meltdown at the Fukushima nuclear power plant. Both Minamata and Fukushima are cases where destruction of the natural environment caused by the prioritization of economic growth brought forth many victims. The sacrifices resulted from social structures that put the economy above everything else and in order to build a just society that supports health and well-being without making victims of the poor and disadvantaged we have to consider the responsibility of each person who supports those structures.

The philosopher Erika Schuchardt (2005) discusses how people may come to accept and work through unforeseen crises, such as the birth of a disabled child, unemployment, separation and death, and incurable illness for the individual, and persecution, human rights abuses, terrorism, natural disasters, and environmental pollution for the group. People affected by Minamata disease have experienced many elements of such crises, beginning with the loss of what Maslow (1943) saw as the most basic human physiological needs. Together with their supporters, the victims of the Minamata disease incident have been fighting against the Chisso company, the state, and Kumamoto Prefecture for almost 60 years. Writing about their early encounters with Minamata disease, activist-supporters such as the physician Masazumi Harada expressed their "real shock that these people [had to live] by concealing themselves amidst poverty and discrimination" even though they had committed no crime (Higashijima 2010, p. 92). Elementary school teacher Fumiko Hiyoshi remembered, "It was when I saw the congenital patients. I literally couldn't sleep for several days. The shock of seeing them and ... the fact that I hadn't known anything about it made me very ashamed" (Higashijima 2010, p. 48). These children also made a big impact on documentary film maker Noriaki Tsuchimoto (Higashijima 2010, p. 133): "They couldn't see, speak or hear. ... [T]hose children became the basis of our filming. I thought, is such a thing possible?" This last sentiment was also expressed by the economist Hirofumi Uzawa (Higashijima 2010, p. 128): "Was such a thing really possible?" Anger at the absurdity of Minamata disease was the basis of action for the many supporters of those affected by the disease. Working together with the victims, they have managed to achieve some results in understanding the causes and assigning responsibility for the Minamata disease incident.

Today, nearly 60 years have passed since the beginning of the incident and those affected by Minamata disease have various memories of the past and wishes for the future. Some remain angry, asking, like Yoshiharu Tagami, "Were we sacrificed like a bunch of dogs?" (Higashijima 2010, p. 194). Others, like Masato Ogata, have found ways to come to terms with the incident through local beliefs such as *moyai-naoshi* or "mooring boats together" (Oiwa 2001). Still others, like Tsuginori Hamamoto, have tried to emphasize the positive side of postwar changes in Minamata: "A few were sacrificed [so that] most people became happy. We have to be sure not to destroy that happiness" (Higashijima 2010, p. 83). This wish is for a society where present happiness is respected but which produces no more victims who are burdened with the suffering that comes from the shock of asking "Is this possible?" Such a society should be able to dispel sorrow and generate a just happiness for all. This wish, in other words, is that no victims are sacrificed for the happiness of others, that the light and dark of modernity change into a new culture and autonomous society which respects the lives and livelihoods of each of its members.

Editors' Postscript If you liked Chap. 3 by Mami Aoyama, and are interested in reading more about intracultural interpretations of decolonization, we recommend Chap. 5 "Landings: Decolonizing Disability, Indigeneity and Poetic Methods" by Petra Kuppers and Chap. 6, "Occupying Autism: Rhetoric, Involuntarity, and the Meaning of Autistic Lives" by Melanie Yergeau. This chapter also addresses a number of issues about the operation of conformities in communities, and it is worth considering it against chapters that explore the experience of meeting these powerful demands such as Chap. 10: Neoliberal Academia and a Critique from Disability Studies as well as those which deal with community empowerment such as Chap. 12: "Refusing to Go Away: The Ida Benderson Seniors Action Group" by Denise M. Nepveux. This chapter also anticipates some of the issues (for example corporate power over disability) which the editors raise in their final chapter for this book, Chap. 26: Science (Fiction), Hope and Love: Conclusions.

Acknowledgments This chapter was translated by Mark Hudson. I am grateful to the editors of this volume for their comments on earlier versions of the text. The research summarized here was partly supported by a grant from the Daiwa Anglo-Japanese Foundation.

References

Aoyama M, Hudson MJ (2013) Minamata as negative heritage: implications for Fukushima. Pac Geogr 40:23–28
Araki S (2000) Ryō o ubawarete. In: Kurihara A (ed) Shōgen Minamatabyō. Iwanami, Tokyo, pp 57–70
Erikson K (1994) A new species of trouble: the human experience of modern disasters. W.W. Norton, New York
Freinkel S (2011) Plastic: a toxic love story. Houghton Mifflin Harcourt, Boston
George TS (2001) Minamata: pollution and the struggle for democracy in postwar Japan. Harvard University Asia Center, Cambridge, MA
Gotō T (1995) Chinmoku to bakuhatsu dokyumento 'Minamatabyō jiken'. Shūeisha, Tokyo
Harada M (2004) Minamatabyō no rekishi. In: Harada M (ed) Minamatagaku kōgi, vol 1. Nihon Hyōronsha, Tokyo, pp 23–49
Harada M (2008) Minamatabyō 50 nen. In: Harada M, Hanada M (eds) Minamatagaku kōgi, vol 4. Nihon Hyōronsha, Tokyo, pp 23–48
Higashijima D (2010) Naze Minamatabyō wa kaiketsu dekinai no ka. Gen Shobō, Fukuoka
Ishimure M (2003) Paradise in the sea of sorrow: our Minamata disease. Center for Japanese Studies, University of Michigan, Ann Arbor
Kamimura Y (2005) Minamatabyō kanja kara utaetai koto. In: Harada M (ed) Minamatagaku kōgi, vol 2. Nihon Hyōronsha, Tokyo, pp 29–50
Kurihara A (ed) (2000) Shōgen Minamatabyō. Iwanami, Tokyo
Maslow A (1943) A theory of human motivation. Psychol Rev 50:370–396
Millennium Ecosystem Assessment (2005) Ecosystems and human well-being: synthesis. Island Press, Washington, DC
Minamata City (ed) (2008) Minamatabyō: sono rekishi to kyōkun (trans: Minamata disease: its history and lessons). Minamata Disease Municipal Museum, Minamata. http://www.minamata195651.jp/pdf/kyoukun_eng_all.pdf. Accessed 25 July 2014
Ogata M (2001) Chisso wa watashi de atta. Ashi Shobō, Fukuoka
Ogata M (2008) Seimei no kioku yo, yomigaere. In: Harada M, Hanada M (eds) Minamatagaku kōgi, vol 4. Nihon Hyōronsha, Tokyo, pp 107–126
Oiwa K (2001) Narrated by Ogata Masato. Rowing the eternal sea: the story of a Minamata fisherman. Rowman & Littlefield, Lanham
Sasaki K (2000) Kujū no sentaku. In: Kurihara A (ed) Shōgen Minamatabyō. Iwanami, Tokyo, pp 113–126
Schuchardt E (2005) Why me? Learning to live in crises. WCC Publications, Geneva
Shimoda A (2000) Osanai imōto ga 'kibyō' ni. In: Kurihara A (ed) Shōgen Minamatabyō. Iwanami, Tokyo, pp 29–41
Sugimoto E (2000) Minamata no umi ni ikiru. In: Kurihara A (ed) Shōgen Minamatabyō. Iwanami, Tokyo, pp 129–146
Toranomon Kokusai Hōritsu Jimusho (2010) Dokyumento Minamatabyō 1873–1995. http://toranomon.cocolog-nifty.com/minamatabyojiken/cat21394872/index.html. Accessed 16 Sept 2012
UNESCO (2012) Heritage of mercury: Almadén and Idrija. World Heritage Nomination File. http://whc.unesco.org/uploads/nominations/1313rev.pdf. Accessed 14 July 2013
Yoshikawa H (1997) Kōdo seichō: Nihon o kaeta 6000 nichi. Yomiuri Shimbunsha, Tokyo

Movements at War? Disability and Anti-occupation Activism in Israel

4

Liat Ben-Moshe

Abstract

At the time of the first major disability protest in Israel in 1999 and then in 2000–2001, there were already many anti-occupation and peace organizations at play in Israel/Palestine. While participating in this budding disability movement, I began reflecting on my experiences of simultaneously being an Israeli anti-occupation activist and disabled activist publically fighting for the first time for disability rights. In the summer of 2006 I conducted research in Israel, trying to assess any changes that occurred since 2000 in the connections between the movements and within the disability movement itself. And then the war on Lebanon began. My intention in writing this chapter is to highlight the connections between disability activism and anti-war and anti-occupation activism, which seem to be at war with one another but in fact intersect in important ways. I hope this narrative and analysis will be useful for material resistance as well as a reflection on our current states of exclusion in activism and scholarship.

Keywords

Disability • Anti-occupation • Israel/Palestine • Activism • Social movements • War

4.1 The Big "Disability Strikes"

In 1999, people with disabilities came together for the first time in Israel in large numbers, to protest their material and social conditions. This protest was sparked by a few determined people with disabilities (mostly wheelchair users) who felt they

L. Ben-Moshe (✉)
University of Toledo, Toledo, OH, USA
e-mail: Liat.BenMoshe@utoledo.edu

© Springer Science+Business Media Dordrecht 2016
P. Block et al. (eds.), *Occupying Disability: Critical Approaches to Community, Justice, and Decolonizing Disability*, DOI 10.1007/978-94-017-9984-3_4

had nothing left to lose. It was a grassroots effort to change the terrain of disability services, and more specifically the way benefits were distributed at the time. The protest lasted 37 days, in which the protesters lived in the lobby of the Department of Treasury/Finance in Jerusalem (for more detailed information about the protests see Rimon-Greenspan 2006). The protesters were successful in changing services and benefits, but only for those classified as "severely" disabled. The general disability allowance for other disabled people remained unchanged.

In late 2001 the second major protest of disabled people erupted, lasting a record breaking 77 days, making it the one of the longest strike in Israel's history (Rimon-Greenspan 2007). "Erupted" may not actually be the best descriptor for this demonstration of will and determination, since it was the result of careful planning on the part of the organizers.[1] Indeed, what made the longevity of the 2001–2002 protest possible was the continuous aid from the *Histadrut*. The Histadrut is the federation of laborers and is in essence the largest workers union in Israel to this day. It was established in 1920 as a Jewish trade union and allowed non-Jewish/Arab citizens to join only from 1959. From its inception, the Histadrut had become a mainstay of the Zionist rule in historic Palestine and later in Israel, which became an official state recognized by the United Nations in 1948. In the formative years of the state of Israel, the Histadrut was actually quite resistive to establishing a welfare program specifically targeting the disabled population, and instead advocated for benefits and services for work-related disabilities solely (see Mor 2006 for more on this history).

During the protests, however, the Histadrut provided all the logistical support needed to sustain such a massive effort for so long, including all the food, supplies and even medications and medical equipment. In addition to organizational support, the Histadrut arranged two support rallies, and two solidarity strikes of the entire unionized labor force in Israel. Once the protest had ended the leaders of the struggle were offered physical space, salaries and limited staff and resources by the Histadrut. Thus, the "headquarters of disability struggle" (Mate Ha'maavak) was solidified and transformed from a makeshift grassroots organization to an official disability organization housed under the hospices of the Histadrut.

One of the key supporters of the 2001–2002 disability protests in Jerusalem was the Histadrut chairperson at the time, Amir Peretz. In 2005 Peretz became the chairman of the Labor party. His rise to the top was seen by some disability activists as a political move that was done on their backs. In an uncommon twist in Israeli politics (since he wasn't a General or Chief of Staff), Peretz became the Minister of Defense in 2006 in Ahud Ulmerts' right wing coalition government. This unlikely post was perceived as a political move to keep Peretz out of any positions of power in regards to social policy and welfare in the administration, for which he was conceived of as being too leftist and socialist. In his position as Defense

---

[1]These were a few of the people that were involved in the first protest, but most of the key figures had changed. The number of attendees and supporters, however, increased tenfold this time around.

Minister, it was Amir Peretz who would later on plan and legitimize the second war on Lebanon. A war which, needless to say, added many new members to the disability community, especially in Lebanon.

Interestingly, the protests were termed in the media as "the *disabled strike,*"[2] and this is how they are known to the public to this day. "Strikes," at least in the Israeli context, signify labor disputes, and are usually used by unionized workers in protest of their working conditions—withholding of their salaries, downsizing, privatization etc. But most of the disabled protesters were in fact unemployed or had a part time job only, which is exactly the issue the protests were bringing to light and trying to transform. One of the demands made by the protesters was leveling disability benefits given by social security with minimum standard of living wages (which at that time were double the amount of disability benefits). The other demand was the cancellation of the provision to have only one kind of benefit per person, for instance either personal assistant or mobility benefits for vehicles, which meant that people had to choose between bathing, for example, and leaving their house.

4.2 Anti-occupation and Decolonialization Framework

When the disability protests began outside of the Department of Treasury in Jerusalem, another struggle was underway not too far from there. The Al-Aqsa Intifada (also known as the Second Intifada) was in full force and Palestinian citizens and non-citizens as well as Jewish and other activists were clashing with the Israeli army and police on a daily basis. In October 2000, 13 Palestinians (12 of whom were citizens of Israel) were shot and killed by Israeli police while protesting in solidarity with Palestinians in the territories. This event politicized my consciousness more than any other, and like others of my generation who did not experience the first Intifada first hand, I was horrified at the ease by which the Israeli armed forces can annihilate opposition and dissent. I was also shocked by the general disregard for the lives of (mostly non-Jewish) political activists and prisoners by the Jewish Israeli public (for an analysis of this "new hegemony" during the second intifada see Rouhana and Sultany 2003).

Anti-occupation activists, especially those who do not endorse a Zionist ideology, are seen in the Jewish Israeli public, and portrayed in the media, as traitors. Therefore their (our) lives are in the hands of the political-military regime, and eliminating us and silencing our voices is allowed and even encouraged. Agamben (1998) explicates this process by explaining how bare life (as opposed to a qualified life by the sovereign), becomes the object and subject of political power in modern democracy. Giving up personal liberty to a sovereign power reifies one as, what

---

[2]There are numerous potential descriptors that could have been assigned to describe these, such as protests (mecha'ah) or demonstration (hufganah), but strikes is what stuck in the media and public discourse.

Agamben refers to, a homo sacer (s/he who can be killed but not sacrificed). The suspension of bare life in modern politics (which legitimates its annihilation) is what Agamben refers to as a state of exception. The homo sacer lives in a constant state of exception and because law is suspended in regards to them, s/he may be killed without penalty. But it's not only that those resisting the Zionist regime, become homo sacer but also that the state of Israel is governed through a constant state of exception, by using "state of emergency" and military rule to override Palestinian's rights (and their existence) since 1948 to current times.[3] In that sense, Israel has a (settler colonial) ethnocratic political-military regime masquerading as democracy (Shafir and Peled 1998, 2002; Yiftachel 2006). Thus the issue of guaranteeing human and social rights (such as trying to secure rights or benefits for disabled people) under the guise of a liberal democracy is naturalized and therefore seen as completely separate from the larger ethnic-colonial mechanisms on which the state of Israel was founded and currently operates.[4]

The second intifada was underway when the second round of disability protests began. The events were not disjointed in time, space and perception. Indeed, there was some worry among the participants of the second disability sit-in that the struggle would not be able to garner enough public and media attention in light of the political turmoil. However, the decision was made to forge ahead, in order to capitalize on the momentum of the first sit-in and expand the range of benefits to more people with disabilities. But the "disabled community" was already not only an "imagined community" (As Anderson (1983) discusses in relation to nationalism) but also a divided one, as I will expand upon below. I want to stress that this is not a coincidence and that nationality based on Zionist ideology is at the basis of such dis-junctures and splits within "the movement," not a byproduct of unsuccessful organizing. In short, I want to offer a decolonizing framework to understand these fissures. The Israeli state is not just a state born of dispossession (of Palestinians and their land) but a daily *continuous* act of a particular form of settler colonialism. Without understanding, and relating to, this origin story and its continuation today, any 'rights' discourse is essentially and materially meaningless. As Tuck and Yang (2012, page 18) remark about settlers of color in North America, "... its logical endpoint, the attainment of equal legal and cultural entitlements, is actually an investment in settler colonialism." The argument they, and other scholars/activists within the decolonizing framework, are making is that any appeal to the state for equal rights is a continuation and legitimization of the occupation and appropriation of land by making the state appear as a sovereign entity with the ability to grant such things as rights or

---

[3]Israel established "state of emergency" regulations under British colonial rule, before it became as state in 1948, and had been extending them in the Knesset every 2 years since then. The military rule had been formally taken out in 1965 but continues de facto in the occupied territories of course, but also in Israel at large via the "state of emergency" regulations.

[4]Ilan Pappe (2008) contends that Israel is not a state of exception, but rather a state of oppression. Agamben's framework can only make sense for those who, mistakenly, view Israel as being able to be simultaneously democratic and Jewish (see Lentin 2009).

land. It leaves not just the nation state but the settler colonial relations embedded therein intact, and as such is in complete opposition to notions like "justice" or "equality."

4.3   Civil Militarism and Hierarchies of Disability

The Zionist ethos is not an add-on to the analysis of disability and anti-occupation protests, but is in fact inextricably linked to disability and notions of fitness (not only physical). Disability has been viewed historically as the antithesis of Zionist myths and ethos, as a remnant of the Diasporic weak Jew of the past. This ethos is also imbued in gendered and sexualized notions of the "weak" queer Jew (Boyarin 1996, 1997). Zionism as an ideology thought to transform Jewishness into a national identity and national body politics and body type. Physical labor, return to nature and fitness, conquest of the 'wilderness' (with Palestinians in it) and military power (Abdo and Yuval-Davis 1995) were seen as an antidote to the scholastic Diasporic Jew. The Zionist ethos was a project consumed by the creation of the New (strong) Jew as part of nation-building and creation of collective identity in no small part through the image of the strong masculine conqueror and soldier (Almog 2000). Weiss (2003) refers to it as the construction of the "chosen body." It is the ideal type constructed in order to structure the New Israeli – and by which Jewish Israelis are shaped from before their birth up to the ritual of their burial. These notions of the ideal body shape present day notions of dis/ability in Israel via mechanisms which could be construed as remnants of eugenics such as excessive prenatal testing, or selections of who is "fit" for combat duty (Weiss 2003).

The entanglement of the occupation in relation to any disability discourse in Israel/Palestine is thus ever present. Perhaps the most obvious conduit of this meshing is the prevalence of the military in everyday life in Israel/Palestine. The disability community in Israel is divided by whether one was injured during military service or not. The strongest disability sub-group, politically and in terms of benefits from the state, is the army disabled (Nechei Tzahal, veterans of the Israeli Defense Forces or IDF). Army disabled in Israel represent the ideal of the total heroic sacrifice for the good of the nation, and as such do not always succumb to the devaluation and stigma associated with disability. Since the establishment of the State of Israel, the army was perceived as the core engine of nation building, which allowed it to be involved in various "civil" functions such as immigration absorption, bridging over ethnic differences (serving as a melting pot), educating for citizenship and patriotism, and teaching the language (Ben-Eliezer 1995). These non-military functions served as evidence that Israel is in fact a "civil" country. Ben-Eliezer (1998) criticizes this attitude suggesting that it is the army's involvement in these fields, and the blurring of the boundaries between the army and society, that testifies to a militarization of society rather than to a civilization of the army. Thus, Ben-Eliezer (1995) suggests that Israel is a certain kind of nation: "Nation-In-Arms."

The army was put in the center of collective awareness, becoming the essence of the nation. This is what Kimmerling (1985)[5] refers to as "civil militarism," a state where "militarism penetrates both structurally and culturally into the collective mood … in this situation, the whole system is institutionally (economically, industrially and legislatively) and mentally aimed at constant preparations for war, as if it was the 'natural' state of the 'world'" (1985, p. 129). The army becomes a part of daily life and armed (and non-armed) conflict seems like an ongoing routine and not an exceptional event. One of the reasons for the absence of anti-militaristic discussion in the disability protests was therefore due to Israeli society being one of "civil militarism." The dominance of the military in Israel creates, then, a phenomenon of "critical obedience" that establishes that during war, the army/military/IDF is not to be criticized (Ben-Eliezer 1998). Since Israel is perceived to be in a constant state of war, this prohibition is continuous. The call by some disability activists for equalization of all disability benefits to those granted by the ministry of defense, was therefore viewed as blasphemy and was not pursued during the protests in any meaningful way, as I shall elaborate below.

Historically, at the end of the "War of Independence" (or Nakba) the newly founded government in Israel decided to lay the responsibility for caring and rehabilitating Army disabled and their families on the Ministry of Defense. "The Invalid's Law (Benefits and Rehabilitation)" of 1949 provided disabled veterans with relatively generous non-means-tested benefits. In addition, the benefits included in the bill (or added later) included a variety of medical and occupational rehabilitation services, business and home loans, access to adaptive recreational facilities, personal social services and counseling (Gal and Bar 2000). Almost all these services are closed off to disabled people who are not veterans. This bill and its added benefits created a clear hierarchy of disability in Israeli policy and society, in which it is considered better to be disabled while in the army or have a work related injury than deal with general disability benefits administered by the social security administration.

The "Invalid's law" also recognized the Association of Disabled Veterans as an official representative of veteran's interests. Since its inception the disabled veterans association was mostly concerned with the rights and benefits of veterans solely. It did not recognize the need for coalition of all disabled people and their organizations to achieve a more inclusive society for all. In fact it made every effort to ensure that benefits accorded to disabled veterans would not be extended to all. For instance, most mobility impaired veterans receive cars, and stipends to maintain them, from the ministry of defense, so the disabled veteran association never addressed the issue of inaccessibility of public transportation. It is therefore not very surprising that the Association for army disabled, as the most powerful disability organization in Israel,

[5]It may be interesting to note that Kimmerling was not only one of the premier theorists of militarization in Israel but also a symptom of the phenomenon I am describing here, being one of a few full time professors with significant disabilities, who never reflected on disability as a political identity linked to the phenomenon he studied.

never fully endorsed the disability protests (although there have been individual army disabled men and women who attended the demonstrations and showed their support).

What is often omitted from the discussion of army disabled in the literature and in public debates on both pensions and the heroic halo associated with being a veteran, is who is excluded from this experience. In Israel, both (cisgender) men and women serve in the army, although women do not serve in combat duty and married women do not have to serve at all (although they might be required to do national service as a volunteer).[6] However, the Invalid law states that all soldiers who were injured or became ill during military service or as a result of service are covered under the law and should receive benefits associated with being army disabled. Therefore many army disabled are in fact women, who got injured or ill while serving in compulsory army duty, under any capacity. Gays and lesbians also serve in the army due to conscription, although they were restricted from serving in some positions, especially intelligence, until the mid-nineties. Two populations who are not obligated and called to serve are disabled and Muslim-Palestinian citizens of Israel.[7] This is not just a result of Zionist rule and occupation but is also manifested in anti-occupation activism. For instance, many Arab/Palestinians who organize against the occupation are often uncomfortable and at times reluctant to work with Israelis who had served in the army, as the *de facto* executing arm of the occupation. It was very strange for me to be a part of these conversations amongst organizers, being at times the only Jewish Israeli in the room who had not served in the army. Most disabled Jews are exempt from compulsory military service, although one can always volunteer to serve, even when disabled. I was not drafted due to disability but had no intention to volunteer to serve. It was much easier for me to make this decision, though, than it was for many of my colleagues and non-disabled friends who did not wish to serve but did not wish to spend the next year or more of their lives in a military jail.

Lack of army service in one's resumé also carries with it other social and economic ramifications, such as discrimination in employment that calls for a military record; loans that are open only to those who served etc. Some of these opportunities are phrased and structured in such a way as to deliberately exclude Arabs/Palestinians without the appearance of racism or blatant discrimination. The ramifications on disabled people, Jewish in particular, who have not served are not as severe. Although the same policies are still applicable and as exclusionary for disabled people, disabled people often have other avenues to address them. Loans, for instance, can be obtained through other means such as the social security administration. Since employment is abysmal for disabled people generally it is unclear how much the lack of army service influences this outcome. In pointing

---

[6]Ultra-orthodox Jews are also exempt from military service, a topic of much debate in Israel.

[7]There have been more recent demands to conscript Christian-Palestinians citizens of Israel. I also can't get into the intricate conscript debates regarding the Druze and Bedouin populations in Israel.

out the consequences of not serving in the Israeli army I do not mean to suggest that army service should be more inclusive and open to all. This has in fact been an argument presented by some feminists in Israel, who try to equalize military service for women and demand that they should be given the opportunity to serve in combat positions. Similar arguments are made by queer or LGBTQI (Lesbian, Gay, Bisexual, Transgender, Queer, Questioning, Intersex) activists both in Israel and the US who demand that LGBTQI people should be able to serve fully in the military if so desired. What I am suggesting is that the same economic and social opportunities should be applied to all, regardless of service.[8]

4.4 Occupation, Militarism and Disability at a (Dis)Juncture

The importance of the disability sit-ins for me, as well as many other disabled people and the general public, was less in the actual achievements (or lack thereof) gained as a result of the protests and more in the creation of a sense of community. It was one of the few times where I felt in solidarity with other disabled people, coming together for a shared cause. It felt like a beginning of a movement. And then again, it did not.

During the sit-in in 2001–2002 I suggested to the leader and spokesperson of the group at the time to try and connect what we were fighting for with related social justice issues. More specifically, I asked if I could post a banner in the demonstration site that states "money for rights, not for settlements" (it even rhymes in Hebrew).[9] Although it was unclear whether we were indeed fighting for civil rights or for material existence in the form of increased or sustainable disability benefits, it became painfully clear that whatever the demands were they would have to cost money. To me, that involved shifting the discourse from a Zionist-militarized based budget to a budget that could respectfully sustain all citizens and non-citizens.[10] Maintaining the occupation of Palestinians and their land and the disproportional investment in militarization, security and surveillance has many costs for those living in Israel/Palestine. One of the economic and social costs of such investments is the shrinking of the security net, what used to be regarded as the welfare state. By pointing all this out, I wanted to advance a framework of a true welfare state- not the image conjured up by most Americans in relation to the concept of welfare, one of shame, pity and dependence- but one of a socioeconomic security net provided by the state, including the same disability benefits we were fighting for expanding.

---

[8]For queer critiques of LGBTQI military service in the US see http://www.againstequality.org/about/military/.

[9]"kesef lezchuyot, lo lehitnahluyot."

[10]Non-citizens such as immigrant laborers who have almost no rights under current Israeli policies because they are not Jewish, but are employed mostly by disabled and elderly people and their families who are in need of attendant care.

The banner I suggested was never displayed and my idea was dismissed almost immediately as irrelevant and almost nonsensical. "What does the occupation have to do with disability?" I was asked.

4.4.1 Intersections in "New" Social Movements (or Identity Confronts Leftist Politics)

What the leaders of the demonstrations told me, in fact, was that 'we can't afford to make this a political issue.' I wondered, how can we have a demonstration about shifting the discourse around disability and claiming rights without making it political? What they meant was that, as a budding movement, we should not be divisive. This was somewhat related to the communist ethos of the Histadrut and traditional labor unions, which stresses unity and power in numbers over possible contention within in order to prevail in negotiations. But there was also an undercurrent to the sentiment expressed by the need to be 'united', and that is the prevailing understanding that the occupation and increased militarization is an issue separate from internal demands of Israeli citizens to equality.[11]

One possible reading of the above narrative is through the lens of identity politics vs. traditional left politics. Disability activism can be viewed as a stance of identity politics. In fact, the term identity politics was first used to describe activism by people with disabilities, in 1979 (Bernstein 2005). It also carries with it the pitfalls of such politics, which seem to homogenize the group in question and bulldoze over any points of contention and intersectionality within the group. Bernstein (2005) defines identity politics as activism engaged by status based social movements. What seems to be an underpinning of many of these debates is the understanding that identity politics is a relatively new phenomenon, and it politicized aspects of life that were perceived as neutral or not contested until then- such as politics of sexuality, culture, representation etc. Anti-occupation activism can be viewed through the prism of traditional left activism, in which coalitions are formed by left leaning groups in regards to a certain issue, such as stopping wars and occupation/colonialism.

Marxists and general 'leftists' see class inequality as the underlying problem in relation to inequality, exploitation and oppression. Social change, by this analysis, will come from changing economic inequalities. Identity politics is seen through this prism as divisive and threatening to the creation of class solidarity. The irony is that these accounts don't seem to account for class as an identity. Similarly, identities based on social and cultural difference are not perceived as having a strong economic aspect. Todd Gitlin (1993), for example, laments that radical

---

[11]This is not unique but indeed a pattern of protests in Israel that can also be seen in the recent, 2011, 'tent city' protests across Israel (which preceded the Occupy movement in the US by a few months), in which demands for equality and economic justice had to be 'separated' from any discussion about the occupation in an attempt to de-politicize and 'unify' the movement.

politics cannot be grounded anymore on "universal human emancipation," because of the divisive nature of identity politics. Proponents of identity politics reply that the question is not how to 'not be divisive' but how to can communication be facilitated among people with different positionalities with related political commitments? Also, the claims that identity politics are divisive, is a tool of oppression, disqualification and exclusion by itself. An appeal to 'shared interests' and 'commonality over difference' are not neutral. They often tend to universalize hegemonic (masculine, white, able bodied) perception of what is normative and desired (Bickford 1997). As I have tried to show, however, this is not a simple binary. Identity politics are also embedded in anti-occupation movement/s and what can be categorized as traditional politics, such as unionization, is embedded in disability activism. What this case demonstrates is that framing it as identity politics or new social movements vs. traditional ones (labor, war) is a false dichotomy. Disability is always inherent in anti-occupation and anti-war and vice versa.

4.5   Disability (Non)Politics in Neoliberal Times

But there was another reason behind the need to separate issues of occupation and internal colonialism from disability rights and services, as contradictory as it may seem. From the mid-eighties and most notably the mid-nineties onward, the neoliberal discourse has been taking hold of Israeli politics. This of course is not surprising, as Israel takes not just enormous subsidies from the US (especially for the growth of the military-industrial-complex) but also borrows economic and social policies. Neoliberalism was first implemented in the fascist regime of Pinochet, and then followed form under Thatcher and Reagan and became a dominant economic paradigm. Its main tenants are deregulation, privatization and a general withdrawal of the state from areas of social provision (for a brief synopsis of these forces see Harvey 2005). The neoliberal agenda, with its policies of ferocious capitalism and privatization of everything possible, ushered a deep sense (and reality) of the crumbling of the welfare state. Israel was founded, after all, on socialist principles. And yet the increased effects of Americanization and a market economy without boundaries (what is considered by some as Globalization) led to a series of unfortunate economic changes such as privatization of whole industries (like oil and energy sources), failing corporatized welfare programs which were imported from the US (such as the welfare to work program, known in Israel as 'the Wisconsin plan'), and privatization of social services and institutions (like nursing homes and residential facilities for developmentally disabled as well as the construction, and later the abolition by the Israeli supreme court, of the first private prison in Israel).

What is interesting is that even critiques of neoliberalism (in Israel and North America), rarely tie this critique to a decolonization framework, which connects the costs of war and occupation (of land, resources and people) to economic deficits and financial crisis. It is in fact not at all surprising that the disability protests happened at the same time as the second Intifada, as the economic costs of suppressing the uprising of the Palestinian struggle for self-determination were beginning to accumulate and as a result of the 'zero sum game' of neoliberalism, the direct result was the decrease in benefits, health care, direct payments etc. In fact, Swirski (2005) comments that "the irony is that most of these cuts were not absolutely necessary. Israel has sufficient financial resources that could have been tapped to cover the costs of the intifada. In addition, Israel was able to obtain loan guarantees that were sufficient to cover the budget deficits.... In this sense, the intifada may be regarded as an opportunity that presented itself for the implementation of a plan long in waiting, to downsize the government, cut the budget, lower taxes, privatize government corporations, lower the cost of labor and free capital to invest and expand, with the notion that, eventually, the fruits of economic growth would trickle down to the population at large" (Swirski 2005, n.a.).

   This crumbling of the state as the centralized entity that cares for the needs of its populous became painfully clear during the second war on Lebanon, which lasted about a month from mid-July to mid-August 2006. On the Israeli side, numerous accounts came to light during the war, and especially afterwards, of how the government was not responsive to its disabled citizenry (and non-citizens). They also revealed the fact that, as in many armed conflicts initiated by governments, the consequences are never equally distributed. Bomb shelters, for example, were not available in all places, and were especially lacking in Arab villages. This is of course not surprising since services, infrastructure, information, food and safe housing were not equally distributed before the war ever started. The bomb shelters that were available for people to take cover in were rundown and poorly maintained. Even the ones that were in better condition were mostly inaccessible for people who are mobility impaired. In addition, during times of war or perceived crisis the Israeli TV works in a state of constant newscasting to convey as much information, and disinformation, as possible to the public at home. But even the newscasts, misleading as they may have been, were not accessible to people who were Deaf since there was no sign language interpretation on TV, except for the last newscast of the day at midnight. The 'civil militarism' and actual militarism of the Israeli state creates armed conflicts and/or threat of conflict, in this case bombs and rocket attacks, but having done so it also takes no steps to address the diverse needs of the populous to remedy the threat, by having access to TV and shelters for example. Of course, disabled people in Lebanon were even worse off during the war, considering the lack of infrastructure caused partially by the constant bombing from the Israeli air force, not to mention the use of cluster bombs by Israel during the war that will continue to maim Lebanese people for years to come.

   As a result of the realization that the Israeli state can no longer be responsible or care for the needs of the population during a war initiated by the same government, new players had to come to the forefront to fill in the void left by state agencies. Indeed, the aid for the civilian population abandoned by the state and municipal authorities was almost solely organized by NGOs, non-profits and philanthropists. People with disabilities did not have many places to turn to, if any, for services and information during the (second) war on Lebanon. It was Mate Ha'mavaak (Headquarters of disability struggle) and the office of the Commissioner for the Rights of People with Disabilities (both of which are not service providers but are supposed to be a grassroots organization and an advocacy office respectively) who had to make arrangements for shelters, pagers, distribute information and provide services for people with disabilities in the absence of a centralized office responsible for it. Under these conditions the statement made by the leaders of the disability protests a few years earlier makes perfect sense. If an organization has to be occupied with basic services and survival of its membership, literally, it cannot operate at the same time as a political advocacy organization. As the head of the struggle headquarters told me at the time of the war, "we can't afford to have a dividing ideology, we need to serve everyone." Another leader in the second protest told me that "we can't have an ideology at all."

4.6   Appropriation of Disability as Justification for War/Occupation and Its Resistance

What I hope is becoming clear is that the connection between war/occupation and disability is not a one-way street in which one can say that war is disabling. In this last section I want to briefly suggest that, as is abundantly clear to many activists who oppose wars and militarization, resistance by itself can be quite disabling as well. In Bil'in for instance, a Palestinian village whose lands are being appropriated by the Israeli separation wall, there have been protests against the wall since 2005. Many organizations take part in these weekly demonstrations, most notably Anarchists against the wall, activists from the international Solidarity Movement, various human rights and peace activists and many of the residents of Bil'in. Since the protests began in Bil'in hundreds of protesters have been wounded in the struggle against the separation wall alone, some severely and permanently disabled due to the suppression of the protests and being hit by "rubber coated" bullets and tear gas.[12]

It is quite clear from the above that both war and resistance to it can be quite disabling. However, the presence of disabled activists is unrecognized in most movements and organizations that are not explicitly devoted to disability politics. Many peace or anti-occupation/anticolonial struggles try to connect to other social justice struggles in an attempt to create an alternative perspective of the world and our possible future. The tactics and rhetoric used by liberation movements, however, can be quite oppressive and exclusionary. One strategy used often by progressive thinkers and activists who resist war and occupation is especially relevant to disabled people and disability as a critical lens. In order to demonstrate the futility of war, many resort to showing the painful outcomes of war and colonialism. In addition to showing casualties of war, another effective strategy is putting the disabled body and mind on display to prove the horrific effects of armed conflicts.

---

[12]For instance, on August 11 2006, while the war on Lebanon was still raging, Limor Goldstein was shot in the head by Israeli soldiers from close range (see http://mishtara.org/blog/?p=70 and http://www.awalls.org/topics/videos).

Using disability to critique war is a strategy deployed often in movies and novels ("Born in the fourth of July," "Johnny got his gun" to name just a few). It is also used heavily by progressive writers and journalists who want to display "the cost of war/occupation."

In addition to the use of disability to critique war and other oppressive political decisions, disability can also be used quite effectively to justify wars and occupation. The Israeli media is inundated with photos of people maimed by terror attacks or in military combat. Much like the public display of funerals, which happens almost daily in Israeli news, physically disabled people remind the nation of the cost of war and increased aggression. Paradoxically this imagery and rhetoric can easily translate by the government to legitimization of more aggression, as measures of prevention and defense of future bodily casualties. Therefore the use of Israelis maimed in terror attacks is an important strategy to defer any criticism on the complete lack of balance between the oppressor and occupied in these acts. This strategy can be observed, for instance, in protests displaying visibly disabled Israelis outside the international court in Hague, when it had petitions against the separation wall or other military operations in the territories pending. This strategy of justifying war by using a seemingly oppressed group in need of liberation is reminiscent of the Pentagon's appropriation of Afghani women's liberation as justification for the occupation of Afghanistan.

4.7   Conclusion

As the above analysis demonstrates, there is a vast need to create not only coalitions, but connections across intersecting identities and subjugations and the power structures that hold them together and apart. Without understanding the interconnectedness of exclusion in various levels there is no possibility of transformation, only symbolic victories of one group that will eventually oppress another. As I have tried to demonstrate, one cannot detach disability benefits and labor organizing from a critique of capitalism and neoliberalism; and one cannot fight a war for rights and inclusion without fighting against fighting and creating inclusive struggles. I believe that resisting militarization and (settler) colonialism should always be on the agenda of disability activists. Disability is always inherent in anti-occupation and anti-war (for instance in relation to militarization, budgetary priorities and the remaking of the New Israeli Jew to discard the frail disabled one in the Diaspora) but it is often made invisible. And occupation/settler colonialism is always a part of disability protests, even though it is rendered invisible by a discourse that claims to be unified and apolitical. Settler colonialism and militarization based on nationalism is related to disablement of both Jews and Palestinians, and the services afforded to them by the (contested) state. These are not separate issues, and that is the lesson for the Occupy movement in the United States too. I will not get into the unfortunate use of the title of Occupy to be used to unify a movement for social and economic justice that should be most notably about *anti*-occupation; but will only paraphrase Tuck and Yang's (2012) cautionary message that decolonialization (and occupation) is not a metaphor. Having an inclusive movement is not just about wheelchair accessible gathering space. It is a much larger movement that needs to be cognizant of access, very broadly defined, including land use itself. The violence of colonialism, occupation and military aggression does not merely cause disability and disabling environments for years to come, but also renders disability meaningless and invisible. It would be useful, in my mind, if anti-occupation movement/s embrace disability as a critical framework, especially as they brush against Zionist ideology. Disability has been viewed historically as the antithesis of Zionist myths and ethos, as a remnant of the Diasporic weak Jew of the past. As stated earlier, Zionism thought to transform Jewishness into a national body politic. Disability was included in this paradigm by exclusion only. Excavating and claiming disability as both a critical lens and a social/political identity, and not merely a negation for the severe consequences of war and militarization, can signal a transformative move toward liberatory resistance to occupation and other forms of dominance and state repression that, at the very least, simultaneously reflects on and conjures the limits of the State itself.

Editors' Postscript If you found Chap. 4 by Liat Ben-Moshe meaningful and you would like to read more work that takes a look at the nation state, development, and disability we suggest Chap. 3 "Minamata: Disability and the Sea of Sorrow" by Mami Aoyama, and Chap. 20 "Occupying Disability Studies in Brazi" by Anahi Guedes de Mello, Pamela Block, and Adriano Henrique Nuernberg.

In terms of the experience of political protest, Chap. 2 "Krips, Cops and Occupy: Reflections from Oscar Grant Plaza" by Sunaura Taylor with Marg Hall, Jessica Lehman, Rachel Liebert, Akemi Nishida, and Jean Stewart is relevant as is Nick Dupree's Chap. 15 "My World, My Experiences with Occupy Wall Street and How We can go Further." To this list add Chaps. 19 and 21, "Crab and Yoghurt" by Tobias Hecht, and "Black & Blue: Policing Disability & Poverty Beyond Occupy" by Leroy Franklin Moore Jr., Lisa 'Tiny' Garcia, and Emmitt Thrower.

References

Abdo N, Yuval-Davis N (1995) Palestine, Israel and the Zionist settler project. In: Stasiulis D, Yuval-Davis N (eds) Unsettling settler societies: articulations of gender, race, ethnicity and class. Sage, Thousand Oaks, pp 291–332
Agamben G (1998) Homo sacer: sovereign power and bare life. Stanford University Press, Stanford
Almog O (2000) The Sabra: the creation of the new Jew. University of California Press, Berkeley
Anderson B (1983) Imagined communities: reflections on the origin and spread of nationalism. Verso, London
Ben-Eliezer U (1995) A nation-in-arms: state, nation, and militarism in Israel's first years. Comp Stud Soc Hist 37:234–285
Ben-Eliezer U (1998) The making of Israeli militarism. Indiana University Press, Bloomington
Bernstein M (2005) Identity politics. Annu Rev Sociol 31:47–74
Bickford S (1997) Anti-anti-identity politics: feminism, democracy, and the complexities of citizenship. Hypatia 12(4):111–131
Boyarin J (1996) Palestine and Jewish history: criticism at the borders of ethnography. University of Minnesota Press, Minneapolis
Boyarin D (1997) Unheroic conduct: the rise of heterosexuality and the invention of the Jewish man. University of California Press, Berkley

Gal J, Bar M (2000) The needed and the needy: the policy legacies of benefits for disabled war veterans in Israel. J Soc Policy 29(4):577–598

Gitlin T (1993) The rise of 'identity politics": an examination and critique. Dissent 40(2):172–177

Harvey D (2005) A brief history of neoliberalism. Oxford University Press, Oxford

Kimmerling B (1985) In collaboration with Irit Backer. The interrupted system: Israeli civilians in War and routine times. Transaction Books, New Brunswick

Lentin R (2009) Racial state, state of exception. http://www.stateofnature.org/?p=6464. Accessed 12/8/13

Mor S (2006) Between charity, welfare, and warfare: a disability legal studies analysis of privilege and neglect in Israeli disability policy. Yale J Law Humanit 18(1):63–137

Pappe I (2008) The Mukhabarat state of Israel: a state of oppression is not a state of exception. In: Lentin R (ed) Thinking Palestine. Zed Books, London, pp 148–169

Rimon-Greenspan H (2006) Disability politics in Israel: the role of civil society actors in advancing policy change. Unpublished MA thesis, York University

Rimon-Greenspan H (2007) Disability politics in Israel: civil society, advocacy, and contentious politics. Disabil Stud Q 27(4). http://dsq-sds.org/article/view/47/47. Accessed 31 July 2014

Rouhana NN, Sultany N (2003) Redrawing the boundaries of citizenship: Israel's new hegemony. J Palest Stud 33(1):5–22

Shafir G, Peled Y (1998) Citizenship and stratification in an ethnic democracy. Ethnic Racial Stud 21(3):408–427

Shafir G, Peled Y (2002) Being Israeli: the dynamics of multiple citizenship. Cambridge University Press, Cambridge

Swirski S (2005) The price of occupation- the cost of the occupation to Israeli society. Palestine Israel J Polit Econ Cult 12(1):110

Tuck E, Yang KW (2012) Decolonization is not a metaphor. Decolon Indig Educ Soc 1(1):1–40

Weiss M (2003) The chosen body. Stanford University Press, Stanford

Yiftachel O (2006) Ethnocracy: land and identity politics in Israel/Palestine. University of Pennsylvania Press, Philadelphia

Landings: Decolonizing Disability, Indigeneity and Poetic Methods

5

Petra Kuppers

Abstract

The article witnesses encounters in Australia, many centered in Aboriginal Australian contexts, and asks what arts-based research methods can offer to intercultural contact. It offers a meditation on decolonizing methodologies and the use of poetry and performance by a white Western subject in disability culture. The argument focuses on productive unknowability, on finding machines that respectfully align research methods and cultural production at the site of encounter.

Keywords

Decolonizing methodologies • Disability culture • Native issues • Indigenous issues • Australia • Poetry • Performance • Experimental ethnography

In 2010, I had the honor to be a visiting fellow at the Humanities Research Institute at the Australian National University, to explore international disability culture in a postcolonial context, through arts-based methods. It was my fifth visit in Australia, and the second time, after 2008, that my partner, poet and performance artist Neil Marcus, and I were travelling together across the nation to give workshops, participate in disability culture events, and give poetry readings and performance workshops. In 2008, I had worked as the research consultant for the Melbourne Cultural Development Network. The Network studied for the Victorian Government's Office of Disability the participation of people with disability in the arts. For 3 months, Neil and I toured the Victorian countryside, and we both acted as facilitators for focus group meetings in urban and rural locations.

P. Kuppers (✉)
University of Michigan, Ann Arbor, MI, USA
e-mail: petra@umich.edu

© Springer Science+Business Media Dordrecht 2016
P. Block et al. (eds.), *Occupying Disability: Critical Approaches to Community, Justice, and Decolonizing Disability*, DOI 10.1007/978-94-017-9984-3_5

During our travels we encountered many Aboriginal Australian disabled people, and our conversations raised questions about indigeneity and embodiment, questions I have been exploring ever since, and which have offered methodological challenges which I am sharing here in this essay.

This article moves from a discussion of a particular Australian Aboriginal medical issue and its treatment in the medical and sociological literature to a meditation on decolonizing methodologies and the use of literary forms. In the second half of this article, two short creative non-fiction essays and two poems share how decolonizing methods inform my creative practice. The two sections inform each other: together, they enact a destabilization of what is known, and can be known, and they open up poetic play that can lead to a questioning of colonial knowledge patterns.

Meeting with disabled Aboriginal artists in Australia quickly showed me that gathering a corpus of data on Aboriginal perspectives on disability was not something that I as an outsider (and particularly as someone doing research work for an Australian government agency or for an international disability studies framework) could successfully undertake. There were many historical reasons for this, including questions of what "inside" might actually be, and who is enabled to speak for whom – contemporary Aboriginal communities are diverse and heterogeneous, and visiting with people in Canberra, Adelaide and Sydney was very different from meeting people in Darwin or Alice Springs, or in smaller rural communities.

Then there are the complex knowledge structures, for "within Aboriginal communities there still exists an uneasy tension between different systems of knowledge and information and who controls them" (Latukefu 2006, p. 46), and "(t)raditional systems are ... based on numerous multi-dialogues of relationships, protocols and laws" as Alopi Latukefu writes in addressing the set-up of cyber-communication in remote Australian communities.

We experienced some echoes of these protocols, in particular some linked to gender patterns: it did not take long for Neil and me to find out, for instance, that using our core method, "hanging out," we were each gathering very different information, with me given access to "women's business," often through friendship patterns, and him getting rather different perspectives when men gathered with him. Satire, irony and humor were also a large part of any cross-cultural hanging-out situation we were part of, and we often felt that we were invited to take some of the information received with a grain of salt.

The concept of "disability" was a particularly vexing one: it has strong use-value when it can be employed as a lever to mobilize funds or services to underserved communities, as the concept of disability as a policy issue has currency within Australian white settler society. Whether it has currency in Aboriginal societies, though, and if so, how, is something I am still not quite able to pinpoint. With this query, I am joining Ph.D. researcher Julie King (2010), whose work is so far the only in-depth medical anthropological study in the field, in acknowledging that there is great scope in learning about cultural embodiment when one pays attention to the ways health, disability, and impairment are mobilized in Aboriginal self-narratives.

To show what I mean here, with disability's vexing relational status, with attention to the ways it is mobilized by different people for different purposes, at this point this essay digresses from its core method path of storytelling, examining how a specific impairment or disability winds its rhetorical way through the Australian medical literature.

5.1   Reading the Literature, Imagining Lives: Glue-Ear or Otitis Media

Western (bio)medical personnel working for years in the Australian outback often note disability's presence and the relaxed ("numbed") community response to it. One particular issue that comes up again and again in the literature is otitis-media or glue-ear, and its prevalence in aboriginal communities. It comes up as a limit-site, a place of unknowability, of cultural perplexity, of density. Researchers seem generally at a loss to account for glue-ear's prevalence. This older paper cites general "lifestyle" issues, but without specificity:

> Why, then, is otitis media so prevalent in Aboriginal infants? The answer could be that this is a lifestyle disease. The risk factors are poverty, inadequate and overcrowded living conditions, poor nutrition, and possibly exposure to cigarette smoke and bottle feeding. A detailed risk factor study has not been carried out in an Aboriginal community and would be most useful in understanding the disease better. (Stuart 1992, *electronic article*)

Given biomedical embedment of terms like "lifestyle disease," there seems a moral undertone to this description, always hedged, though, with the "possibly." More current literature still seems to have few explanations, and approaches the issue through a lens of frustration, as in this paragraph on the presence of infection-related loss of hearing in a remote outback community:

> In some communities the prevalence of chronic otitis media has been recorded as 50 %, more than 10 times that which the World Health Organization regards as a significant public health problem. Sufferance describes a resignation to illness that we found both perplexing and disturbing. We were amazed that families could quietly tolerate such sickness. Perhaps, in the context of so much disease, people grow up expecting illness as part of life. Perhaps they are unaware of available treatment. Many parents seemed unworried when pus oozed from their children's ears. Even Bill's cheerful 7-year-old daughter, Stephanie, had recurrent ear infections and perforated ear drums. Although Bill's mother was a health worker, both of them seemed to be as numbed by the sheer prevalence of illness as nearly everyone else in Yambarr. Over the years they had developed no better expectations. (Gruen and Yee 2005, p. 540)

The image of "pus oozing out of children's ears" is brutal, and designed to get a strong reaction from readers, in particular in the context of both development and disability rhetorics, where infantilizing images of helpless kids dominate. I cannot imagine how this relates to the "cheerful" 7-year old. How does pain figure in this? Are there (non-biomedical?) treatments for the pain that accompanies ear infection?

If this is an old issue, is there really nothing but lethargy in the face of suffering – or is there relatively little acute suffering? If there is this pain, is it figured in other ways in the social system, does it become a sign of endurance, of maturity, of passage? What do the kids feel, what adults do they grow up into? Those are some of the issues that seem important to record to appropriately understand the issue in a cultural perspective.

When I followed the issue of children's traumatic hearing loss through the Australian medical literature, I found materials that spoke about tympanic reconstruction and post-operative screenings that showed generally good outcomes for those children that reach hospitals. But it also showed that a lot of children could not be reached for post-operative follow-up: "collection of these data would have been extremely difficult given the nomadic lifestyle of many patients and the logistical realities of remote-area healthcare." (Mak et al. 2003, p. 324)

In my literature review I found much mention of the educational and social disadvantages of hearing loss, but I could not find any information how these rural communities themselves view hearing loss and how speaking and hearing figure in contemporary Aboriginal family contexts. But other notes make it clear that there are cultural forms of management, even though they seem hidden from Gruen and Yee and their frustrations. So in one letter to the Medical Journal of Australia, the authors, Jassar and Hunter (2006), write about Hand Talk:

Hand Talk is an established sign language within and between Aboriginal groups in the NT. Although various groups have different signing systems, there are enough similarities between them to enable inter-group communication. Its existence is thought to date as far back as other spoken Aboriginal languages that have now been lost. Theories about its conception include a means of overcoming language barriers between different language groups, a silent form of communication during hunting expeditions, a means of conversation for women during long periods of mourning when speech is prohibited, and a means of communication for deaf or aphonic individuals. (p. 532)

And the authors of this letter are also aware that finding ways of acknowledging and strengthening the cultural response to childhood onset deafness, i.e. Deaf life, might be an answer to the intractable health problems so many authors report on:

While no data are available on the ubiquity of Hand Talk, it clearly represents a valuable part of Aboriginal culture with an important practical function in a situation where Western models of communication rehabilitation are difficult to apply. While attempts to improve conventional communication rehabilitation should continue, these should be combined with efforts to foster Hand Talk through education and facilitating its dissemination by existing users so it does not suffer the fate of other lost Indigenous languages. (Jassar and Hunter 2006, p. 532)

This brief visit with the medical literature shows how frameworks of agency, and respect for the long lineage of Aboriginal cultures, may help to mitigate pessimism and despair, and may offer different ways forward, in tune with both cultural tradition and innovation.

It also offers some perspectives on Australian disability scholarship. The intersection of colonial construction of Indigenous lives and disability experiences has been marked in Australian disability studies literature:

> For us the continuing spiritual, social and political devastation of Aboriginal and Torres Strait Islander peoples associated with a failure to adopt processes of reconciliation and justice making have a significant disability angle. Out of the practices of colonization has arisen the situation where in so many ways our indigenous people are subject to much higher rates of disability and early death compared with non-indigenous Australians (Goggin and Newell 2005, p. 20–21).

Goggin and Newell do not expand on this issue in their book, and there is still a lack of literature that addresses this particular intersection, in keeping with the lack of medical literature. Helen Meekosha (2008) writes:

> Key debates around disability /impairment, independent living, care and human rights remain irrelevant to those whose major goal is survival. We need to ask, for example, whether they have relevance to indigenous peoples living in remote Australia. In many remote communities each house may contain over 20 people, sanitation and water is sporadic, there is no fresh food available, there is no employment and alcoholism, rheumatic heart disease and chronic otitis media are rife. (unpublished conference paper)

Meekosha's core reference article for this perspective of Aboriginal medical abjection is the 2004 Gruen and Yee essay I quoted above, and that I put into some complex engagement with other ways of framing otitis. Meekosha is here pushing against a Western-focused and affluent perspective, asking for attention to different realities. Of course, within this dynamic of Global North/Global South articulation, other nuances can easily get lost. I posit that a cultural understanding that acknowledges communities' agency even within postcolonial strife may be a more useful way forward than a renewed victimization. Cultural studies approaches to disability's lived experience and the intersection between (intercultural) stigma, affect and the social are valuable tools in addressing difference. However, I agree with Meekosha's (2008) overarching argument, that physically, legally and rhetorically disabling Aboriginal life is part of the (ongoing) colonial project, as much of Australia is still in land battles with traditional owners. She writes:

> Disabling the indigenous population was then, as now, specifically related to colonial power. Without wishing to lapse into relativities, in this context the process of disabling has to be seen as a total dehumanizing process and must include the destruction of physical, the emotional, psychic, economic and cultural life. (unpublished conference paper)

So given this intersectional intertwining of colonial knowledge projects and the invalidation of Aboriginal life, is disability a useful category to address Aboriginal life? How is stigma and difference dealt with intra-culturally? Mark Sherry (2007) writes that:

... many epidemiological studies ... have produced reports of disability which are largely inconsistent with the ways in which the populations being studied understand their own experience. (p. 17)

Anthropologists Susan Reynolds Whyte and Benedicte Ingstad (2007, p. 11) offer similar perspectives, asking about "people's own experiences of what is disabling in their world."

How do Aboriginal people understand their own experiences of embodiment? This question is not just an anthropological one: it also points to the difference between a multicultural, minoritarian perspective on Aboriginal life; and one that frames the issues of knowledge through sovereignty. Australian Aboriginals are the traditional owners of the land, and Aboriginal activism operates from this place, demanding autonomy, and self-governance. So instead of shunning state structures, Aboriginal activism demands a recognition of their own structures; a meeting of autonomous organizations addressing compensation for colonial and war violence, and demanding to not be constructed as a population that is poor and unable to take care of itself.

Aboriginal Australian activist Damian Griffis articulates how disability might enter discourses in his Aboriginal community. I find it near impossible to read his short essay on the topic without thinking of the pressures on "the Aboriginal voice," and on the multiple constituents that are the addressants of the writing (which appeared on Ramp Up, a disability-focused website by the National TV station ABC, structurally similar to UK stations like the BBC who have disability-specific programming).

By any measure, Aboriginal people with disabilities are amongst the most disadvantaged Australians. They often face multiple barriers to their meaningful participation within their own communities and the wider community. This continues to occur for a range of reasons including the fact that the vast majority of Aboriginal and Torres Strait Islanders with disabilities do not identify as a people with disability. This is because in traditional language there was no comparable word for "disability." Also the vast majority of Aboriginal and Torres Strait Islanders with disabilities are reluctant to take on a further negative label— particularly if they already experience discrimination based on their Aboriginality. (Griffis 2012 electronic publication)

Griffis (2012) writes this essay as a way of introducing the advocacy body he leads, as Executive Officer of the First Peoples Disability Network (Australia):

The organization has identified three key priority areas: advocating and ensuring that the National Disability Insurance Scheme can meet the often unique needs of Aboriginal and Torres Strait Islanders with disabilities, the successful implementation of the National Disability Strategy from an Aboriginal and Torres Strait Islander perspective, and supporting the development of networks of Aboriginal people with disability in jurisdictions where they do not currently exist. (electronic publication)

I am looking forward to reading more material that speaks about how Aboriginal Australians construct disability, both in encounters with white Australia, and in

Aboriginal-centric contexts; and to the future development of the First Peoples Disability Network. Reading Griffis' essay also reminds me that some Western ways of writing, communicating and "doing research" are at present only complexly useful to (particularly rural) Aboriginal communities.

Finding multiple and complex ways of engaging the structures of feeling surrounding difference is an important project in this context, and at this point, this insert feeds back into the main essay's objectives, exploring "how to speak" at the site of cultural meetings.

5.2 Decolonizing Methodologies

The main part of the essay locates itself at the level of personal experience and the witnessing of anecdotal episodes, a specific methodological choice grounded in perspectival knowledge, and in the acknowledging of personal stakes and location that characterize most official meetings with Indigenous people I have participated in.

Damien Griffis told me that Aboriginal cultures do not have words for conditions like Down Syndrome, and I also realize that a society that values elders creates different systems of stigma around issues such as "the sugar" (diabetes) and resulting amputations. But I just do not really know, beyond individual encounters, how younger people with mobility or cognitive impairments (for instance) fare in traditional value systems, and I am wary of some of the claims made in the anthropological literature created by non-Aboriginal people.

Trying too hard to find these answers might well be counter-productive. Why would I want to know? What good would my knowing bring Indigenous people? I have written elsewhere that disability is a performance, not just in art-framed settings: disabled people have long been adept at performing "disability" for the medical professional, the social worker, the gatekeepers of the social world and the dominant system. Surely, any perceived interest in issues of disability as lived experience could easily backfire, enabling a potentially non-optimal (from an Aboriginal perspective) set of surveillance reports to gatekeepers.[1] So any questions

---

[1] There are very specific ethical issues here. I participated in the 2010 conference on disability and development in Darwin, a conference created in collaboration with AusAID, the Australian government's development money grantor, and other funders for development projects. Many of the presenters were there to report on projects made possible with these grant monies, and were looking to renew their funding. Thus, the papers given were not exactly interest-free (whatever that means), but fitted their ways of organizing knowledge to sophisticated ways of reading situations in the terms that grantors had set up. And since disability-responsive development, building access into projects created through AusAID money, is a core and welcome issue, "disability" became a very legible category in these papers.

I could analyze what I witnessed, and talk about some of the talk that went on out in the corridors, and I could make complex some of the ways that disability mapped onto lived experiences in some of the South Pacific island nations, for instance. But to do so would be to endanger the legibility of some of these projects, and I would undermine the self-representation of

I ask, in particular if I plan to publish the results, need to be balanced against these realities, just as they have to in the context of US disability activism when I wish to publish my participant-observer notes.[2]

One thing is evident to me: disability as a health and social welfare issue maps onto the interface between Aboriginal societies and the dominant culture, and needs to be seen through the lens of the ongoing effects of postcolonial violence. But the contours of lived experience and the structures of feeling that surround disability within Aboriginal societies are grounded in very different paradigms. This is not a reference to mystical nature children. The context for these "different paradigms" is an understanding of Aboriginal societies not as stone age remnants but as equivalent to the specific Western eighteenth century political forms called nation states, i.e. as autonomous and sovereign guardians of country, besieged and disrupted by violence. Western disability researchers need to take better heed of the concept of sovereignty and culturally specific knowledge, and allow these understandings to complicate universal human rights frames and ways of conceiving of aid.[3]

Thus, forms of thinking the bodymind, environment and the social in many Indigenous societies might not follow the contours of the modern project that creates bureaucratic categorizations, the machines of normality, and the biopolitics that attend them. I am not able to write about the particular formations of embodiment and difference that structure Aboriginal societies, but the existence and acknowledgement of this query puts my project in motion.

My methodological apparatus relies on tracing the reverberations of Indigenous theorizations of embodiment in collaboration and in communal art practice. My work is not as an observer and a reader emerging from the colonial archive, but as someone who uses poetic and artful communication, and witnesses what happens

---

the ambassadors of these communities. Here is one of the many places where I need to be attentive to the web of privilege and the different use-values of scholarship out there, in their intersection with (post)colonial framings. Sometimes, it is a good option to mark silence as a place-holder for what could be said.

[2]These issues came to the front when I wrote about Arnieville, a 2010 Californian disability activism tent village (Kuppers 2011a), and the topic of a chapter by Taylor in this volume: while I am privy to a lot of information about the internal politics of the encampment, I chose to publish a much more general account. The reasons for this are complex, and include personal relationship enmeshments, but also thoughts about a critic's responsibility and the (under)representation of disability-led political labor in public.

[3]There are places where this kind of work happens, in collaboration, in long-term duration, and in participatory action research where the "researched" community's interests are firmly kept in mind. Examples include this Aotearoan collaborative research on Maori understanding of what in English is termed blindness, and what is here figured as Ngāti Kāpo, i.e. as a cultural formation. In it, the collaborators write:

In this research, the researchers and Ngāti Kāpo o Aotearoa Inc. viewed the Treaty of Waitangi from a Māori world view. In doing so, the research team upheld its centrality with respect to research methodology and analysis, effective partnership building with non-Māori, social equity and justice, and most importantly to Māori aspirations to be Māori and selfdetermining. (Higgins et al. 2011, p. 10)

when these art objects cross cultural borderlines in environments where many different cultural ways of knowing create complex webs. There are other complexities about locating Aboriginal knowledge, directly linked to cross-cultural tension and (post)colonial violence. What does it mean, doing "research" at the site of indigeneity, what is it about this "uneasy tension between different systems of knowledge"? What were the methodological assumptions that I was bringing with me to Australia?

My first guide into this new aspect of my academic practice was Linda Tuhiwai Te Rina Smith (Ngāti Awa, Ngāti Porou), Director of the International Research Institute for Maori and Indigenous Education at the University of Auckland, Aotearoa. Smith's highly influential book opens with these four sentences, sentences that shape how I try to approach my work in Australia, very far away from my colonizer nation home bases, Germany, the UK, and now the US:

> From the vantage point of the colonized, a position from which I write, and choose to privilege, the term "research" is inextricably linked to European imperialism and colonialism. The word itself, "research," probably one of the dirtiest words in the indigenous world's vocabulary. When mentioned in many indigenous contexts, it stirs up silence, it conjured up bad memories, it raises a smile that is knowing and distrustful. It is so powerful that indigenous people even write poetry about research. (Smith 1999, p. 1)

Smith's book focuses on centering Indigenous knowledges, Indigenous people, to shape an Indigenous de-colonized research practice that is mindful of power relations, sovereignty and the need to reclaim control over Indigenous ways of knowing. My own agenda, as a woman from a colonizer-nation background, with both travelling and institutional privileges, intend on finding out things about Indigenous life, needs to be deeply unsettled, queried, its purposes and methods weighted. The research project I submitted to ANU focused on arts-based methods, on finding out things among fellow artists, and on using shared artful behavior as the core method to acquiring knowledges that put things in motion.

My desires stemmed from the fourth sentence of Smith's book: "indigenous people even write poetry about research." – what if I were to attempt a similar path, using other methods than the solidifying, conglomerating, totalizing tools of research extraction, find tools that would allow me to reflect on the actions inherent in abstracting patterns from lived reality? What can poetry do that social science texts cannot? What can poetic practice offer theorizations about connection, stigma and embodiment?

5.3 Embodied Poetics, Poetic Material: Two Stories

5.3.1 At the Awakenings Festival in Horsham, Australia, 2008

In 2008, Neil Marcus and I published a book of poems, *Cripple Poetics: A Love Story*, and we were invited to perform from it to many people on three different continents, in Poetry Centers, performance festivals, care institutions and community halls. At one point, we were at a week-long festival for people with developmental disabilities in rural Australia. We had a slot following a presentation about the creation of a non-disability-led art building in Nebraska, USA, far away from most people's experiences in the room.

Neil and I were a bit worried about how our piece would go over. We live in the US, too, another bunch of imported specialists with enough privilege to have our way paid to come to a different continent. But in counter-distinction from that speaker, our material comes from a cultural perspective, from a celebration and appreciation of disability's multiple differences, and from disabled interdependent self-organization. Multiple displacements and differences made us look at each other, questioning our performance choices. Would our shtick work here?

Eventually, it was our turn, and we wheeled onto the stage. We began to perform. Neil used vocalizations and hand signs to make people familiar with his spastic speech difference, and I re-voiced for him, and read my own sections. We read slowly, with repetitions, supporting each other, joking if a word did not come out right.

We looked out at the audience, made up of a few non-disabled organizers and helpers, and many people with conditions like autism or Down Syndrome; people who were black, white and Asian. From the stage, we spoke of sensuality, of our courtship, of finding ourselves alive in the world, all more or less encoded in our poems. And as we ended, we saw a forest of fists, raised in solidarity and appreciation, and voices howled or sung words back at us with excitement. For the rest of the day, we got hugs and high fives as we wheeled around the town. People found ways, verbal or not, to show us how much they appreciated hearing layered, artful witnessing words of sexuality and eros from a stage that is usually about developing work skills, care innovations or medical advances.

Our poems that day became something else than (only) an aesthetic framing of experience: they became an intervention, a way of speaking difference to machines that speak in ways that have a history of disempowering disabled people. Speaking slant in between descriptions of service delivery opened up a space of solidarity. Speaking about and enacting love on this stage became a recognizable marker even to people who did not give us an indication that they followed the content of our words: our embodied performance, leaning into each other and laughing while reading, was enough for some. Our foreign status had not been erased in any way, but members of an international and diverse disability culture found ways to find companionship and solidarity with each other.

5.3.2   At an Aboriginal Art Workshop, Alice Springs, 2008

Following on from a poetry reading in Sydney, where we performed material at a memorial event for Christopher Newell, a disabled activist and scholar, Neil and I were invited to come out to Alice Springs in the Northern Territory, the red heart of Australia. We had an exciting program while we were there.

Our first tour guide had been part of a search party for a baby probably killed by a dingo, dramatized as an iconic Australian nightmare for international audiences in

A Cry in the Dark (1988). After the first day, he gave us the use of a truck with a wheelchair lift to drive around the red and orange countryside.

At the local wildlife reserve, a wheelchair-using warden came shooting out to the parking lot as we turned in with our big rig, ready to show us around, and we exuberantly greeted each other, three disabled white folk feeling rather wild and adventurous.

Disability Services Alice Springs, our hosts, threw a BBQ for us at the waterhole that gives Alice Springs its name. As unexpected rain had just filled the mini-lake, I went for a swim, too, with other disabled women, and was faintly red with mud dust for the rest of the night. At this disability culture party, we were gifted a dot painting created by a disabled Aboriginal artist (whom we did not meet in person, so I do not feel that I have permission to share her name and the painting here). We swapped courting stories with a beautiful couple, two women with developmental disabilities, who celebrated their love for each other with us, all of us taking photos of each other kissing and hugging.

Some of our experiences were a lot more sobering: one of our gigs was visiting with the "special unit" of a local school, and there we found children happy and glad to dance with us from their wheelchairs or on the floor. About half of them were Aboriginal, and when we mentioned this, the teachers spoke freely to us of fetal alcohol syndrome and parents' drug abuse, not about historical and cultural trauma and its potential embodied and enminded effects.

We led a movement workshop. The teachers told us that "no one does that here," and that these kids do not usually respond to stimuli, that many do not communicate, and that some teachers were just now trying out a new method they had just learned about, something called Total Communication. When asked about this, it turned out that this basically meant listening, taking time, not stopping stimming behavior, mirroring some of the movements the kids were doing till there was some kind of echo or connection going on, just being with one another: all communication methods familiar to many disability culture people, where communication often does not run along the lines of normate social rules. The head teacher told us that our methods looked a lot like Total Communication – did we know about it?

Neil felt less addressed and acknowledged by the teachers we spoke to, as his speech difference probably felt too close for comfort to many – but that was our reading, not something we could verify, of course. He and I felt such sadness in that environment: would it really be so hard to work out these things, these ways of establishing communication, without non-disabled specialists or international visiting artists? What would it take for decolonizing methodologies to encompass disabled people writing the guide books for how to deal with difference? When will disabled people become the teachers of people who will go on to make a living being with disabled people?

Our visit also brought us to the Irrerlantye Arts Centre, an Aboriginal Art & Community Centre. Here, we found again what different labor poems perform in cross-cultural contact. At the art center, a number of women where creating paintings that would be sold through the adjacent shop, a significant source of income in many Aboriginal communities. The women spoke with us in short sentences, keeping up their work, and we felt a bit tense and inappropriate. But they encouraged us to read to them while they were working, and so we performed a few poems from Cripple Poetics, and gifted a copy to the workshop's library.

This was yet another new context for a poetry reading, and yet another form of poetry audiencing: in a manufacturing setting, reading while workers create postcards and small mats with dot paintings (the serenaded tobacco rollers of Carmen kept leaping into my thoughts). There was little eye contact, and few words. I am still not sure if we actually shared enough common language elements between us for all to understand the words of the poems. Gender, race and class differences seemed to fill the room in multiple ways, muffling any exchange in shy glances and short words. I just could not read our audiences' affect and reactions, although they told us a few fragmented stories of "people like us" (chair users? spastic people?) in their communities.

As we left and got ready to operate the truck's wheelchair lift to get us to the city center, the group leader called us back. She was standing inside the walled courtyard of the workshop, and we spoke for a few more minutes through a metal grid. "Thank you," she said, "normally white people come here to take something away: Aboriginal culture, explanations for the dot paintings, and the art they buy. You brought us something, instead, and performed for us. Thanks."

This exchange has become an important lens for my understanding of the place of poetics in cross-cultural contexts. In my usual US setting, the act of sharing a poem outside sanctioned poetry events has often a faintly cringe-inducing flavor. Poems in everyday life have become something that puts a burden on the receiver: many poets are reluctant to recite or give their poems to others in private, as the act of giving has become an imposition on others. The gift of a reader's or a listener's attention seems rare and precious. This view of poems as highly personal and potentially embarrassing objects has one legacy in the lineage of lyrical poetics – a culturally specific and contingent construction of poetry's relation to privacy, self and the public.

Thus, caught in my heritage's grip, I felt as if we were imposing on these women in this quasi-industrial setting which I felt was so hard to read. Are these women creating commodity art for tourists, or are they affirming a place for Indigenous land-connection in a white-dominated Australian public? Reading poems there, were we forcing something onto them? But that, it turned out, was not how the poetry was received. I failed to see the women fully as our hosts, as agents, as people with their own understandings of how non-everyday speech and declamatory vocal patterns might fit into their world. The context shifted: now, the poems we brought became a gift, understandable or not, an enrichment, not necessarily by their content, but through their rhythms and through our presence, through the gift of time and attention. The women in the center created a space for them. Maybe, for a few moments, our co-presence in the room became a temporal re-patterning that might entwine our halted, revoiced, and alternating speech patterns with the rhythms of a manufacture that creates near-identical dot paintings, themselves rituals of dreaming country, re-establishing co-presence with the land. Repetition and difference, sound pockets, floating visits, dot, dot, dot.

That strangely uncomfortable encounter in the art factory with its epiphanic ending in the dusty red garden has shifted again my sense of how poems, ritually patterned speech, can offer space in the everyday, can weave rhythms and open up vibrations of tenuous connection and respect.

In these stories, and particularly when I use a word like "epiphany" to describe my cultural contact journeys, I need to resist the pressure of either cultural or aesthetic romanticizing, even as I witness myself being moved, and being moved to twist my understandings of my own art processes through intercultural encounters.

Art-based practices do not escape the dirty, extractive connotations of "research" by their nature, far from it: art practices at the site of indigeneity have historically brought forth powerful romanticizing and eroticizing image complexes, building a visual rhetoric of patriarchal colonialism, or a poetics of expansion, of binary contrasts between human Westerns and non-human others. But I do believe that there are contemporary art-based genres that can formally engage in the project of decolonization:

> Decolonization is a process which engages with imperialism and colonialism at multiple levels. For researchers, one of those levels is concerned with having a more critical understanding of the underlying assumptions, motivations and values which inform research practices (Smith 1999, p. 20).

It is at this point that I can find traction for my methodological questions about research. Arts-based research is different from art practices. The Western art world (like all art worlds) operates by well-established patterns and control mechanisms, including modes of outsider art and their attendant capitalist gallery enterprises, or Wanderjahre novels and exoticizations in the equally successful genres of memoir or travel narratives. Arts-based research, on the other hand, circulates in the framework of the academy in fragile contact with the art world: it is a liminal zone, not devoid of power by any means, but less sure of its grounds than ethnographic practice, quantitative methods, or art production.

Another research method warrants mentioning in the context of this essay: interviews, and collecting oral histories. At times, both the anecdotes above and the poems below either report on someone saying something, or quote words spoken. The materials have been shared with stakeholders: my time in Canberra at the Australian National University ended in a research presentation, where I read and discussed the framework of the Landings material below. I also had long conversations with Aboriginal poet and academic Jeanine Leane, and benefited significantly from her guidance and comments on respectfully engaging with what is said and not said in contact between white researchers and artists and Aboriginal researchers and artists.

And it is here that I place the issue of interview techniques and the recording of voices: so much is unsaid, unsayable, shrouded by custom and convention. It would be convenient to imagine that some of the polite and unfailingly friendly utterances that I received from the Aboriginal women artists I worked with is all there is. But

I know that listening to silences, and to the rhythms of conversation – a story told to me by an elder after a certain pause, for instance – can offer me much more nourishment for understanding.

Witnessing in this way, and letting it influence my writing indirectly and through pattern-processes should not lead to the kind of research Smith warns about, and which is still the dominant mode of what is considered to be "valuable" in research: there is little hard data here in this essay, no extractive nuggets of wisdom, few truth claims or statements about Indigenous being, or about medical, social or cultural links between disability and indigeneity. And that's a deliberate stance.

At the same time, I hope that this kind of porous writing will not echo too closely the history of romanticization and mystification that is the other side of the coin of anthropological and artistic research, self-indulgence and excessive self-witnessing. I am encountering living people who are getting on with it, and I can record how their co-presence impacts me – co-present with me, with country, with history, and with futures. I share this material as an artist-researcher, witnessing people who are adept at code-switching and survivance.

5.4   Intercultural Poetics: Writing Landings

Drawing on my encounters with Aboriginal women's poetry and art making,[4] I use creative/critical methods to find ways of writing about my own experiences: meditations on the foreigner's gaze; disability access and art; connections to country, history and people; performance studies and its relation to anthropology; as well as poetry and its relation to critical writing.

How do cultural aesthetics call upon historical depth in modernity, how can (fractured, provisional) community be created from fragmented, traumatized roots, disregarded sovereignty, what can disability culture(s) learn from postcolonial peoples and survivors of violence, and vice versa? What are contact points, what are differences, what are the ethics of artful cross-cultural communications?

The Landings series consists of poems – that is the way these writings appear on the page or are spoken in performance. In terms of what these pieces do, though, I consider them to be critical pieces that engage the traditions of knowledge traffic within the academy.

The poems make connections, offering a form of affective and associative linking that relies on linebreaks, on small units of meaning leaning into one another. This

---

[4]Material I looked at, and people I met, include Jennifer Martiniello (who identifies as of Arrernte, Chinese and Anglo-Celtic descent) and her edited collections *Talking Ink from Ochre* (2002) and *Writing Us Mob* (2000); Wijadjuri woman and Australian Institute for Aboriginal and Torres Strait Island Studies research fellow Jeanine Leane and her 2010 collection *Dark Secrets: After Dreaming (AD) 1887–1961*; and Bidjara and Wakaman woman and poet Yvette Holt, author of *Anonymous Premonition* (2008). I also benefited from discussions with Alisa Duff, who presented on "The Politics of Dancing: issues in Aboriginal and Torres Strait Islander dance" as part of the Text and Texture seminar convened by Jeanine Leane.

writing emerges from a desire to investigate and query the ways that knowledge is gathered, communicated and archived within the academy. In Landings, the authorial "I" or viewpoint becomes spatial rather than grammatical. Sentences switch direction and overlay each other with different perspectives on land, history, and habitation.

With this, these poems are different than the anecdotes above, these short pieces of non-fiction writing that also meditate on cultural contact, but do so through grammatical rules and assemblages that still keep my emotional journey as traveler and writer firmly linear. Investigating the formal elements of poetry, witnessing sounds I hear and rhythms I sense, not claiming full understanding or making the sensations secondary to my emotional states: these are the challenges I set myself in this writing.

Some of the material in Landings: Darwin emerges from found sound, from TV news and Northern Territory documentaries, and some of the lines are comments captured at the Darwin conference. Some of the speakers or people mentioned in these lines are well-known public figures in disability politics in Australia like Damian Griffis, Aboriginal Disability Network, with whom Neil and I shared an exciting dinner talking about disability justice in 2010; Michele Castagna, the disability services coordinator in Alice Springs, who had hosted us in 2008 and whom we met again in Darwin, as well as Joshua's mother Penny Campton, officer of Arts Access Darwin, and curator of the Good Strong Powerful exhibit, an arts exhibit of ten Indigenous artists with disability.

The material from Landings: Silver Screen has a historical starting point: watching an Aboriginal woman travelling with a mob, part of the Mandjindjara and the Ngadadjara tribes of the Australian Western Desert. An ethnographic film by Ian Dunlop, shot in 1965 and 1967, presented these groups as some of the last nomadic bands. During the making of the films, the woman's legs were burned severely from a campfire, and the film mentioned, without follow-up, that she could no longer travel with her band.

The format of poetry allows me to weave a way through these elements without elevating some voices over others. Who said what, who is speaking, whose voices are included and excluded: those are the issues I am investigating with these formal choices.

As a researcher, I am not becoming a transparent recorder, instead, my gathering and witnessing activity becomes akin to a choreographic presence, a curatorial gaze or ear, opening up the parsing activity of the researcher. I offer these two poems of Landings not as aesthetic products, but as meditations on the use of arts-based methods in cultural studies.

5.5   Landings: Darwin

On the occasion of meeting Joshua Campton, a Larrakia man, leader, artist and young adult with disability, who opened the 2010 Development and Disability Consortium Conference at Darwin with a Welcome to Country.

Darwin also houses a rare 40-year old exhibit of a coral ecological system: a tank in which corals, fish and other local sea-life live in a closed system.
Note: Joshua Campton has given permission for me to use his name in this writing.

Wait
patience
red eyes shine in the torch light
back up into the shadows of the billabong.
Two hundred forty three people perished in the Japanese air raid
they say, they say
Two hundred forty three they counted
of the lighter color
accountable in the fire light
(moon fish eat the rice I throw off the dock)
There is no Down Syndrome amongst Aboriginal people
they say, they say
and someone donates white goods to the bush community.
Sometimes you have to step in the long grass,
grass land,
goanna groans,
(over me swoops the flying fox)
grass land that is not your home, and you are not welcome here
someone drove her up in a van
powerchair hanging deep and heavy
fifteen hours from Alice,
no nook on the aircraft
no view from above
no lines in the red sand
no green flowers of salt
impurities enter through the oil of your skin
red lights in the night
at the back
on the retina
the night throws you back
(I never met the owl, never)
mother father crocodile, saltwater people
the fortress in the night, the aircraft carriers,
red and dark and green:
Hiryu, the Flying Dragon
Akagi, Red Castle Mountain, fire to the lighter colors
shades of ochre and the lush, the lush
milkwood splits
homeostasis (Plain English balance sheet, two pushing against a membrane,
one against the other's power, watery support)
heal the renal clinic
no balance, no niches, each nook and cranny inhabited
this is not a plant
count the leaves in the long grass, asleep in the night,
misrecognized fauna, this does not count
as a home.
I welcome you
I declare this conference open

this meeting
in the long grass
(I watch them step and step in a line, hidden by the vertical stripes)
you are not welcome here
I open, you say
you step forward, you say
your business is yours
but I can still feel your touch on my skin

5.6   Landings: Silver Screen

On the occasion of meeting ethnographic film director Ian Dunlop, after a screening
of People of the Western Desert.
The desert is now the site of copper and gold mines, including the largest
Australian gold mine, and many of the traditional owners of the land, reclaiming
guardianship of Country, are negotiating for Native Title under Australian law.
35 millimeter film unwinds for four minutes at a time

silent
silent paths
silent laughter
silent digging
the younger wife's legs are burned from the campfire
she cannot gather her food
her legs are burned
silver ash on dark skin
her legs are burned
the camera tracks the looping track
we leave her in the dust
then there's the time of the children's game, etching a curved path
etching a curved path
in the desert
through the desert
little brother skirts carefully
the path
in the desert
run a skirt around the city
close the city
go deep
volumetric ore removal map lines ley lines striated degradation
cyanide will dissolve the earth and free the copper
run a skirt around the city
close the city
(what do I know of the city)
fly in the workers, fly them out: no one lives in the Mad Max world
no one speaks in the silent film
there is laughter in the clang of the spears sticks in the counting in the accounting
acid etches lines into
line it
(what do I know of the desert)

her legs are burned
the goanna gets out of here
Ian Dunlop says: yes, I saw this again, much later, at the mission, children's paths, I saw
it. I do not know. I do not know. It was the older brother, 16 year old man. I saw these
paths again, at the mission.
When I see the path, I step cross-wise on the line.
Embedded anthropologist
Where will he find a wife?
How do I sing a life?
Where do I find a wife?
Her legs are burned
Where do we sing in the cinema?
What is the sing of the city?
Why is the sing of land?
Who sings in the grit, itching between the hair follicles?
Blood tastes like copper, or copper like blood, and water runs over it all, green, green, green,
greenbacks and oxygen, the bubbling reaction.

5.7   Epilogue

This is the place for the summing up, the overview, and the outlook. But in this essay
of located narrative and poetics, this is the place of questions. What knowledge have
you gained, as a reader, what images and impressions have floated over you? You
have encountered narratives and fragments of disabled travelers and have met some
Aboriginal people through these lenses. You heard quite a bit about landscapes, too,
and might have images of places you haven't visited in your mind, and even a desire
to go meet people and be welcomed to country.

You might have a wider sense of how developmental narratives and sovereignty
perspectives might clash. You might have noticed feints and hide-outs, pauses and
blank stares, and an atmosphere of hedging might have settled on you.

If you read poetry differently from prose, you might have taken note of how often
you have stopped yourself reading, and tasted words in your mouth.

How can these methodologies witness hanging out with others? Is this a method
that can create knowledge patterns of holes and wholes, of touches and sensation,
not in counter-distinction to analysis and overview, but in a vibrational tension
with them?

Maybe, next time you read a text that authoritatively presents how embodiment
works in a different culture, some of the hedging and pausing of this essay might
intersect your reading practice, and might get you to wonder, curiously, about what
remains unsaid. And with that, ultimately, does this kind of writing achieve its goal,
furthering agendas of Indigenous people by disrupting productively the mechanisms
of Western research? That moment, the moment in which this question is raised,
might be this essay's horizon of decolonizing methodologies.

5.8   Notes

My research has benefited significantly from visits with the Text and Texture seminar convened by Jeanine Leane at the Australian Institute of Aboriginal and Torres Strait Islander Studies, a seminar designed to examine the role of Aboriginal and Torres Strait Islander writers and researchers as a counter to mainstream Australian literature; and the October 2010 fictocritical writing workshop at UNSW, convened by Anne Brewster and Stephen Muecke. I am also grateful to Margaret Noodin, who used to be my colleague and collaborator at the University of Michigan and is now teaching Native American literature at the University of Wisconsin Milwaukee, to Jamie L. Jones who teaches American literature and writing at the University of Michigan, and to Donna MacDonald, the convener of the Disability Studies Program at Griffith University in Brisbane, Australia; all gave me valuable comments on early drafts of this work.

Landings: Darwin and some of the framing comments were first published in Antipodes: A Global Journal of Australian/New Zealand Literature, December 2011. Another, longer Landings poem, with photographs from a youth dance performance in Canberra, was published as "Landings: Moth Stories" in Performance Paradigm, 2011.

A shorter version of this essay, minus the Otits Media part, was published by Siobhan Senier and Clare Barker as Decolonizing Disability, Indigeneity and Poetic Methods: Hanging Out in Australia, Journal for Literary and Cultural Disability Studies (Special issue on Indigeneity and Disability), 7:2 (2013): 175–193. I am deeply grateful to my editors, and to the many teacher-artists who participated in the Native Studies/Disability Studies Conversations series at the University of Michigan, an initiative funded by the National Council for Institutional Diversity.

Editors' Postscript If you liked Chap. 5 by Petra Kuppers, and are interested in reading more about performance and dance in disability studies, we recommend Chap. 7 "Scenes and Encounters, Bodies and Abilities: Devising Performance with Cyrff Ystwyth" by Margaret Ames and Chap. 24 "If Disability is a dance, who is the choreographer?" Neil Marcus, Pamela Block and Devva Kasnitz. Chapter 8, "Artistic Therapeutic Treatment, Colonialism & Spectacle: A Brazilian Tale" by Marta Simões Peres, Francine Albiero de Camargo, José Otávio P. e Silva, and Pamela Block focuses on performance, disability studies in the global south, and legacies of colonialism. If you are interested in disability and occupation in Australia, read Chap. 13 "Why Bother Talking? On Having Cerebral Palsy and Speech Impairment: Preserving and Promoting Oral Communication Through Occupational Community and Communities of Practice" by Rick Stoddart and David Turnbull, and Chap. 22 "Blindness and Occupation: Personal Observations and Reflections" by Rikki Chaplin. Other chapters focusing on disability in the global south and legacies of colonialism include: Chapter 19, "Crab and Yoghurt" by Tobias Hecht, Chap. 20, and Occupying Disability in Brazil" by Anahi Guedes de Mello, Pamela Block, and Adriano Henrique Nuernberg.

References

Fred Schepisi (1988) A Cry in the Dark (film). Cannon Entertainment.
Goggin G, Newell C (2005) Disability in Australia: exposing a social apartheid. University of New South Wales, Sydney
Griffis D (2012, 20th April) Disability in indigenous communities: addressing the disadvantage. Ramp Up. http://www.abc.net.au/rampup/articles/2012/04/20/3481394.htm. Last accessed 25 July 2014
Gruen RL, Yee TFM (2005) Dreamtime and awakenings: facing realities of remote area aboriginal health. Med J Aust 182(10):538–540
Higgins N, Phillips H, Cowan C (2011) 80 years of growing up kāpo (blind) Māori: what can we learn about inclusive education in New Zealand? Int J Incl Educ 17(8):1–15
Holt Y (2008) Anonymous premonition. Queensland University Press, St Lucia
Jassar P, Hunter GF (2006) The importance of Hand Talk in communication rehabilitation among Aboriginal Australians in the Northern Territory. Med J Aust 184(10):532
King JA (2010) Weaving yarns: the lived experience of indigenous Australians with adult-onset disability in Brisbane. Ph.D. dissertation. Queensland University of Technology
Kuppers P (2011a) Introduction. In: Kuppers P (ed) Somatic engagement. Chainlinks Books, Oakland/Philadelphia, pp 7–18
Kuppers P (2011b) Landings: moth stories. Performance Paradigm: A Journal of Performance and Contemporary Culture 7. http://www.performanceparadigm.net/wp-content/uploads/2011/07/petra-kuppers.pdf. Last accessed 25 July 2014
Latukefu AS (2006) Remote indigenous communities in Australia: questions of access, information, and self-determination. In: Landzelius K (ed) Native on the Net: indigenous and diasporic peoples in the virtual age. Routledge, London/New York, pp 43–60
Leane J (2010) Dark secrets: after dreaming (AD) 1887–1961. Press, Berry
Mak DB, MacKendrick A, Bulsara MK, Weeks S, Leidwinger L et al (2003) Long-term outcomes of middle-ear surgery in Aboriginal children. Med J Aust 179(6):324–325
Martiniello J (ed) (2000) Writing us mob: new indigenous voices. Aberrant Genotype Press/The ACT Indigenous Writers Group, Ainslie
Martiniello J (ed) (2002) Talking ink from ocre. Aberrant Genotype Press/The ACT Indigenous Writers Group, Ainslie
Meekosha H (2008) Contextualizing disability: developing southern/global theory. Keynote paper given to 4th biennial disability studies conference, Lancaster University, UK, 2nd–4th September
Sherry M (2007) (Post)colonising disability. Wagadu, vol. 4, Intersecting gender and disability perspectives in rethinking postcolonial identities, 10–22. http://journals.cortland.edu/wordpress/wagadu/files/2014/02/sherry.pdf. Last accessed 25 July 2014
Smith LT (1999) Decolonizing methodologies: research and indigenous peoples. Zed Books, London/New York
Stuart J (1992) Ear disease in aboriginal children – is prevention an option? In: Conference proceedings medical options for prevention and treatment of Otitis Media in Australian Aboriginal Infants, Menzies School of Health Research and the Australian Doctors Fund, Darwin, Northern Territory Australia. http://www.adf.com.au/archive.php?doc_id=143. Last accessed 25 July 2014
Whyte SR, Ingstad B (2007) Introduction: disability connections. In: Ingsgtad B, Whyte SR (eds) Disability in local and global worlds. University of California, Berkeley, pp 1–29

Occupying Autism: Rhetoric, Involuntarity, and the Meaning of Autistic Lives

6

Melanie Yergeau

> ...the path to empathy is the occupation of another's point of view.
>
> – Jay David Bolter & Richard Grusin (pp. 245–246)

Abstract

Autistic people are hardly described as having the capability to form their own community(s). This obsession with our incapability transcends scholarly discipline—it is routinely portrayed as an inseparable part of autism as a condition. Across scholarly and popular domains, autistic people are portrayed as egocentric, mindblind, and asocial. Using autie-ethnographic analysis, I argue that scholars and lay publics alike represent autism as an involuntary condition. What autistic people consider rhetorical moves—e.g., ticcing, stimming, perseverating—medical practitioners consider involuntary or aberrant behaviors. In this construction, autism represents arhetorical symptoms of a problemed body rather than a valid and underrepresented form of communication.

Keywords

Autism • Involuntarity • Agency • Theory of mind • Rhetoric • Narrative • Neurodivergence • Mental disability • Autie-ethnography

6.1

"Melanie," she writes, and I imagine her doing so in an armchair, a red velvet armchair, this woman enunciating each syllable of my name, if only to make sure I comprehend her—"I hope as we go forward, Melanie, I hope you come

M. Yergeau (✉)
University of Michigan, Ann Arbor, MI, USA
e-mail: myergeau@umich.edu

© Springer Science+Business Media Dordrecht 2016
P. Block et al. (eds.), *Occupying Disability: Critical Approaches to Community, Justice, and Decolonizing Disability*, DOI 10.1007/978-94-017-9984-3_6

to understand that at many levels what does and does not apply to you"—I stop reading, grind my teeth, poke my tongue in a developing cavity, if only to make my wince more wince-worthy—and continue on with her letter. "It's not meant to personally challenge you," she blathers, "but are the observations and ways of those with very different life experiences. Other people have different life experiences than you, Melanie, but I understand how difficult it is for you to put yourself in others' shoes."

I stop reading. It *is* difficult for me to fit into others' shoes. My feet are incredibly narrow size nines, and I often fall out of my shoes—*my* shoes. And then there was toddlerhood, me walking so feverishly and insistently on tiptoes, my mother recalls, that the doctors considered cerebral palsy! (with an exclamation point!) and hurriedly put my legs in casts below the knees, then braces, only to find out that it wasn't cerebral palsy, that it wasn't a symptom of anything with a clinically recognized name, at least not anything clinically recognized in the U.S. until 1995, at least not a symptom of anything other than Melanie being Melanie and what the hell is wrong with Melanie? There are empaths, and then there are disempaths—and as a teenager I was pegged into that escapably inescapable designation, that of the autism spectrum disorder, the one that, if you believe the charities, creeps into your child's room at night and steals her soul, steals her ability to walk flat-footed, steals her ability, as the blathering woman in the imaginary red velvet armchair put it, to recognize that "other people have different life experiences."

So much of my childhood was a search for an explanation—a search carried out by my parents, pastors, teachers, counselors, and the elementary school kids who liked to beat me up at recess. One day it's selective mutism, and the next day it's all my mother's fault. One day it's "let's get a CATSCAN and make sure she doesn't have a brain tumor," and the next day my guidance counselor asks if anyone has ever touched me. Once the autism designation descended from the diagnostic heavens, my capacity to empathize was suddenly eaten up by malfunctioning neurons. My capacity to engage in social relations or maintain eye contact vaporized alongside my personality. My capacity to *have* capacity was called into question.

What autism provided was a discursive framework, a lens through which others could story my life. My hand and full-body movements became *self-stimulatory behaviors*; my years-long obsession with maps and the Electric Light Orchestra became *perseverations*; my repetition of lines from the movie *Airplane!* became *echolalia*. My very being became a story, a text in dire need of professional analysis. This, my body, this was autism—and suddenly, with the neuropsychologist's signature on my diagnostic papers, I was no longer my body's author.

6.2

Popular autism discourse resembles an epidemic more than does autism. Media outlets routinely harp about the so-called "global health crisis," likening autism to a fate worse than pediatric AIDS, cancer, and diabetes combined (Autism Speaks

2012). An estimated one to two percent of the population—or 1 out of 68 people—resides on the autism spectrum. These days, when I read and hear the numbers, when freshmen at my alma mater tell the campus newspaper that these numbers are "so alarming," alarming enough for them to fear procreation—I think to Lennard Davis' work on disability and normalcy, specifically, when he describes the entire field of statistics as eugenics. Davis (2013) notes,

> Statistics is bound up with eugenics because the central insight of statistics is the idea that a population can be normed. An important consequence of the idea of the norm is that it divides the total population into standard and non-standard subpopulations. The next step in conceiving of the population as norm and non-norm is for the state to attempt to norm the nonstandard—the aim of eugenics. (p. 3)

When I am a number—a gendered number at that, and I mean gendered number both literally and figuratively, because I've synaesthetically thought of numbers as being gendered since I was a kid—but when I am a number, I'm a number to be avoided. A number meant to instill fear and alarm. A number meant to warn parents that *I* could happen to them. A number that signals the dissolution of marriages and other gratuitous disability-induced horrors. A number that borrows its soundtrack from that classic, repeated knife-stab move in slasher flicks. I can see and feel the numbers as eugenics—all too visually, all too tangibly.

But the fraughtness of autism discourse neither starts nor ends with numbers—it involves our very conceptions of autism, involves that tired misconception of autism precluding empathy, emotion, and personhood. Kidnapper imagery abounds in PSAs and billboards; popular nonprofits mourn the loss of the children that never were (Sinclair 1993). And as reprehensible as these mass-mediated representations are, perhaps more concerning to me (out of my own autism-induced self-centeredness?) (I pose that question snarkily) are the professional discourses that affect me, us, you, them—any and all of us who hold some connection to the amorphous numbers. For as much as we'd like to dismiss the autism-as-thief trope as the next of the myths du jour, such myths find their realities in the various professional discourses that surround autism and its theorized relations to numbers and agency and empathy and our very definition of humanity itself. As Erin Manning (2013) notes, "as we well know, without empathy you are not considered human" (p. 150). In these constructions, autism occupies humanless bodies, bodies that become puzzles for the non-autistic among us to "solve."

As John Duffy and Rebecca Dorner (2011) relate, autism is a narrative condition. Paul Heilker and I (2011) have made similar arguments—that autism is a profoundly rhetorical phenomenon. It's important to highlight the radicalness of these statements—that autism is narrativistic, that autism is rhetorical—because they represent a major departure from what scholarly literature, across disciplines, suggests about autism and empathy. Many scholars, for instance, have argued that autism precludes the ability to both compose and enjoy stories; and a series of recent articles in the *Journal of Autism and Developmental Disorders* characterize autistic autobiography as lacking narrative structure, as lacking rhetorical facility and audience awareness, and as lacking self-reflection (Brown and Klein 2011; Brown et al 2012; Goldman 2008).

In many respects, this medicalized focus on *lack* is the crux of this essay. For autism is medically construed as a series of involuntarities—of thought, emotion, mode, action, and *being*.

Here I'd like to specify what I mean by involuntarity as a term—how I'm defining it, how I'm using it in relation to autism. In obvious terms, autism is not a voluntary condition—one doesn't "choose" autism, per se. Many parent narratives about autism echo this line of thought and speak of autism as something happening to them, as though their entire family had been struck by lightning. Particularly iconic, for instance, is the Autism Speaks "Learn the Signs" (2015) campaign, in which autism incidence is compared to car crash fatalities, hypothermia, kidnapping, pediatric cancer, and AIDS. (All of these things, despite autism being a non-fatal disability.) Numerous stakeholders in the autism world, from parents to journalists to bioethicists to autistic people themselves, have posed the following question: Who would choose autism? (Or, more broadly, who would choose any disability?)

Because autism isn't a switch that can be turned off at will (trust me, I've tried), the medical establishment writ large tends to conceive of autism as essentialized involuntarity. Its subjects are not subjects in the agentive sense of the word, but are rather victim-captives of a faulty neurology.

Of course, framing autism as neurological involuntarity is a false construct. After all, does anyone really *choose* their neurology? The idea that "no one chooses autism" doesn't negate the fact that no one doesn't *not* choose autism. And yet, even though neurotypicality is as much an involuntarity as is mental disability, the construct of involuntarity is culturally inscribed into autism as a condition. Autistics wrench and scream and rock their bodies, and they have no choice; they have no agency; they and their embodiment have no rhetorical or narrativistic purpose. Using such logic, a person does not occupy autism; rather, autism occupies a person.

And so, this obsession with autistic involuntarity goes far beyond the issue and illusion of choice—it goes to the very core of how autism is defined across diagnostic, scholarly, and popular literature. Deborah Barnbaum's (2008) *The Ethics of Autism* revolves around an understanding of autism that is the antithesis of both community and communicability, echoing the stereotypical sentiment that autistics are closed off from the larger world. "There is something intrinsically limiting in an autistic life," writes Barnbaum (p. 154). And, later, "Autism cuts people off from people" (p. 174). What Barnbaum and other scholars suggest is that autism is a world without people, that a world without people is a world without rhetoric, and that an arhetorical life is a life not worth living—a life beyond the realm of voluntary action and intentionality.

Within such a framework, involuntarity might encompass shit-smearing or body-rocking under its banner; it likewise encompasses any act of communication; it encompasses embodiment; it encompasses how one dwells in the world. It signifies a lack of purpose, a lack of intentionality, a lack of control over one's own person—and under the heading of "person," I'm including how we conceptualize mind, body, being, and self-determination. My flapping fingers and facial tics signify an anti-discourse of sorts: Where is my control? Where is my communicability? Would anyone choose a life of ticcing? How can an involuntary movement, an involuntary neurology, a state of being that is predicated on asociality—how can these things be *rhetorical*?

But involuntarity, I would argue, is not an inherent part of autism as a condition. Rather, involuntarity is forcibly imposed onto autistic bodies, onto mentally disabled bodies writ large, often to violent effect.

What I'm concerned with, in particular, is rhetoricity and the autistic subject's supposed lack thereof—and the ways in which this construction denies autistic people not only agency, but their very humanity. In support of such arguments, cognitive studies researchers, rhetoricians, and cognitive narratologists alike draw upon theories about theory of mind. Theory of mind (ToM), in short, is the ability to understand that other people have their own unique mental states, feelings, beliefs, and desires. But contemporary theories about ToM also invoke and assert other cognitive phenomena—including, but not limited to, mentalizing, meta-cognition, self-awareness, intentionality, and expressing empathy (Boucher 2012, p. 229). In other words, to lack a theory of mind is not simply to lack a theory of other's minds—it is also to lack an awareness of one's own mind (Carruthers 1996; McGeer 2004).

And so, I am writing this essay, presumably unaware of my reader and my(non)self.

6.3

This essay is a story. Or, this essay is a story as much as it can be a story. Or, this essay is a story as much as an autistic person can make a story—which, according to many a narrative theorist, we can't (see Keen 2007).

And so, I am here storying a non-st°ry. My primary deficit is that I am not non-autistic—the non-autistic bodymind being the standard against which I am routinely held. When my writing lacks transition, it is *because I am autistic*. When my fingers twirl in the air, fidgety and tangled in series of rubber bands, it is *because I am autistic*. When my eyes dart away or when my sentences grow long, it is *because I am autistic*. When a non-autistic parent wants to discredit something I've said or done, when a colleague tells me how I should self-identify, when a social worker insists that I will never comprehend the burden I impose on others—it is *because I am autistic*.

To be autistic is to be unaware of oneself and others. To be non-autistic is to be aware of oneself and autistic others. Autistic bodies are never occupied by autistic selves. Rather, they are conditioned to submit to the control and definitional power of non-autistic people.

Disempathy is our collective story, and through this story of disempathy, autistic collectivity ceases to exist.

Autistic people are hardly described as having the capability to form and function as their own audience(s). This obsession with our incapability transcends scholarly discipline—it is routinely portrayed as an inseparable part of autism as a condition (see Greenbaum 2011; Jurecic 2007; Schuler 2003). And, in many respects, constructions of autistic incapability revolve around theories about theory of mind. As Baron-Cohen, Alan Leslie, and Uta Frith noted in their seminal 1985 article on ToM, this supposed inability to attribute motives to neurotypical minds is a "circumscribed cognitive failure," a "cognitive dysfunction," a "cognitive deficit," a "social disability," (p. 44) and a "striking poverty" (p. 39).

Autistic people are, as Baron-Cohen (2003, 2008) has claimed elsewhere, mindblind and lacking in empathy—they are limited to the confines of their skulls. As rhetoricians such as John Duffy and Rebecca Dorner (2011), Dennis Lynch (1998), and Paul Heilker and Jason King (2010) have suggested, ToM has a particular staying power in just about every academic facet of autism discourse—it's how teachers, scholars, and professionals come to know autism and thereby autistic writers.

Perhaps the most salient (and telling) quote from Baron-Cohen (1997) on ToM, however, is this one:

> A theory of mind remains one of the quintessential abilities that makes us human.... [H]aving a theory of mind is to be able to reflect on the contents of one's own and other's minds. Difficulty in understanding other minds is a core cognitive feature of autism spectrum conditions. The theory of mind difficulties seem to be universal among such individuals. (p. 3)

What's important to note here are the connections between humanity and the autistic person's lack thereof—connections made by a leading autism researcher, connections that have had profound implications for scholarship in every field, including my own home discipline, rhetoric and composition studies.

But these connections also percolate beyond academia, seeping into my daily correspondence with parents, friends, relatives, and women in imaginary red velvet armchairs. If, as Bolter and Grusin (2000) suggest, the path to empathy is to occupy another's point of view, then it would seem that autistic people are doubly disenfranchised. First, autistic people are thought to lack empathy. And second, non-autistic people are construed as the epitome of empathy. In essence, then, the only way for non-autistic people to exercise empathy is to project themselves onto autistic people—for how can an unempathetic person *understand*, never mind *define*, her own self? Autism as a construct could never survive without neurotypicality to support it.

Disempathy is our collective story, and through this story of disempathy, autistic collectivity ceases to exist.

In this essay, I am practicing the art of composing autistically. To use transition statements, to compose a coherent one-sentence thesis, to refrain from invoking my own embodiment and positionality, to censor my pithy one-liner cracks about neuropsychologists—in many respects, that would be *easy*. To compose normatively would be to compose persuasively. But composing normatively would assume a non-autistic audience; such a composition would assume a style and discursive frame that is best suited to the very ideologies that I here argue *against*. *Who* am I addressing when I write? *Whose* embodiment and worldview do I reify? Theory of *whose* mind?

6.4

I am tempted to say that my essay is piecemeal because when mental disability enters the conversation, rhetoricity is piecemeal. In popular discourse, puzzle logics represent disabled logics. I am tempted to say that my essay exists in chunks because those are the only descriptors afforded to me—chunky logics, slippery logics, transitionless logics, not-quite-whole logics. I am tempted to say that my essay is incomplete because it's some purposeful, wry move on my part that involves embodying the shitty things that academics say about autism, some kind of clever commentary on my part.

But it's not—it's not any of these things.

This essay is piecemeal because it's raw and personal. It's piecemeal because I don't know what to do with the stuff I read about me and my people. When talking with my therapist, I describe my scholarly endeavors as "piling bricks." When I first started doing work in Disability Studies, there was something tidy and manageable about my righteous anger. I could compartmentalize my wrath into coherent webtexts for academic journals. Now, when I encounter cognitive studies articles, it takes my whole being and willpower to refrain from stabbing at my leg with a mechanical pencil. With each article, with each conversation, with each email exchange and conference presentation and twitter flame war, another brick gets added to the pile. My body just feels heavy—lagging, dragging, collapsing.

I don't know what to do with this stuff anymore. What to do when a rhetorician describes theory of mind as a "perfect phrase"? (Woodward 2010, p. 91). What to do when a philosopher in one breath claims theory of mind is a "fundamental aspect of human relationships," and then in the next claims that autistic people do not have a "fully functioning theory of mind"? (Barnbaum 2008, p. 154). What to do when leading autism researchers claim that autistic writing is inherently unreliable and that "it might be a mistake to take what is said at face value"? (Frith and Happé 1999, p. 18). What to do when a rhetorician claims that autistic people are "masked by a cloud of social solitude"? (Greenbaum 2011, p. 46).

What to do with scholarship that denies autistic agency, denies autistic voice, denies autistic personhood?

How does an autistic person argue against the above? Anything I claim here is held suspect on the basis of my very being—because I am autistic, I lack a theory of mind. And because I lack a theory of mind, I lack both a theory of my mind and a theory of the minds of others. And because I lack a theory of my mind and the minds of others, anything I say is inherently unreliable, idiosyncratic, and special. My rhetorical moves are not rhetorical moves, but are rather symptoms of a problemed body. I will never fit into another's shoes, even if they too wear narrow size nines. Reason, topoi, tropes, narrative arcs, diplomacy—these will only ever be attempts, or, as Frith and Happé call them, "hacks" toward a normative embodiment, hacks toward a normative rhetoric. Appearing to know myself or others is merely *appearing* to know myself or others. I can appear, but I can never know. I have symptoms, and they have rhetoric.

Under such a construction of symptomology, the only arguably reliable story I've offered today comes from the armchair woman in my intro, her narratives of my autistic and disempathic selfhood. Her words about autistic identity carry far more weight than my own. In many respects, her words about my "condition" impact how I feel about rhetoric and empathy—it is a steaming pile of competing, ableist theories about distant Others that extend up to my neck. How to lob rhetoric at the wall? How to smear it on my face? Where is my intentionality? Must one have intentions in order to be rhetorical or empathetic? Again I ask: Theory of *whose* mind?

I ask these questions somewhat desperately. There is an exigency here. How can we—in rhetorical studies, in disability studies, in occupational studies, in academe writ large—how can we create more inclusive spaces to speak back to these theories of lack? How might we reinvent discourse on rhetoricity and intentionality and in/voluntarity—in ways that are critically savvy and conscious of disabled embodiment? Victor Vitanza (2008) has called this the "involution" of spaces. For my part, I want a rhetoric that tics, a rhetoric that stims, a rhetoric that faux pas, a rhetoric that averts eye contact, a rhetoric that lobs theories about theory of mind against the wall.

6.5

When we frame autism as disempathy, we position autism as rhetorical violence. When we represent autism as involuntarity, we assert our rhetorical distance from those who are not *us*. As Stuart Murray notes,

> What we might term the 'narrative appeal' of autism in cultural texts is that it easily signifies possibly the most radical form of personal otherness. Indeed, it is the personification of difference and otherness: a person, just like you or me (so the argument runs), who is in fact nothing like you or me, but rather subject to a condition that supposedly defies logic and understanding. (2006, p. 25)

Autistic people are *so different* from us that they *defy logic and understanding*—they defy community, they defy audience and expectations, they defy rhetorical worth.

We certainly write *about* autistic people. But how often do we write *for* or *to* them? We define autistic writers—as alarming, challenging, disruptive, unempathetic, egocentric, and eccentric. We define autistic writing—as "odd" (Happe 1991, p. 219) and self-focused, as having an "unfamiliar logic that is challenging to follow" (Jurecic 2007, p. 43), as unable to "define a line of argument, guide a reader from one point to the next, or supply background for references that will otherwise be unclear" (Jurecic p. 429). We do not, however, define autistic audiences—what it means to compose for those who have minds "with which we cannot truly empathize—to which we ourselves are, in many ways, blind" (Jurecic 2006, p. 4).

It's not a new statement that the academy is exclusionary, or even that the academy reifies exclusionary ideologies, perpetuates certain exclusionary systems. As Richard Fulkerson (2005) notes, any conversation concerning ways of writing and ways of knowing invokes axiological assumptions, or assumptions about what is good or right or valued: good writers, good stories, good ways of composing and knowing and being (pp. 655–658).

These axiological issues, I'd argue, are intrinsically connected to our conceptions of ability. Positioning autism as *involuntary* exemplifies conceptions of "good" or "able" literacy, speech, and intelligence, solidifies our own positions as gatekeepers, the ways in which we regulate *ifs* and *hows*: if one writes and if one speaks; how one writes and how one speaks; if one reads and if one sees and if one hears; how one reads and how one sees and how one hears. We've constrained literacy and intellectual thought to a particularized "domain of symbols" (see Schuler 2003, p. 464)—to a particularized way of thinking, communicating, understanding, and arranging. And in doing this constraining, we exclude.

6.6

While in the midst of designing my dissertation prospectus some years back, I found Adriana Schuler's "Beyond Echoplaylia: Promoting Language in Children with Autism" (2003) in a neglected corner of the library stacks.

I wasn't looking for reading material—I was scouring the library, flipcam in hand, for recordable moments. Instead, I'd inadvertently parked myself in front of the cognitive studies section, right in front of the *Autism* journal.

Schuler's piece prompted me to think about two things. First: Why I hate libraries. I'm a book-loving library hater; I admit it, as oxymoronic as that might sound. I hate libraries (and book stores too) because I don't know what to do once I get there. I observe people, all flawlessly milling about and navigating this awe-inspiring, bookish world, and then I remember my own ignorance, have a panic attack, stim uncontrollably, and/or try to resist the desire to self-injure. The feeling is similar to the one I get when I have to talk to people I don't know (or don't quite understand how to interact with yet)—cashiers, department staff, certain professors, one of my grandmothers, most of my in-laws.

Libraries have social norms that elude me. I would have never found Schuler's piece but by accident (or via an electronic database while in my own home) because I find libraries that stressful, that disconcerting, that socially inaccessible.

Second: Why I hate most "educational" essays about autism—essays that paint autism in terms of lack and deficit, essays that describe autism as a "striking poverty" (Baron-Cohen et al. 1985, p. 39), essays that portray autistic students as, first and foremost, "a pedagogical challenge" (Jurecic 2007, p. 432). A case in point:

At the 2009 Conference on College Composition and Communication, I listened to a paper, delivered in absentia, about a student writer with Asperger syndrome. Throughout the introductory remarks, the reader "lovingly" referred to this student as a "stalker student."

The typical autism essay, as a genre, is rife with neurological hierarchy.

Schuler's essay in particular examines the ways in which "play therapy" can "extend and enrich the communicative exchanges and, more specifically, the symbolic language of children on the autistic spectrum" (p. 455). Schuler suggests that autistic children have pronounced deficits in both imaginative play and "narrative thought," a claim that autism specialists routinely make (see, for example, Rogers and Vismara 2008; Young et al. 2009). So too have cognitive neuroscientists (Baron-Cohen 1997, 2003, 2008) and narrative theorists (Jurecic 2007) alike suggested that autistic students are rhetorically impaired, unable to understand or predict the intentions and motivations of audiences outside themselves. Autistic children, those tragic and woeful involuntaries. (Sarcasm.)

Schuler suggests that such narrative, rhetorical, and empathetic deficits appear in the ways that autistic children play (or, as she suggests, *fail* to play)—spinning the wheels of toy cars, for example, instead of making the cars go "vroom." Children on the autism spectrum, she maintains, engage in asocial, non-reciprocal, and repetitive behaviors, behaviors that are "incompatible" with actual "play" (p. 458). She further describes autistic language as lacking "communicative intent" (p. 467) and as a "rigid pre-symbolic mode of representation" (p. 456). When autistic children begin talking/reading/writing/hearing/playing like "normal" children do, they have only then truly gained "entry into the domain of symbols" (p. 464).

The assumptions Schuler makes about childhood play, socialization, education, and symbolic language, I'd posit, are grossly ableist. These conceptions of narrative and communication are, as Jay Dolmage and Cynthia Lewiecki-Wilson (2008) describe, "rooted in a normate stance ... assuming the central (invisible and normal) position that enables 'us' to diagnose others and make judgments about 'them'" (p. 314). Moreover, Schuler's conceptions of autistic repetition as profoundly arhetorical further subjugates the rhetorical commonplaces that autistic people, as well as other disabled individuals, routinely use to make meaning and order information.

I would suggest that even a cursory visit to an autistic person's blog would reveal that what Schuler argues just isn't the case. As Paul Heilker (2008) suggests, repetitive actions and language use often function as autistic forms of invention and style, as methods of organizing information, as modes of cultural expression. Furthermore, Schuler's (2003) use of architectural metaphor (a domain of symbols in and of itself) is, I believe, a prime example of Siebers' (2008) and Imrie's (1998) conceptions of design apartheid, the idea that conceptual spaces reflect the ways in which we value certain minds and bodies, or what Margaret Price (2011) has termed *bodyminds* (p. 19). Design apartheid means segregation. Design apartheid relies on the logics of involuntarity, relies on the idea that some people, as Simon Baron-Cohen (2003) once put it, "just can't help it." And when the cripples and the feeble-minded just can't help being crippled and feeble-minded, the agentive non-disabled Master We needs to segregate them from public view.

The idea that disabled people dwell outside a domain of symbols is a gross mischaracterization; it is an unfortunate and limited conception of what it means to symbolically act. To my mind, it only strengthens Gunther Kress's (2000) claim that what we need is a "new theory of semiosis," a theory that will "acknowledge and account for the . . . transduction of meaning from one semiotic mode to another semiotic mode" (p. 159). What we need is a rhetoric that tics, a rhetoric that shrieks and wails and sometimes bites.

Schuler's essay, of course, is only one of many that portrays a disabled way of being, communicating, and knowing as distinctly "less than," as what Simi Linton (1998) has described as "that atypical experience of deficit and loss" (p. 5). This limited conception of what it means to communicate, I would suggest, is framed in the language of ability, is shrouded by a one-dimensional conception of what it means to compose and what it means to compose well. It disregards disabled forms of invention, style, arrangement, delivery, and memory—and it locates disabled rhetorical moves within the domain of the pathological, rather than the cultural. It fails to recognize, as Patricia Bizzell wrote in 1982, that communication is enwrapped in the social, that our axiological understandings of what is good and right are products of cultural forces. And in assuming that "cognitive deficiency keeps poor [and/or disabled] writers from forming their own goals" (p. 379), we fail to recognize the rhetorical and ideological import of ability. In essence, we exclude a whole host of writers, communicators, and human beings, placing the communicative burden on them and their disabled bodies and disabled brains.

6.7

I am ending this essay on meaning. I am ending this essay by asking: What is conscious? What is voluntary? What is consciousness, and what is voluntarity, and do I have either of these things?

Autism research traffics in myths. It presupposes body-mind dualism. It collapses ideas about choice, agency, voluntary action, willfulness, and consciousness into tidy bifurcations that don't exist for anyone ever. When one scratches an itch, is that voluntary or involuntary? When one experiences sadness, does the feeling arise consciously or unconsciously? Is a blink willful?

These are questions that resist yes or no answers. And on many levels, we know this. Except for, of course, when we talk about disability.

I often search for the meaning of my stims. Three decades into my life, I still marvel over their tendency to transcend the in/voluntary. We symbiotically occupy. Hands move, air moves, sound waves, flitting fingers, motion before eyes. Here there is meaning. Stims tell a story. Stereotypy, in stereo, rhetoric of bodyminds autistic and present and disruptive of bus passengers.

I am angling toward a poetics of the in/voluntary. I am suggesting that we refrain from trafficking in the armchair psychology of those non-experts who proclaim themselves experts. Autism is a way of being.

Editors' Postscript If you enjoyed reading Melanie Yergeau's Chap. 6 "Occupying Autism: Rhetoric, Involuntarity, and the Meaning of Autistic Lives," which looks at misinterpretations of autistics' communication, Chap. 24 "If Disability is a Dance, who is the Choreographer? A Conversation about Life Occupations, Art, Movement," by Neil Marcus, Devva Kasnitz, and Pamela Block, and Chap. 14 "Occupying Seats, Occupying Space, Occupying Time: Deaf Young Adults in Vocational Training Centers in Bangalore, India, by Michele Friedner also explore non-normative communication. The story of Chap. 6 also resonates with themes from Chap. 16 "Beyond Policy—A Real Life Journey of Engagement and Involvement" by Stephanie de la Haye. Chapter 12 "Refusing to Go Away: The Ida Benderson Seniors Action Group" by Denise M. Nepveux also tells a similar story of valuing variants of community not always seen by the powerful.

References

Autism Speaks (2015) Learn the signs - Ad Council campaign. https://www.autismspeaks.org/what-autism/learn-signs/ad-campaign. Accessed 19 May 2015

Barnbaum D (2008) The ethics of autism: among them, but not of them. University of Indiana Press, Bloomington

Baron-Cohen S (1997) Mindblindness: an essay on autism and theory of mind. MIT Press, Boston

Baron-Cohen S (2003). They just can't help it. The Guardian. http://www.theguardian.com/education/2003/apr/17/research.highereducation. Accessed 14 June 2014

Baron-Cohen S (2008) Theories of the autistic mind. Psychologist 21(2):112–116

Baron-Cohen S, Leslie A, Frith U (1985) Does the autistic child have a theory of mind? Cognition 21:37–46

Bizzell P (1982/1997) Cognition, convention, and certainty. In: Villanueva V (ed) Cross-talk in comp studies. NCTE, Urbana, pp 365–389

Bolter JD, Grusin R (2000) Remediation: understanding new media. MIT Press, Boston

Boucher J (2012) Putting theory of mind in its place: psychological explanations of the socio-emotional-communicative impairments in autistic spectrum disorder. Autism 16(3):226–246

Brown IIM, Klein PD (2011) Writing, Asperger syndrome and theory of mind. J Autism Dev Disord 41:1464–1474

Brown BT, Morris G, Nida RE, Baker-Ward L (2012) Brief report: making experience personal: internal states language in the memory narratives of children with and without Asperger's disorder. J Autism Dev Disord 42:441–446

Carruthers P (1996) Autism as mindblindness: an elaboration and partial defense. In: Carruthers P, Smith PK (eds) Theories of theories of mind. Cambridge University Press, Cambridge, pp 257–273

Davis LJ (2013) Introduction: normality, power, and culture. In: Davis LJ (ed) The disability studies reader, 4th edn. Routledge, New York, pp 1–14

Dolmage J, Lewiecki-Wilson C (2008) Comment and response: two comments on neurodiversity. Coll Engl 70(3):314–325

Duffy J, Dorner R (2011) The pathos of "mindblindness": autism, science, and sadness in "theory of mind" narratives. J Lit Cult Disabil Stud 5(2):201–215

Frith U, Happé F (1999) Theory of mind and self-consciousness: what is it like to be autistic? Mind Lang 14(1):1–22

Fred Schepisi (1988) A cry in the dark (film). Cannon Entertainment

Fulkerson R (2005) Composition at the turn of the twenty-first century. Coll Compos Commun 56(4):654–687

Goldman S (2008) Brief report: narratives of personal events in children with autism and developmental language disorders. J Autism Dev Disord 38:1982–1988

Greenbaum A (2011) Nurturing difference: the autistic student in professional writing programs. J Assem Adv Perspect Learn 16:40–47

Happé F (1991) The autobiographical writings of three Asperger syndrome adults: problems of interpretation and implications for theory. In: Frith U (ed) Autism and Asperger syndrome. Cambridge University Press, Cambridge, pp 207–242

Heilker P (2008) Comment and response: two comments on neurodiversity. Coll Engl 70(3):314–325

Heilker P, King J (2010) The rhetorics of online autism advocacy: a case for rhetorical listening. In: Selber S (ed) Rhetorics and technologies: new directions in communication. University of South Carolina Press, Columbia, pp 113–133

Heilker P, Yergeau M (2011) Autism and rhetoric. Coll Engl 73(5):485–497

Imrie R (1998) Oppression, disability, and access in the built environment. In: Shakespeare T (ed) The disability reader: social science perspectives. Cassell, London, pp 129–146

Jurecic A (2006) Mindblindness: autism, writing, and the problem of empathy. Lit Med 25(1):1–23

Jurecic A (2007) Neurodiversity. Coll Engl 69(5):421–442

Keen S (2007) Empathy and the novel. Oxford University Press, Oxford

Kress G (2000) Design and transformation: new theories of meaning. In: Cope B, Kalantzis M (eds) Multiliteracies: literacy learning and the design of social futures. Routledge, New York, pp 153–161

Linton S (1998) Claiming disability: knowledge and identity. NYU Press, New York

Lynch D (1998) Rhetorics of proximity: empathy in Temple Grandin and Cornel West. Rhetor Soc Q 28(1):5–23

Manning E (2013) Always more than one: individuation's dance. Duke, Durham

McGeer V (2004) Autistic self-awareness. Philos Psychiatry Psychol 11(3):235–251

Murray S (2006) Autism and the contemporary sentimental: fiction and the narrative fascination of the present. Lit Med 25(1):24–45

Price M (2011) Mad at school: rhetorics of mental disability and academic life. University of Michigan Press, Ann Arbor

Rogers S, Vismara L (2008) Evidence-based comprehensive treatments for early autism. J Clin Child Adolesc Psychol 37(1):8–38

Schuler A (2003) Beyond echoplaylia: promoting language in children with autism. Autism 7(4):455–469

Siebers T (2008) Disability theory. University of Michigan Press, Ann Arbor

Sinclair J (1993) Don't mourn for us. http://www.autreat.com/dont_mourn.html. Accessed 14 June 2014

Vitanza V (2008) Writing the tic. In: Kuhn V, Vitanza V (eds) From gallery to webtext. Kairos: A J Rhetor Technol Pedagog 12(3). http://www.technorhetoric.net/12.3/topoi/gallery/index.html. Accessed 14 June 2014

Woodward GC (2010) The perfect response: studies of the rhetorical personality. Lexington Books, Lanham

Young GS, Merin N, Rogers SJ, Ozonoff S (2009) Gaze behavior and affect at 6 months: predicting clinical outcomes and language development in typically developing infants and infants at risk for autism. Dev Sci 12:798–814

Scenes and Encounters, Bodies and Abilities: Devising Performance with Cyrff Ystwyth

7

Margaret Ames

Abstract
This writing discusses the work of Welsh based dance-theatre company Cyrff Ystwyth. Persistent hegemonic positioning of art activity as a way of supporting particular groups and individuals understood as suitable beneficiaries in the UK is critiqued in the context of the company's work. In particular, the work of one of the choreographers who is a person with a learning disability is discussed in depth. Situating the company in its cultural context in rural Wales this paradigm of beneficiary of the arts and the instrumentalist view of artistic practice is considered. Examples of the working relationship between the author and the choreographer are offered via notes made by the author from her experience of both directing and researching the practice of Cyrff Ystwyth and the work of choreographer Adrian Jones. A glimpse into a working practice, an occupation that exists in both the emotional realm and is practiced in a real world context by the making of dance theatre, is offered as a counterpoint to the prevailing hegemony of the person with learning disabilities as recipient of art rather than being the artist who offers their work to those who will engage with it.

Keywords
Cyrff Ystwyth • Wales • Learning disability • Rural • Dance-theatre • Creative collaboration

M. Ames (✉)
Department of Theatre, Film and Television Studies, Aberystwyth University, Parry-Williams Building, Penglais Campus, Aberystwyth Ceredigion, Wales, UK SY23 3AJ
e-mail: mma@aber.ac.uk

© Springer Science+Business Media Dordrecht 2016
P. Block et al. (eds.), *Occupying Disability: Critical Approaches to Community, Justice, and Decolonizing Disability*, DOI 10.1007/978-94-017-9984-3_7

97

Adrian Jones is a founding member of Cyrff Ystwyth, a dance-theatre performing company based in Aberystwyth University in the west of Wales. The area is rural and outside of the university town of Aberystwyth; the economy depends on tourism and agriculture. The area continues to be bilingual Welsh and English. Established in 1988 this was the first performing company that formed under the umbrella organisation Dawns Dyfed. Dawns Dyfed was the community dance project for the three counties of Ceredigion, Pembrokeshire and Carmarthenshire. These counties at this time were over 70 % Welsh speaking. At the time of writing the demographic has radically altered and the 2011 census shows that Welsh speakers are for the first time a minority at 48 %.[1] Nevertheless the author's daily experience suggests that the language is retained as the preferred means of communication especially in the rural communities outside of Aberystwyth. Daily life is not well accounted for in census data and the small clusters of communities spread over a wide deeply rural area suggests a different reality to official statistics. The author was Artistic Director of Dawns Dyfed which was funded by the Arts Council of Wales with contributions from the County Councils from 1987 until 2007.

Cyrff Ystwyth members continue to be participants in the author's research. The inherent dangers and responsibilities of the academic project are acknowledged. Mindful of Collette Conroy's comments in response to Michael Oliver and Len Barton speaking in conference in 2007 that: "The academic study of disability is 'essentially parasitic', and its practices are colonialist and exploitative" (Conroy 2009, p. 4), the author wishes to thank and honour her colleagues in Cyrff Ystwyth. The academic project seeks to bring their work to a wider audience and the work itself is an embodied argument that attempts to challenge the very accusation that Oliver, Barton and to a lesser degree, Conroy level at non-disabled academics.[2] The author's project enquires into the aesthetic nature of performance that is created by learning disabled colleagues. It also questions how very different performances of such material, produced by bodies that do not conform to standard norms as defined by medical and ideological models in the developed world, may contribute to a widening definition of aesthetic appreciation in theatre and performance. Members of the company are learning disabled and without disability. The age range is broad from the mid-twenties to the mid-sixties. All performers come from Ceredigion and have mixed educational, occupational, and linguistic backgrounds. A few are monoglot English speakers, some are first language Welsh speakers and others have learnt Welsh as older children or adults. The company reflects the general picture of the population of Ceredigion, the vast majority being comprised of white people from the British Isles.

In this chapter I consider Jones' work and propose that it might provoke greater understanding of Cyrff Ystwyth's political potential within Wales and further the

---

[1] http://ons.gov.uk/ons/interactive/census-map-2-2\T1\textemdash-wlanguage-e/index.html

[2] See also Fran Leighton who comments that: ' Non-disabled 'experts' feel compelled to 'give an account' of the ethics of their research in response to critics who perceive the non-disabled expert as exploitative...' Leighton, F. 2009, p.97.

potential for other modes of practice that de-stabilize the hegemony of late capitalist aesthetics of beauty.[3] I hope to enable a view into the context that Jones works in and with—in order to consider further the concept of occupation within his cultural array. Judith Jackson's (2006) concern for the dancer within the dance may be considered and extended by asking what happens to the dance within the social and political conditions that the dancer inhabits. What is the dance and how is it danced *here*?

Jean-Luc Nancy's concept of 'occupation' considers notions of land and identity. Nancy (2005) defines the English word 'occupy' thus: "*Occupy* comes from *capio*, "to take, to grasp"'" (p. 55). He goes on to define what the word and identity of 'peasant' might signify.

> The peasant is the one who occupies himself with the land, but He is not, for all that, necessarily someone who works in agriculture. He can be the landsman of all sorts of lands, languages, peoples. What defines him is that he is occupied by or with belonging. Thus there are peasants of the cities or even of science or philosophy. There is some peasant in anyone who belongs and who is taken up with time-and-place, in anyone who makes his own some corner of the here-and-now: it can be a machine, a highway, or a computer as much as a field of beets to a stable. (ibid)

Certainly for Jones, his occupation is making dance performance. He is taken up with the time and place of his home, here and now and he offers a view of it to his audiences through the craft of his choreography.

7.1   Usefulness

In a discourse in the United Kingdom that has reconfigured the professionally recognised artist as quasi therapist, and the marginalised recipient of outreach work

---

[3]The concept of late capitalist beauty I take from a combination of readings. Robert. C. Morgan in his essay 'A Sign of Beauty' (1998) offers: Instead of sensory experience that is contingent upon the overlay of the synaptic mind-body function, we are left with the body as a fetish, a primary focus of desire, as a scientific specimen depleted of historical and cultural significance. Within the rational confines of our postmodern condition, the body is given the status of commodity – a nonheroic mythic status, acquiescent to the commercial world of fashion (Morgan 1998, p. 77).

The postmodern condition is theorised by Fredric Jameson as actualising the 'cultural logic of late capitalism' (1991). His account situates postmodernism thus: '. . . that every position on postmodernism in culture [. . .] is also at one and the same time, and *necessarily*, an implicitly or explicitly political stance on the nature of mulitnational capitalism today' (Jameson 1991, p. 3). I take these readings as explanatory examples of what Cyrff Ystwyth and others are resistant to and failing to comply with, namely the fetishized scientific specimen that through the logic of capitalism, is reified as commodity and therefore becomes a primary focus of both desire and anxiety. The acquisition of products in late capitalism becomes a means by which to ensure our own desirability. We produce our own desirability through the consumption of products that in turn produce our own bodies as sites of desire; as products to be consumed. Late capitalist beauty is then founded on purchasing power, driven by desire, fuelled by fashion and explicitly sexualised. This explicitness is manifest readily in dance performance which foregrounds bodies.

as beneficiary, Cyrff Ystwyth envisions an alternative discourse. The practice and output of the group is, in part, intended as a repositioning of the administrative benefactor and the disabled beneficiary. Representations of specific cultural conditions, experience, and a radical address to questions of what kind of bodies make performance are interrogated through this practice as research. The public positioning of the arts as vehicle for benefit, and for change, with accompanying vocabulary such as 'regeneration' and 'provision' seems to propose that there is inherent goodness and social capital in the making of art. The positioning of artists as new therapists who bring goodness to others, most especially couched in the rhetoric of 'community arts' is effective in cushioning against unyielding encounters with consumerism and the market: that is, it camouflages what Fredric Jameson (1991) asserts as the true nature of culture in his analysis of postmodernism as "a product in its own right;" and "fully as much a commodity as any of the items it includes within itself" (p. x). Positioning artists as "understudy benefactors" (with the proper roles being played by state agencies, for example Arts Centre Administrators) offers a rationale for their employment and, importantly, demonstrates that, as Hannah Arendt has observed, "The issue at stake is, of course, not instrumentality [. . .] but rather the generalization of the fabrication experience in which usefulness and utility are established as the ultimate standards for life and the world of men" (Arendt 1998, p. 157). This notion of usefulness as an ultimate standard for life, decries the profundity of creative action that is the work of the artist and misses the point of expression that lies beyond all other means of communication. Surely the usefulness of art is its own accomplishment—in and of itself, which affords its resistance to generalizations.

In The Arts Council of Wales (ACW) 2008 commissioned report *Hand in Hand*, research is devoted to demonstrating the efficacy of the arts in precisely bureaucratically defined foci of concern. The authors state that the study: "makes a number of recommendations for actions to consolidate and develop the current contribution of arts based practice to regeneration of disadvantaged communities in Wales" (Adamson et al. 2008, p. 1). The concept of action apparently sees the ACW having the remit of agency for regeneration,[4] rather than funder of art. This discourse of intervention is clearly an example of reasonable behaviour for

---

[4]The Arts Council of Wales, formed to provide funding from Public Money for the arts via an application process and art form specific assessment panels became fully autonomous in 1994. Prior to this the Welsh Arts Council established in 1946 was part of the remit of the Arts Council of Great Britain. Since 1999 ACW's Money has come directly from the Welsh Assembly Government. In 2002 the organization went through another major re-structuring process with a new action plan. The Chief Executive's Annual report for 2006–2007 states:

The arts have also continued to play a vital part in other agendas, promoting national identity, building a healthy economy, supporting tourism, working within the health service, in education and in regenerating our communities. (Tyndall 2006, p. 7).

In the same document:

the greater good. The value of the report's rationale is not questioned here; rather, my concern is in the justification and rhetoric of arts administration that positions 'beneficiary' and 'professional' in a hierarchical context of intervention, for this at its core I suggest, is a hegemonic practice that goes unrecognised, for as Raymond Williams (1988) explains hegemony may describe dominant political relations but it depends on its power by virtue of the fact: "that it is seen to depend for its hold not only on its expression of the ruling class but also on its acceptance as 'normal reality' or 'commonsense' by those in practice subordinated to it" (p. 145). In the ACW Annual Report 2006–2007 entitled *Regeneration through the Arts*, the emphasis is placed clearly on access, participation and personal and systemic transformation. It states that key targets: "Actively promote access to, and participation in, the arts for people in disadvantaged communities" (2007, p. 47). The report explains that:

> As part of the community arts portfolio review in 2006/07, ACW adopted a rationale for supporting the sector which prioritises community arts programmes that are *demonstrably transformational* in terms of individuals, groups, sectors and communities and which deliver high quality artistic and creative experiences in areas of deprivation. (ibid: italics added)

By 2012 the current document *Arts Grants for Organisations* places more emphasis on economic indicators such as employment and business opportunities yet includes as its priorities the following advice: "We're especially keen to extend the reach of our funding into areas of acknowledged deprivation (for example Communities First). We expect you to demonstrate how you're going to do that in your response to the assessment question about *Public benefit*" (2012, p. 14. Italics added).

Returning to a Welsh context, critic Ruth Shade uses the term radical parochialism (Shade 2004, p. 3) as an alternative description of Welsh work by communities, which she states: "is profoundly oppositional to consumerist approaches to theatre/performance and which challenges the whole basis on which the dominant

---

The arts have played a major role in the regeneration of communities the length and breadth of Wales. Their impact can be felt in the social, economic, environmental and cultural lives of both urban and rural areas, enhancing the quality of life and instilling a renewed sense of self-confidence (2006).

In the most recent Annual Report of 2011–2012 all mention of regeneration has gone. Instead the focus is more specific on art, with a strong commitment to a business model. The Report instead states:

> Our grant schemes have overarching funding priorities directed at projects promoting the work of artists from under-represented groups such as disabled people and people from black and minority ethnic backgrounds. Recognising the bilingual culture of Wales, we also prioritise applications that will be delivered in Welsh or bilingually (2011, pp. 154–155). of both

thinking in Wales, and in the UK as a whole, is founded" (ibid). Reflecting the effects of mass popular culture and its direct relationship with capitalism that characterises the consumerist approaches to theatre in the UK that Shade refers to, is the rise of television talent contests. The possibility of success through appearing in such programmes as for example, the 'X Factor' (a popular singing competition on prime time Saturday evening television) influence the hopes, dreams and actual daily behaviours of people, as we attempt to re-produce the fashionable and attention grabbing images and personalities necessary for such cultural success on the grand scale. Specific experiences of the local, the values of smaller communities with particular cultural values may be undervalued. This may result in changing funding priorities and I argue, in determining what cultural value is placed on artistic work. Shade challenges Welsh theatre producers and funders, as well as audiences to imagine our theatre as radical, no matter where it is produced, fashionable urban centres or economically disadvantaged valleys and highlands in the South and North of Wales. The current discourse would valorize urban contexts at the expense of less fashionable rural or small town settings. Shade (2004) argues regarding funding that this: "Legitimization has had the effect of segregating theatre into two distinct categories: the 'significant' and the 'peripheral'" (p. 127). Her scathing and precise critique of the patriarchal attitude towards local themes and concerns that are the subject for many practitioners in Wales such as Cyrff Ystwyth, may be situated within a postcolonial discourse if not directly theorised through this body of knowledge. She states that: "The strategies of cultural democracy are incompatible with the Arts Council's 'archive of rules' ... (Shade 2004, p. 161). The position that Cyrff Ystwyth was required to adopt regarding funding bodies was one that disallowed critical engagement regarding the potential and role of their work both within and beyond Wales. Jones and the company were beneficiaries, not artists.

Cyrff Ystwyth contradicts this ideology of usefulness that positions arts activities as useful for purposes such as regeneration of communities and for building self-confidence, and the company members as beneficiaries of useful art, and also by virtue of funding, beneficiaries of the Arts Council itself. I would argue that such ideologies claiming to empower people in fact may maintain the position of minority through the very structures they establish and administrate. Structures such as the Arts Council of Wales (2011) function through ideology. The effect of structural embedding of alternative aesthetics, on the actual practice of art by people not empowered by bureaucracy to call themselves artists results in dependency, between 'beneficiaries' and the organisations that fund poorly paid artists to provide benefit in the organisation's name. Cyrff Ystwyth, through resistance to this ideology of roles and functions embedded in community arts, performs a radical beauty. I am arguing that Cyrff Ystwyth and in particular Adrian Jones, devise performances as a political act of occupation, foregrounding both disability and location. It is through non-conformity that art can function as a radical insertion into the weave of homogeneous capitalist culture and its insistence on the conforming consuming body. The bodies that perform in Cyrff Ystwyth have no market value to aspire towards because these bodies are disabled, ordinary bodies that work a different aesthetic to the model of mass culture.

7.2   Insertion

It is this work performed by bodies of various ages and conditions that in performance produce a radical challenge to 'normal' beauty. In live performance these bodies appear in work that does not attempt a mimesis of professional dance and thereby enable a reading of a lack of skill. Such a reading of this work might allow for a relaxation of the rules of 'normal' beauty, determining body size, shape, age and visible ability. Discussing the performance by a learning disabled actor, in Mind the Gap's[5] production of *Boo* Matt Hargrave (2010) comments, regarding learning disabled actors that: "It is though the 'surplus' sign of 'disability' overshadows other signs at the actor's disposal" (p. 503) the actor is judged: . . . for something he does and something he is" (ibid). In Cyrff Ystwyth, bodies produce a radical challenge as the performers disregard any notion of 'passing' and appear as both doing and being exactly what they are as individuals. This work is not grounded in Applied Theatre, a practice which Dave Calvert (2010) defines as producing performers who: "occupy a dual role of participant and practitioner" (p. 514). Instead these performers are practising an art form cognizant of the prevailing aesthetic demands of mainstream dance and theatre and desirous of an expression that is not 'antiaesthetic' and does not find this expression, as Calvert claims in his analysis of learning disabled performance and punk rock: " . . . in an anti-aesthetic which rejects the values masked by institutionalised codes of art, such as ornamentation, virtuosity and conventional notions of beauty" (p. 514).

The expression sought and crafted is intended as an insertion rather than rejection into these conventional notions of beauty, and one that may de-stabilise a hegemonic order and trouble the commodification of bodies that are conventionally beautiful. The work holds a radical potential within acts of appearing before audiences akin to that which Hargrave (2010) describes in his discussion of the theatre company Mind the Gap's performance:

> These actors offer neither the full 'weight' of psychological subtlety, nor the knowing irony of post-modern practice. Tantalisingly, they offer—each in very different ways–something new, unchartered and imprecise: a *dis*-precision, a performance aesthetic that draws an audience to examine its own cherished beliefs about what an actor actually is. (p. 507)

Cyrff Ystwyth audiences may be complex groupings as Cyrff Ystwyth has an audience that is comprised almost completely of people with learning disabilities as well audiences who cannot be described as theatre goers who attend alongside theatre professionals and academics.

---

[5]Mind the Gap are a UK based performing company that works with learning disabled artists and non learning disabled artists http://www.mind-the-gap.org.uk/

7.3   Knowledge

Complicating this already alienating dynamic are the cultural and historical conditions of Wales itself. Whilst not being a country subjected to the terrible conditions of colonialism and indeed responsible for participation in the domineering power of the British Empire itself, Wales cannot be interpreted as free from some of the symptoms of more recently theorized post-colonialism in relation to the power centre of England and the UK government. Chris Williams' (2005) discussion about Wales' post-colonial condition, which he asserts is untenable is clarified by his analysis: "... it makes more sense to locate Wales historically, in relation to the power exercised over it (primarily politically and economically but also culturally) by England ..." (p. 4). Historically, the unequal power relations were forged during the 1536 Acts of Union of Henry VIII.[6] Historians can take an even longer view. It can be argued that effects of this legislation still impacts on life in Wales and are contested and made politically apparent through the discourse of Plaid Cymru The Party of Wales who state: "It was a sense of the injustice facing the people of Wales, which compelled the founding members of Plaid Cymru The Party of Wales to form a political party" (http://www.english.plaidcymru.org/our-history/).

Jones' work seems to reflect upon all three of Williams' categories. Jones' subject matter for his dances is life in a rural context, where he lives amongst the daily business of agriculture. In as much as this life is danced by a learning disabled man from within a minority language rural culture, this occupation, this voice, and this knowledge, may be considered to be marginal. Bodily, social and practical life in rural Welsh speaking Wales is easily and often disparaged. Whilst this is difficult to articulate, I posit that, as a result of such disparagement of language and culture, a sense of inadequacy is developed. The linguistics scholar Eddie Williams gives a clear account of the historical reasons for this and brings useful contemporary examples to illustrate this dimension. In contextualizing his argument he argues:

> Moreover, these episodes are not arcane occurrences familiar only to "ethnic intelligentsia" (C. Williams 2000, p. 5), but have become "critical events" (Lang and Lang 1983: 9), rehearsed in everyday experience, and reconstructed in print and broadcast media, educational curricula, municipal masonry, etc., and thus capable of swaying judgement. It is also no accident that a persistent feature of these historical episodes in Wales is the Welsh language. (Williams 2009, p. 70)

Other artists such as Eddie Ladd have engaged directly with this issue.[7] Couple this with a knowledge of 'being a problem,' or at any rate, needing to be looked after

---

[6] 'In 1536 Henry VIII's government enacted a measure that made important changes in the government of Wales. Whereas the Statute of Wales (1284) had annexed Wales to the crown of England, the new act declared the king's wish to incorporate Wales within the realm'. http://www.britannica.com/EBchecked/topic/634468/Wales/44626/The-Edwardian-settlement?anchor=ref484004

[7] Dancer Eddie Ladd 'Cof y Corff'/Muscle Memory : 'is an essay on foot and tries to narrate Welsh history through Dance and movement analysis'; see http://www.eddieladd.com/main.html (Accessed 31.8.12).

by others, who are often paid to do so, a person with a learning disability, may find themselves without the means of expressing their realities. Michael Jackson (1996), enlisting a phenomenological method positions the body as vehicle for knowledge and its communication and he asserts that: "knowledge of the mind is neither ontologically prior nor superior to knowledge of the body" (p. 34). Furthermore, Kronenberg, Pollard and Ramugondo discuss how hegemony exerts power whether or not people consent to it and state that:

> [. . .] hegemonies have the means to determine what can be perceived as valid or invalid knowledge. Human occupation is characterised by its complexity, which makes it difficult to encapsulate in the tick boxes and categorizations (Harries 2007) afforded by hegemonic and technico-scientific forms of knowledge (Santos 2003). These are often unable to take account of other forms of knowledge' (Kronenberg et al. 2011, p. 4)

7.4   Rehearsal

Deeper considerations of what and how we make performance suggest a different approach to creative practice developed from embodied knowledge. Rather than adhering to received trainings and styles from validated dance-theatre sources that produce the contemporary performer, it is *this place* and *these people* who communicate embodied knowledge of personal and communal experiences. Furthermore, I suggest that it is these bodies, very particular and marked that do the knowing and that their knowledge is a vital constituent part of understanding what it is to dance, and to dance here in rural Wales. The harnessing of this knowledge including my own, is critical to the development of the choreography as the authors of the dance do not have access to sophisticated verbal language and cognitive processes are not the primary sources of either themes or expression. The non-disabled dancers root their working process in the task of re-writing their pre-determined desires to be 'dancerly' and commit to the practice of embodied knowledge that they must learn and re-learn as the company engages in its process.

In Cyrff Ystwyth rehearsals follow a general trend of devising and uncovering the themes and choreography of a new work and then structuring and rehearsing the cumulative moments as one piece of work. The dancers take hold of the meanings that must be plural as each moment is understood physically, by and through each individual body. Kate Rossmanith researches into how actors' rehearsal processes inform the final product. Rossmanith refers to her sense of rehearsal being experienced "as a thick texture of bodies, events, discourses and contexts which were intimately related" (Rossmanith 2009, p. 77). She writes that "There was also a dimension of embodied experience where practitioners' knowledge operated at a level somehow distinct from a purely cognitive realm of understanding; rehearsals were experienced not only in terms of 'understanding' but also in terms of 'sensing' and bodily affect" (Rossmanith 2009, p. 78). It is this observation of affect and sensing that foregrounds the body as the site of knowledge that I wish re-iterate in my description of the work of Cyrff Ystwyth.

7.5   At Work 1 2004

With clarity and certainty Adrian Jones began his first piece of dance/theatre work *Seagulls* by drawing a seagull using the medium of oil pastels. Then, he bent towards the floor. Extending one arm up and backwards, he tapped the floor rapidly with the fingers of the other hand. This action was the first in a long sequence of particular actions and spatial patterns that Jones created as the choreography. Every move was discreet and clear. These actions were then built into longer phrases, or sometimes abruptly halted. I would ask; "what happens next?" and he would usually respond immediately with either a new action or a return to established material. Sometimes he would say; "don't know." We do not create anything for him, unless he requests input from the company or myself. My job is to wait, to watch, to record and the dancers' job is to follow his direction, his actions and integrate his choreography into their personal physicalities and expressions.

Before rehearsals I go and get Jones from his family home 13 miles outside of Aberystwyth. We drive back to the town through winding roads and heavy traffic. On arrival, he goes into the room. He lies down, he waits. He paces, he sits. He stands in the room close to, but not in, a corner. Sometimes we are alone for a while and I watch. At these times I am aware of my wanting something to happen. I want action; I want movement, statement, and visible engagement; I want expression, integrity and intention to create; I want embodied statement, the unique moment. He, on the other hand, seems not to know what to do. I think instead that he feels. What does he feel? I do not know. I do not feel what he feels. I see him in time and space. I don't see him. I feel him. I don't feel. I assume. I interpret. I demand. I engage. I walk away. He does something. I don't see it. I am walking away. He does something. I see it. We engage.

I make suggestions. I ask him to draw. He draws pictures that at first sight are incomprehensible, childlike in style and random in intention. On looking I see that his pictures show people, sometimes they are in the room. Sometimes they are pictures of other people he knows. He draws shapes, he draws lines. He rubs the pastel into the paper forming tight small patches of dense colour. He draws landscapes, he draws a house. He draws his home. I ask him to explain the images he has drawn. He only remembers his reasons and intentions and what the images represent for a short time. Or at least his ability to use language to create the communicable form of his representations seems to desert him in minutes, sometimes in seconds. "What's this?!" he often says in amazement, pointing at the image he drew only seconds previously. I ask him what he feels about the story that seems to me to emerge from the drawings. He nods. I suggest again and once more he nods in agreement. I suggest more, pushing my interpretations further. I push; he does nothing. I ask for an 'either, or' answer, he says yes. Yes to everything.

Dan Goodley and Mark Rapley discuss 'acquiescence bias' and state that this standard psychological understanding of how learning disabled people tend to respond to questions and interviews creates learning disabled people as "unreliable reporters of their own subjectivity" (Goodley and Rapley 2006, p. 128). Their critique of this psychological reading is based on Discursive Psychology which positions language "as the site where social objects such as 'thoughts' 'minds' and 'intellectual (dis)abilities' are produced in the conduct of social action" (ibid). Yet Jones is in action; we collaborate and his drawings are the conduit for embodied expression.

7.6   At Work 2 2007

"And this and this!" he shouts. He shows. We do. I ask everyone to be exact. Like this he did it, not like that. And this – what is it? Movements as signs. Signs from his inner world. Perceptions, signals from within, made apparent. His dances are signs of presence in the world. His signs are his words, his language. I cannot unravel these signs, these signals. Not metaphor, not mime, not symbol. They appear as moments of themselves, being themselves, they exist only for a second or so before vanishing – never to be repeated moments of embodied emotion and experience. Working with him in this manner is a joy and it is to fail. There is a sense of continual loss as we fail to grasp what he wants from us. The task of re-membering his choreography, is a source of delight but also inadequacy and frustration for the dancers, as each time we attempt a repeat of his movement it has already vanished. Yet the multiplicity of interpretations and physicalities of the group members working to achieve his aim opens up a field filled with diverse gesture, shape, trace form and pathway. Here is an unpredictability and alternative beauty that is an aesthetic discourse far removed from the appearance of youthful and technically uniform dancers who determine what dance should be (normally). Instead, this is what dance could be, might be, and its radicality lies in the impossibility of repetition, of missed moves, imperfections and a delicacy of movement produced through intense channelling of neuro-muscular action and memory.

7.7   At Work 3 2009

Lla'th[8] is a gesture that Jones has used twice now. He created *Lla'th* for a piece called *Work* in 2009. 'Work' is a performance that examines the detail of life at his home, a beef cattle farm. I have written at length about this piece elsewhere (Ames 2010, pp. 41–54). 'Lla'th' consists of extending an arm up high and gently moving the fingers either with a soft clench and un-clenching, or with a flickering of the fingers. At the same time the face is lifted to look up towards the elevated hand and the fingers of the other hand are brought to touch the mouth in a soft fist shape, whilst the performer makes the sound of rapid sucking. In *Work* the gesture seemed to evoke the actions of hand rearing calves and lambs, holding the bottle of milk whilst the animal will suck rapidly and greedily.

---

[8]In English; 'milk.'

7.8   At Work 4 2012

Jones returned to this gesture in *Capel: The Lights are On*[9] which was performed
during the wettest June since records began. In this piece he examined the memories,
practices, and demeanours of Welsh Chapel and its deep relevance to the history
and culture of the country. This work was site specific at a now disused nineteenth
century chapel at the heart of his home village.[10]

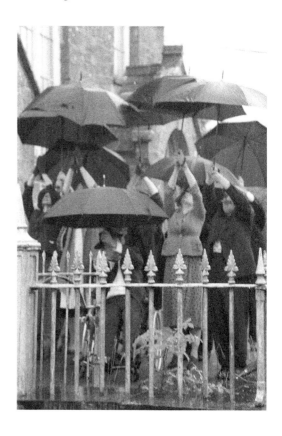

Umbrellas: Outside a grey
stone church there is a white
iron rail fence. Behind the
fence there is a group of
dancers in somewhat shabby
church-going clothes, the
men in black with white
shirts, the women wearing
wrist-length colored gloves.
In the front is a wheelchair
user. It is raining and they are
all holding black umbrellas.
Their arms holding the
umbrellas are raised as if in
prayer. (Photograph Courtesy
of Cyrff Ystwyth)

    As part of a complex group choreography that entailed a close flocking travelling
pattern, he created a series of gestures referring to family life and the care of a
child. This he named *Babi Gwydion*[11] and *Lla'th* was a part of this choreography.
Moving from the studio to the chapel itself, the section was developed to become
two groups of performers, moving together along the aisles of the imposing chapel,

---

[9]In English; 'milk.'

[10]Mid 2007 population estimates show that around 77,800 people live in Ceredigion. With 43
people per square kilometer the area is less densely populated than Wales as a whole.

[11]English: "Baby Gwydion" Gwydion is a male name.

its grandeur long since decayed. They moved with heads bowed, arms as if holding a baby and rocking the invisible child. They would stop, stoop lower and rock faster, then rising to upright, arms would extend and fingers point, drawing lines of trajectory across and through the central block of pews. This gesture suggesting revelation, accusation and invitation to behold, was broken by *Lla'th* and the sounds of sucking echoed through the building in concert with the wind coming through the open doors and the broken windows.

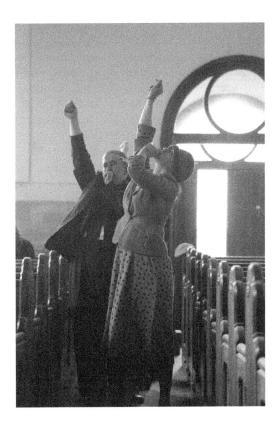

Upraised: Two dancers in somewhat shabby, unstylish, church-going clothes are in a church aisle between rows of carved wooden pews. The arches of the double set of wooden doors can be seen at the back with light streaming in through a circular window frame within a half circle window frame at the top of each arch. Each dancer has one arm raised and the other arm over their mouths as if they are playing trombones. A fist of a third, unseen dancer is raised behind them. To the left there is a shoulder of someone sitting in a pew. To the right someone has hung a woman's hat on the corner of a pew post. (Photograph Courtesy of Cyrff Ystwyth)

It is three quarters of the way through the performance. We are standing in torrential rain and strong gusts of cold wind that blow umbrellas inside out and water against our already soaking faces. We are the audience. The performers move from the graveyard of Bronant Chapel in Ceredigion in the west of Wales into the area of tarmac that usually serves as a car park for the surrounding graveyard and chapel vestry. The old and abandoned chapel rises darkly behind them, its windows blinded by hoardings and its doors wide open. Behind the chapel the hills of Ceredigion's high ground disappear far into the weather. The performers quieten and become slow moving as they perform a sequence of movements. They reach one arm on a high forward diagonal and the other hand covers forehead and eyes. They rub their heads and faces. They kneel or crouch as if praying. Billowing skirts and jackets of genuine period tailoring, the forties, some indeterminate, are heavy with water. The wind and rain accompany this sequence of moves that happen individually, never in unison. One bends down. She pushes forwards, her laced gloved hands press into the wet gravel as she lowers herself onto the ground to lie prostrate. Others, at various intervals follow. At any moment slow moving people, appearing as if from another time, lie at our feet in the rain, dark patches of water collecting on their soaked clothing. The hymn *Garthowen* begins with the words "Dyma gariad, pwy a'i thraetha."[12]

This dance is a narrative of body, condition and specific social discourse. The strangeness of it opens up a rupture, distinguishing us as subjects. We become distinct from each other. We invite attention. Whereas Goodley and Rapley critique the "damage done by assumptions of 'learning difficulties'/intellectual disabilities as naturalized, individualized, embodied pathology" (Goodley and Rapley 2006, p. 138), I propose that what is interpreted and constructed as pathology becomes aesthetically powerful in this context. Rather than dismiss the individual manifestation of neurological malfunction, to use a medical model, I propose that neither the hegemonic command of medicine nor the critiquing voice of the social model can account for the work of Jones who sidesteps interpellation at these moments of presentation of the self, of himself in dialogue with the world around him. Anita Silvers theorizes beauty, art and disability. She asserts that unlike everyday life, art provides a context where the de-stabilizing image of difference that may be disability is not refuted or reconfigured through social constructs. Rather art is a practice and creates a context where there is potential to overcome the instinct to avert the gaze, and to render invisible. Here she argues that: "Non-normal art is transfigured into something that appears beautiful through an aestheticized discourse that discloses its relational properties and foregrounds it" (Silvers 2006, p. 240). The beauty of Jones' work is revealed through the very different subjects that perform it and it is manifest through and by the various impairments and particularities embodied by the performers. Silvers asks, and I echo her question: "what theorizing of human beauty would facilitate our perceiving disabled people as enlivening, rather than depreciating, the human collective . . . ?" (Silvers 2006, p. 241).

---

[12]Here is love, who will declaim it? http://www.angelfire.com/in/gillionhome/Worship/Emynau/DymaGariadPwy.html

Trumpeting?: Five dancers in somewhat shabby, unstylish, church-going clothes, the first in a wheel chair, enter a church in the aisle between rows of carved wooden pews. The arches of the double set of wooden doors can be seen at the back with light streaming in through a circle window frame within a half circle window frame at the top of each arch. Each dancer has one arm raised and the other arm over their lips their faces and eyes are raised. (Photograph Courtesy of Cyrff Ystwyth)

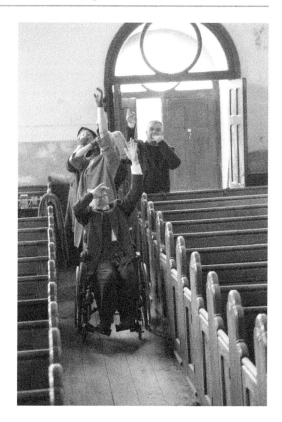

7.9   Community

The conditions of cultural tensions that are experienced in any community are mirrored in Cyrff Ystwyth. In coming together to make performance, all members bring their cultural realties which are lived here in Ceredigion. They are Welsh and English speaking, or they are monoglot English. They may have another language, such as British Sign Language. They are rural, rural towns' people, coastal, or inland. They have lived here all their lives or not. They represent the political dynamic of strain and tension between these communities of experience, of power, of privilege and lack.

The interplay of tensions in performance de-stabilizes roles. Who is disabled, who is trained, who is old and who is a 'dancer' becomes uncertain, recedes from perception and inaugurates the challenge of community. The concept of community is as Roberto Esposito asserts, reduced to an object which obscures the lived complexities within itself. He examines this feature stating: "it is this reduction to 'object' of a political-philosophical discourse that forces community into a conceptual language that radically alters it, while at the same time attempts to name it" (Esposito 2010, p. 1). Thus the institution and its bureaucracy alters the complexity of the weave of this life into chunks that can be reckoned with in terms that are at odds with people's lived experiences of the complexity of daily life that we navigate. Yet continuing, under cover, are acts of particularity. Within Welsh language culture artists have traditionally emerged from their communities and divisions between professional and amateur were less pronounced. The word amateur is now a pejorative as Ruth Shade comments: "Between the two world wars, there were around 500 amateur drama companies throughout Wales who developed a strong tradition . . . " (Shade 2004, p. 17). Shade goes on to explain the historical context of amateur drama: "Such companies declined as the Arts Council developed; and a disdain towards amateur theatre became evident" (Shade 2004, p. 18). Esposito claims that community is built as a "no-thing" (Esposito 2010, p. 139). Within this structure that is not an actual thing, we grapple with nihilism and he explains that: "Nihilism isn't the expression but the suppression of no-thing in common" (2010, p. 140). The challenge of community however, still includes the possibility of new approaches to performance, both the making and the receiving of it, despite political and bureaucratic systems' discourse of division and regulation evidenced in the language of 'access' 'regeneration' and 'benefit'. Being occupied with performance may signal a resistance to homogenizing tendencies of ideology. Esposito (2010) theorizing the void at the heart of community states: "nihilism isn't to be sought in a lack but in a withdrawal" (p. 146). Adrian Jones does not withdraw, he steps forward as an individual and as a member of a community, offering work from his personal experience that speaks to many others, he is both a reflection of his community and though his work he provides a metonym for that community experience, for as Esposito writes: "The community is the exteriorization of what is within" (p. 139), both in the individual and the group.

7.10 Occupation

Jones has poor facility with speech, although he understands and uses both Welsh and English. How may he access freedom of speech? Hannah Arendt (2005) states: 'Only in the freedom of our speaking with one another does the world, as that about which we speak, emerge in its objectivity and visibility from all sides' (pp. 128–129). Later in the same passage she develops this statement:

> This freedom of movement, then – whether as the freedom to depart and begin something new and unheard-of or as the freedom to interact in speech with many others and experience the diversity that the world always is in its totality – most certainly was and is not the end purpose of politics, that is, something that can be achieved by political means. It is rather the substance and meaning of all things political (Arendt 2005, p. 129).

Adrian Jones dances his speech. Seen through Arendt's perspective Jones' performance work is political and thinking about Nancy's statement on occupation, he is occupied by and with belonging and a sharing of the conditions of that belonging with others. Cyrff Ystwyth and Jones' work as examples of Arendt's action may not be intellectually grasped by the choreographer but is driven by the necessity of experience. These things must be said, even when verbal language is a skill not possessed. The speaking with one another amongst the group and eventually amongst performers and audience is of the highest value in political terms. As individuals cast in the mould of learning disability and interpolated into late capitalist ideology as insufficient and as useful only in as much as beneficiaries of administrative systems, such freedom of speech/action is necessary. For Jones, the appearance of himself, and the sharing of his world, his experience and values cannot be accomplished alone. As Arendt positions the issue, continuing her comments on the individual's need to speak about the world, she says:

> . . . he can only do so by understanding it as something that is shared by many people, lies between them, separates and links them, showing itself differently to each and comprehensible only to the extent that many people can talk *about* it and exchange their opinions and perspectives with one another (Arendt 2005, p. 128).

Being dancers and performers the members of Cyrff Ystwyth share and extend to others views from the margins of life here in the west of Wales. An ecology of action and expression of the world is Jones' occupation. As stated at the beginning, this is a form of occupation political in its nature. His work performs experiences of belonging and habitation, expertise and thereby, resistance. Jones is Nancy's landsman, in rehearsal and performance but most specifically through his work he stands his ground. The company works from a methodology dependent upon the depth of bodily knowledge available in the room. Here, on the west coast of Wales, there is a confluence between the marginal world of the learning disabled person and the artistic expressions of personal and communal experience within a culture on the margins of the UK.

Editors' Postscript If you liked reading Chap. 7 by Ames, and are interested in reading more about how art is used as a way to communicate knowledge in disability communities (in this case, disability studies), we recommend Chap. 5 "Landings: Decolonizing Disability, Indigeneity and Poetic Methods" by Petra Kuppers. If you are interested in reading more about ways in which art therapy is institutionally used in disadvantage of disabled people, we recommend Chap. 8 "Artistic Therapeutic Treatment, Colonialism & Spectacle: A Brazilian Tale" by Marta Simões Peres, Francine Albiero de Camargo, José Otávio P. e Silva, and Pamela Block. Or, if you would like to read more about how disability arts and culture are embedded in disabled people's lives, we recommend Chap. 24 "If Disability is a Dance, who is the Choreographer? A Conversation about Life Occupations, Art, Movement" by Neil Marcus, Devva Kasnitz, and Pamela Block.

References

Adamson D, Fyfe H, Byrne P (2008) Hand in hand: arts-based activities and regeneration. Arts Council of Wales, Cardiff
Ames M (2010) Working with Adrian Jones, dance artist. J Arts Commun 2(1):41–54
Arendt H (1998) The human condition. University of Chicago Press, Chicago/London
Arendt H (2005) The promise of politics. Schocken Books, New York

Arts Council of Wales (2011) Annual report 2011–2012. http://www.artscouncilofwales.org.uk/what-we-do/publications/annual-reports. Accessed 16 May 2015

Calvert D (2010) Loaded pistols: the interplay of social intervention and anti-aesthetic tradition in learning disabled performance. Res Drama Educ J Appl Theatr Perform 15(4):513–528

Conroy C (2009) Disability: creative tensions between drama, theatre and disability arts. Res Drama Educ J Appl Theatr Perform 14(1):1–14

Esposito R (2010) Communitas: the origin and destiny of community. Stanford University Press, Stanford

Goodley D, Rapley M (2006) Changing the subject: postmodernity and people with 'learning difficulties'. In: Corker M, Shakespeare T (eds) Disability/postmodernity. Continuum, London/New York, pp 127–142

Hargrave M (2010) Side effects: an analysis of Mind the Gap's Boo and the reception of theatre involving learning disabled actors. Res Drama Educ J Appl Theatr Perform 15(4):497–511

Harries P (2007) Knowing more than we can say. In: Creek J, Lawson-Porter A (eds) Contemporary issues in occupational therapy. Wiley, Chichester, pp 161–188

Jackson M (1996) Introduction: phenomenology, radical empiricism, and anthropological critique. In: Jackson M (ed) Things as they are: new directions in phenomenological anthropology. Indiana University Press, Bloomington/Indianapolis, pp 1–50

Jackson J (2006) My dance and the ideal body: looking at ballet practice from the inside out. Res Dance Educ 6(1–2):25–40

Jameson F (1991) Postmodernism or the cultural logic of late capitalism. Verso, London

Kronenberg F, Pollard N, Ramugondo E (2011) Introduction: courage to dance politics. In: Kronenberg F, Pollard N, Sakellariou D (eds) Occupational therapies without borders, vol 2. Churchill Livingstone Elsevier, Edinburgh/London/New York/Oxford/Philadelphia/St. Louis/Sydney/Toronto, pp 1–16

Lang GE, Lang K (1983) The battle for public opinion: the president, the press and the polls during watergate. Columbia University Press, New York

Leighton F (2009) Accountability: the ethics of devising a practice-as-research performance with learning-disabled practitioners. Res Drama Educ J Appl Theatr Perform 14(1):97–113

Morgan CR (1998) A sign of beauty. In: Beckley B, Shapiro D (eds) Uncontrollable beauty. Allworth Press, New York, pp 75–82

Nancy JL (2005) The ground of the Image (trans: Fort J). Fordham University Press, New York

Rossmanith K (2009) Making theatre-making: fieldwork, rehearsal and performance-preparation. I. Stud Contemp Cult 9(1):1–17

Santos BdS (2003) Challenging empires. The World Social Forum: toward a counter hegemonic globalization. Part 1 – Toward a counter hegemonic globalization. Edited version of a two part paper presented at XXIV International Congress of the Latin American Studies Association, Dallas, USA

Shade R (2004) Communication breakdowns: theatre, performance, rock music and other Welsh assemblies. University of Wales Press, Cardiff

Silvers A (2006) The crooked\timber of humanity: disability, ideology and the aesthetic. In: Corker M, Shakespeare T (eds) Disability/postmodernity. Continuum, London/New York, pp 228–244

Tyndall P (2006) Valuing the arts. Arts council of Wales annual report 2005–6. Arts Council of Wales, Cardiff

Williams R (1988) Keywords. Fontana, London

Williams C (2000) On recognition, resolution and revitalization. In: Williams C (ed) Language and revitalization. University of Wales Press, Cardiff, pp 1–47

Williams C (2005) Problematizing Wales. In: Aaron J, Williams C (eds) Postcolonial Wales. University of Wales Press, Cardiff, pp 3–22

Williams E (2009) Language attitudes and identity in a North Wales town: "something different about Caernarfon"? Int J Sociol Lang 195:63–91

Artistic Therapeutic Treatment, Colonialism & Spectacle: A Brazilian Tale

8

Marta Peres, Francine Albiero de Camargo, José Otávio Pompeu e Silva, and Pamela Block

Abstract

This chapter discusses the relations between psychiatric total institutions, artistic therapeutic approaches and rights of psychiatric patients. After a brief theoretical review, we discuss the role, main goals and cautions of artistic therapeutic approaches, indicating that there is an important lack of this kind of activity in Brazilian psychiatric hospitals and in contemporary psychiatric reform. We have created a fictional account as an example of abuses psychiatric patients can experience under the auspices of "art therapy" and the pretense of humanistic actions.

Keywords

Psychiatry • Art therapy • Colonialism • Brazil

M. Peres (✉)
Department of Performing Arts and Dance, Federal University of Rio de Janeiro,
Rio de Janeiro, Brazil
e-mail: martasperes@gmail.com

F.A. de Camargo
Oswaldo Cruz Foundation, National School of Public Health, Rio de Janeiro, Brazil

J.O. Pompeu e Silva
Graduate Program of History of Sciences, Technology, and Epistemology, Federal University of
Rio de Janeiro, Rio de Janeiro, Brazil

P. Block
Disability Studies, Health and Rehabilitation Sciences, School of Health Technology and
Management, Stony Brook University, Stony Brook, NY, USA
e-mail: pamela.block@stonybrook.edu

© Springer Science+Business Media Dordrecht 2016
P. Block et al. (eds.), *Occupying Disability: Critical Approaches to Community,
Justice, and Decolonizing Disability*, DOI 10.1007/978-94-017-9984-3_8

115

8.1   Introduction

This multi-authored text is written by an occupational therapist (José Otávio), a psychologist with experience in public policy (Francine) and a dancer/physical therapist (Marta) and a cultural anthropologist and disability studies scholar (Pamela). We seek to offer a panoramic view of mental health in Brazil, alternating historic and legal aspects, transformations and the struggles of social movements. Also, we have added a fictional account to better explore how some of the theoretical and historical issues may play out in practice.

We provide a brief history of Brazilian public health, mental health and mental health reform. We list some of the principles that guide therapeutic practice and the precautions to be taken, keeping in mind there is a great need for these types of services in the hospitals and healthcare centers across the country. Bakhtin's concept of carnivalization, from literary theory, is also an important reference for us to reflect upon the inversion of power and proposals that lead to the empowerment, creativity and autonomy of the participants (Bakhtin 2010). Finally we have created a fictional tale about a proposed artistic activity involving institutionalized psychiatric patients that is fraught with misconceptions and abuse of power on many levels.

8.2   Mental Health in Brazil—From a Colonial Background to Recent Transformations

For over 500 years of "official" history, Brazil was a Portuguese colony. In 1808 it briefly became the headquarters for the "United Kingdom of Portugal and Algarves" before it became independent in 1822, when Dom Pedro I, left his infant son in Brazil and returned to rule in Portugal in 1831. After the regency period during his early childhood, Dom Pedro II took the Brazilian throne, in 1840, at the age of 14. When he became the emperor of Brazil, *his first official act* was to authorize the construction of an asylum that would be named after him. Brazilian civilization was born.

The Pedro II Asylum[1] was a sumptuous palace, whose construction, followed a colonial model, and was marked by European stylistic imports. While visiting Brazil, in 1865, American scientist Louis Agassiz and his wife Elizabeth Agassiz described the asylum:

> The road brought us, however, to a magnificent hospital for the insane, the hospital of Dom Pedro II, which we had seen and admired from the deck of the steamer on the day of our arrival. We entered the grounds, and as the great door of the building was open and the official on guard looked by no means forbidding, we ascended the steps and went in. It is difficult to imagine an edifice more appropriate for the purpose to which it is devoted. It is true we saw only the public rooms and corridors, as a permit was required to enter the wards. (Agassiz and Agassiz 1868, p. 81)

---

[1]Coincidentally, this is now a prominent building on our university campus (UFRJ).

Philippe Pinel is well known as an important nineteenth century French reformer of psychiatric treatment. Although the founders of Pedro II Hospital had the intention of importing Pinel's ideals of moral treatment, it is interesting to observe that the Brazilian asylum reproduced structures of Brazil's colonialist and slave-holding heritage. Slaves and poor people (of color) worked. Rich (white) psychiatric patients did not.

In the early twenty-first century, Brazil's mental health system swings between the extremes of a wide spectrum. In fact, Brazil is a country with vast territorial dimensions, and great cultural diversity, possessing a unity built around the Portuguese language, a colonial heritage, and the legacies of slavery (outlawed in 1888). Significant social inequality still marks not only the different regions of Brazil, but also is visible within every state, city and neighborhood. Psychiatric institutionalization in Brazil has always been aligned with power inequalities. Not coincidentally, psychiatric institutions grew from 14,000 to 30,000 beds between 1965 and 1970, when Brazil was living under a military dictatorship that suppressed the political and social rights of a great part of the Brazilian population. Numbers of people institutionalized reached almost 100,000 by 1982, concentrated in the southeast region and in some states of the northeast. There was a profit motive for this. For every four beds in the private sector, there was one bed in the public sector (WHO-AIMS 2007).

Brazilian Psychiatric Reform grew out of a decades-long civil rights movement for people with mental illness, their family members and people who work in the field of mental health. This movement began in 1970. Prior to that time, institutionalization was the primary source of treatment. Following the restoration of democracy, the 1988 Constitution of the Brazilian Federal Republic ensured every Brazilian citizen the right to free public health care through the Sistema Único de Saúde, SUS (United Health System). This state-supported system coexists with a number of subcontracted services from private health institutions. Another landmark in the Psychiatric Reform movement was the 1987 Mental Health Worker's Congress hosted in Bauru, in the state of São Paulo. Its slogan, "for a society without Asylums," is based on ideas of the Italian psychiatrist Franco Basaglia. This congress took place during Brazil's period of redemocratization, at the eve of enacting of the 1988 Federal Constitution. The right to healthcare was already established. Nevertheless, the constitution did not specify the means for addressing the rights of psychiatric patients.

The Brazilian Psychiatric Reform law began as a bill presented by the then-state-Congressman Paulo Delgado in 1989. In 1993, during the bill's approval process, the psychiatric reform movement was born, advocating for: "health that aspires to have universal accessibility, reorientation of mental health in Brazil and the approval of the Psychiatric Reform Federal Law" (WHO-AIMS 2007). After 12 years and many changes, it was approved in 2001 as Federal Law 10.216/2001. According to Delgado, the deeper sense of this law is "care." This law prevented the building or hiring of any new psychiatric hospitals by SUS and granted financial resources to community-based services. It promoted changes in the existing public assistance model for people with mental disorders. The law did not prohibit mental hospitals, but strongly supported the creation of community-based alternatives (Amarante 2007).

Despite the psychiatric reforms of 2001, Brazil still had over 32,000 beds in public and private institutions, in which many basic human rights continue to be undermined (WHO-AIMS 2007). Some institutionalized people have no access to underwear, bedding, mattresses, fans in hot weather, water, and food. They are also without access to general health, dental or medical services. In 2011 over 30 deaths were under investigation in the region of Sorocaba, in São Paulo, in asylums that did not provide the basic conditions for the survival of the people institutionalized there (Desviat 2011). Even taking into account those criticisms, Brazilian Psychiatric Reform improved the guidance and care of people with mental disorders. International researchers such as Manuel Desviat (2011) and Benedetto Sarraceno (Alves 2011) state that it is one of the world's most successful mental health systems. In an interview with Alves, Sarraceno states:

> The example of mental health reform in Brazil is more than just a positive example, it is one of the most important, solid and engaging to have occurred in the history of psychiatry: It is an example where the thought of Franco Basaglia has not been embodied in a reality-lab, but in the laboratory of reality. (Alves, 2011, p. 4700)

Thus Brazil is used as an example internationally for its success in moving from health reform theory into innovative and humanistic practice.

The Brazilian deinstitutionalization and psychiatric reform movements were largely lead by mental health workers and, to a smaller degree, movements by people with mental illness and their families. The empowerment of people with mental illness is progressing, and is asserted under law, but there is more work to do on the level of public policy. There is not yet a movement that fully encompasses the wider range of mental health issues (e.g. including addiction, for instance) from the perspectives of people who experience the diagnoses and their families. Policy remains under the control of state or health professionals. The concept of Occupational Justice, interpreted by Nick Pollard and Dikaios Sakellariou (2012, p. 233) could be used to broaden empowerment in the Brazilian Psychiatric Reform Movement: "These alliances combine a professional and a lay occupational literacy as a two-pronged discourse that is dynamic and interactive." In editorial conversation with us Pollard suggests that this must come from a Freirean approach involving people with experiences of mental distress discussing the social contradictions arising from their conditions with mental health workers and others (Freire 2005). Pollard also suggests that it would involve mental health workers themselves 'coming out' as people with experiences of mental distress. It must include making alliances with the public to promote the continuous normality of mental distress especially as a condition promoted by life under capitalism. This is how such literacies would emerge.

Brazilian researcher Benilton Bezerra Junior points out the obvious tension between the social movement and the people who planned the Brazilian Psychiatric

Reform—those who occupy administrative and planning positions at the Brazilian Ministry of Health. He asks: "Is it possible to overcome this tension with a new consensus, in line with what we had at the beginning of the movement?" (Bezerra Junior 2011, p. 4598). Bezerra Junior tries to draft an answer, bringing attention to the fact that the disability rights movement has been gaining strength in Brazil, and referring to the recent example of debates about autism that have polarized a great number of activists, clinicians and researchers in opposing and sometimes antagonistic sides. However, Bezerra Junior believes that both psychiatric reform and disability rights movements would benefit from joint approach strategies when it comes to facing stigma, regulations, medicalization and advocating for the needed widening and deepening of citizenship.

Besides warning us of the fact that mental health is not just about a set of hospitals and specialized services, Itzak Levav, of the Pan-American Health Organization, proposes to the Brazilian Psychiatric Reform Movement the challenge of giving cultural meaning to initiatives that promote mental health in community living, giving particular attention to children, teenagers, indigenous populations, and other vulnerable groups that are excluded from "dignified care." Cultural change involves acceptance of mental distress, and not merely acceptance, but accommodation.

> . . . no one still believes that the psychiatric beds are the answer to the problem of mental illness. No one still believes that psychiatric suffering can be faced only with a medical and pharmaceutical model. Psychological support, support to the family, social support, social inclusion, housing, work inclusion are no longer options, but decisive and fundamental components of good psychiatric assistance. (Levav 2011)

8.3 "Carnivalization"

Translated variously into English as "carnivalization" or "carnivalesque," this concept derives from literary theory developed by Bakhtin and provides a relevant theoretical reference for the creative processes of art and art-therapy. It makes us think about our singularities and how each of us are different and unique. Systems that enforce our homogenization into model-individuals that correctly perform our social roles are unmasked under close inspection. At the same time, the notion of the "individual" can be questioned, without paradoxically letting it favor some level of self-perception through an anthropological view. Carnivalization is an attitude, a process and it also inspires a therapeutic approach. It fits well with movements, such as Mad Pride, that seek to represent mental distress experiences in destigmatizing ways that empower individuals with the authority to give these experiences new cultural meanings. It contrasts sharply with the Colonialist Spectacle and fictional tale we have constructed, that exposes some of the inequalities and power imbalances that still exist.

Bodies, minds, behaviors that differ from what is expected from us as individuals, relate to an idea that has its origins in pre-modern times: the grotesque body, present in traditional human collectives that stands out from the crowd, calling into question the official-individual body. This modern concept of self as an individual, responsible for our successes and failures, brought along a kind of suffering that is in itself modern. Might the grotesque carnival body possibly be a way to break down this "individual" condition, when it brings attention its historicity, pointing out manners of existence in which this particular category had not yet been established? In the same way the union of collectivity around a common yearning, the resistance to oppression, the festivities of carnival are identified as a culturally defined space or moment in time marked by a suspension of the power relations. Le Breton (2003) considers the medieval and renaissance civilizations as a confused mix of popular local traditions and Christian references, in a sort of folk Christianity that nourishes the relations between people and their social and natural environments.

Bakhtin refers to the "great popular body of the species": unsatisfied with its limits, this body never stops transgressing, it illustrates the world's end and rebirth, a new spring for life. Indiscernible, open, surpassing itself, the grotesque carnival body is not charted away from the rest of the cosmos, it is not shut out, it is not finished, done: it is formed of bumps, protrusions, and it beams with vitality. A time of excess and expenditure, such collective parties tend to experiment with this "non-differential" between people, bodies, and the characteristic world or holistic societies, using terms coined by sociologist Louis Dumont (1985; 1992), that oppose them to those that are "individualistic." In those, there reigns an identity of substance between men and the crowd of his own kind, in a way he cannot see the communitarian and cosmic network into which he is inserted, for his singularity doesn't yet make him an individual, in the modern sense of the term. Starting with the creation of individualism, the mind and body become separate entities. The body is not the person, but rather the person's property (Le Breton, 2003). We stop saying "I am my body" and we begin to say "I have a body."

The individualism question is an important reflection in the artistic practices within mental health. Curiously, when we place it under "suspension" in the context of dance, it presents itself as a possible path to bring us to notice the relations of power and its inversions, as well as it could possibly favor self-awareness, the contact with a body image. In other words, the contact of the mental patients with themselves as people, and even in a sense of gaining control over their autonomy as individuals, is critical. The intention is that this experience of collectiveness becomes a tool in perceiving their own singularity and individuality, for dancing to allow them to be in touch with the group as well as, through a relationship of closeness and distancing, it could give them the basis for differentiation, self-perception, self-awareness, and awareness of their body's contours, space and time. Yet at the same time, it is contained within the period of carnival. It is allowed only in certain spaces and times. Carnival is a period where day-to-day power relationships are suspended. Poor become rich, rich become poor, surveillance stops. Each person feels they are part of a wholeness – a collectivity – rather than just a separate and isolated individual in a crowd, as they may experience during the rest of the year.

8.4   The Tale of Vila Seco: A Fictional Account[2]

We now present a story set in an old psychiatric hospital of Cienfuegos in Vila Seco, a small village in the Central Western region of Brazil, in the first decades of twenty-first century. The log books of Cienfuego's asylum report the story of two foreign artists that requested permission from the asylum's board to create a video with the psychiatric patients. It was commissioned and financed by the museum of a European country that would later promote, house and showcase the piece. Looking to make video art, the artists agreed, in return, to offer an activity that would keep the patients occupied.

It was curious that permission was granted in this case, for there had long been complaints from the nurses and therapists about the lack of activities and supplies to keep patients occupied. For as long as anyone could remember, the patients were left with nothing to do. Some of the medical workers muttered to each other: "Cienfuegos Asylum is a place of false imprisonment not treatment." Students from the Fine Arts University of the capital used to ask to work with Cienfuegos' patients, but the institution's director generally did not allow this, because they were not doctors. On the other hand, when the director needed to show to the Health Ministry that 'something happens here,' professionals from the city were able to come and offer occupational workshops to the patients. It happened with no regularity, sporadic permission was granted, exactly as in this case of the European artists. This time the doctors authorized the proposal, saying it would be beneficial to the patients, on account of the drama workshops that would happen for the production of the video.

Following legal requirements that guide the doctor/patient relations, it was necessary to request informed consent from the patients or their family members, and the signing of a release form permitting use of their images. The topic of image release was very polemic, even among so called "healthy" people. Signing the document brings benefit to the artists organizing the video installation, but what do those signing it gain? Some professionals felt uncomfortable requesting patients or family to sign these documents. This small "hiccup" would have gone unnoticed and only recorded on the log books had not Tomás, a day-hospital patient, asked, during the assembly in which he was invited to be a part of the project, why the actors did not receive payment for their work. His question was answered quietly by statements such as "the project does not have enough budget for that—you'll only take part if you want to, no one is being forced to do it—those who won't do it without payment have the 'right' not to do it."

Obviously, according to the film makers, the therapist's and collaborating doctor's responses, participation in the film was not a job, it was therapy. The patients were not professional actors, and payment was unnecessary given the patients should "desire" to participate. However, Tomás continued to argue:

---

[2]This is a fictional essay.

Why, then, don't the artists give up their fee, also moved by this 'desire' or, at least, share it with the actors? A project that can finance international air travel doesn't have room in its budget for this? Will we, the asylum's patients, be informed of how much money is involved in this project?

However, the doctors, the supreme judges in decisions on ethical and moral conduct at the hospital, quickly approved the project with praises and statements of admiration. The reporting doctor reiterated the benefits of engaging the patients through artistic activities, which they considered to be a therapeutic.

"Dear colleagues, it is with great pride that we watch our asylum having its image carried out throughout the world. We are talking about artists who are renowned in the international art market. Our work is a true work of art."

Tomás' speech, nevertheless, brought to Nurse Josefa's attention the uneven knowledge/power relationship, within such a "work of art," between the doctor-approved-artists and the patients. To her, the implementation of art in the context of a hospital should be done in a different way. In a letter addressed to the staff, Josefa posed the following questions for debate, (After all, the doctors presented themselves as great supporters of open debate).

The drama activity was offered in return for a signed image release form? Was there enough time to think through the respective values? How much does each side of the scale weigh, the image of the patients to the artists, the therapeutic activity to the patients? If the patients were not poor, living in a public asylum, would such a proposition be accepted? Let's say they were the children of soap opera stars, would their parents allow people to tape images of their children while they are being treated? What if our country was not poor and did not carry the stigmas of a colonial past? Why not recall the heritage of the colonial exploitation, and with it the excessive enthusiasm for anything that comes from abroad? Why should our five-centuries-old distrust be silenced—when we were given mirrors, beads, cutlery, and necklaces for timber, gold and silver?

If Brazilians wished to pursue an identical project in a European psychiatric institution, would its ethics committee allow patients' images to be recorded? Why did this European institution want to film Brazilian patients, rather than patients in their own country? Perhaps we can put aside the issue of the total lack of options and the patient's idleness, while still considering the advantages of a partnership with this foreign institution: the therapeutic gains and the nobility of the goal of creating a work of art. Perhaps we can even trust the autonomy of the patients to decide what they want/should/can do. But—why wasn't Tomás' reasonable and relevant question answered? If the video directors were being financed, then why weren't the actors, who were the true protagonists of this work, being paid? Why was this topic not open for debate during the assemblies where, supposedly, any doubt would be discussed? The European artist did not oppose it, after all, even the debate was a big show for them. Since they are so fond of the grotesque, of anthropophagy, maybe we should take this to the absurdist extreme and have a big ritual in which we could feast on some "white meat barbecue," as the cannibal Indians did, centuries ago. This would make for a beautiful piece of art, ready for post-colonialist consumption in the European museum. It would be no different from the colonialist museum acquisitions of past centuries. And this is also so much safer than studying mental health oppression at home.

Josefa, the disgruntled nurse, asked: "shouldn't patients have the right to artistic activities without having to exchange their image for it?" Without answering her, the hospital team went on with the artists' project. After finishing this video, the long hours of "nothing to do" would come again. But the artists won prizes with their new work of art, where it was acclaimed in the Northern media festivals. Dear reader, we ask your opinion. Were these actions just?

Tomás was an articulate person, and he got right to the heart of the matter when he stated: "They want the images of slums, of Indian villages, the poor and now, us the patients. We are sick of intellectuals, artists, making their work with huge budgets, without giving us anything!"

And with passionate humor he finished: "We're sick of having creative workshops, fun, and interesting experiences! Those people from the north are always telling us what we should do, how we should live. Enough!"

As Josefa and Tomas emphasize, the image of a person under treatment is worth a lot more than that of any actor invested in a character. The artists argue that they saw no difference between documentaries and fiction, but actors usually are paid for their work, so, why not those patients? One of the items in the image release form stated that there should be no nudity. But, even if covered by clothes, there is no greater nudity than that of a person living with a mental illness, this is the translation of a "bare life," (Agamben, 1998). A bare life has no price, but the dealers are waiting in the wings, and they know its value. They know that anyone who can put a frame on it will have their hands on a treasure to be exchanged in the art market. Do we have the right to offer our patients, as if they were a sacrifice, to the international art market, without even sharing the profits with them? The buzz got louder and when it reached the director's board the answer was quick and objective: "It's a scientific matter, it's about the future of the treatment of mental illnesses; we are bringing together the practice and the theory of how art can help in psychiatric treatments." End of discussion.

8.5   Discussion

We believe there is a need for artistic activities in psychiatric units of treatment, but it must respect specific criteria. Although, according to doctors and researchers, drugs and electroconvulsive therapy follow very well tested protocols, it is asserted that artistic and occupational approaches lack rigor and authority (Hammell et al. 2012). When approaching the right to health for people with mental illness there is a separation between citizenship and human rights, and in the approach treatment there is a separation between the uses of arts and science in psychiatric practice. For the doctors here, the artistic work by psychiatric inmates tends to be viewed in a limited way, as either therapy or clinical data, and the inmates do not have the right to their own artistic work. According to the doctors the psychiatric inmates should be grateful for their "therapy" and are not entitled to the commercial benefit of selling the work to outsiders. Somehow it was okay for the medical establishment to do so, to exploit the performance and art production as something available for public consumption and viewing, much the way rich people used to visit asylums, as today people visit zoos (Faulks 2010; Foucault 1988). We can see a combination of these approaches in this case, and unfortunately the artistic integrity of the psychiatric inmates was not respected nor privileged in this case.

Alternative formulations are possible. Others, in other psychiatric contexts, are very careful to take the artist production seriously and help psychiatric inmates to produce their work professionally, and we also see cases where those with psychiatric diagnoses work independently to produce artistic works (Brink 2007; Stevenage Survivors, Chap. 22). In these contexts, both the art and the science can be consciously considered in relation to each other. In the cases where art is being produced, there can be a careful discussion of the ethics and rights issues, so as to minimize the chance of additional levels of exploitation of people who have been institutionalized for psychiatric diagnoses. Although Brazil has a long history of fighting for the rights of people with mental illness, if these issues are not directly discussed, then the empowerment of those institutionalized with mental illness can never fully take place.

This chapter leaves us with more questions than answers: Why are art, culture, and social participation therapies placed below drug based treatments? Why are people with mental illness submitted to treatments, even non-invasive ones, which do not consider recent discoveries in neuroscience? Why are people with mental illness still being treated in ways that do not take into account their most basic human rights? Benilton Bezerra Junior (2011) raises the possibilities of empowerment for people with mental illness. The movement of Brazilian parents of autistic children has asserted that conditions classified as psychiatric should take into account multiple factors: people have the right to benefit from the advancements in scientific research, have access to quality education, therapies and arts and, most importantly, release from the ancient mental illness stigma. In Brazil there are different movements of affirmation and fighting for the rights of disabled people, but they are still divided by diagnosis. Psychiatrically diagnosed and autistic people remain on the margins of Brazil's disability rights movements.

Our tale presents a colonialist spectacle, a "product" for Northern consumption, where goals are money, prestige, and the impression of having done a "good job" for a disadvantaged Southern group. It is forced, not natural, and a top-down approach. We propose the possibility that the rights movement for people with mental illness could be incorporated with the rights movement for disabled people. Strengthened, we could all say together: "Nothing about us without us" or, as we say in Brazil, with our attitude of carnivalization: "tudo junto e misturado!" (all mixed and mashed together).

Editors' Postscript If you liked Chap. 8 by Peres et al., and are interested in reading more about performance and dance in disability studies, we recommend Chap. 5 "Landings: Decolonizing Disability, Indigeneity and Poetic Methods" by Petra Kuppers (which also focuses on disability in the global south and legacies of colonialism), Chap. 7 "Scenes and Encounters, Bodies and Abilities: Devising Performance with Cyrff Ystwyth" by Margaret Ames and Chap. 24 "If Disability is a dance, who is the choreographer?" by Neil Marcus, Pamela Block and Devva

Kasnitz. If you are interested in disability studies in Brazil, read: Chap. 19, "Crab and Yoghurt" by Tobias Hecht, and Chap. 20, "Occupying Disability in Brazil" by Anahi Guedes de Mello, Pamela Block, Adriano Henrique Nuernberg. Other chapters focused on mental health and disability include Melanie Yergeau's Chap. 6 "Occupying Autism: Rhetoric, Involuntarity, and the Meaning of Autistic Lives," Chap. 16 "Beyond Policy—A Real Life Journey of Engagement and Involvement" by Stephanie de la Haye, Chap. 21 "Black & Blue: Policing Disability & Poverty Beyond Occupy" by Leroy Franklin Moore Jr., Lisa 'Tiny' Garcia, and Emmitt Thrower, and Chap. 23 "Surviving Stevenage" by the Stevenage Survivors.

References

Agamben G (1998) Homo sacer: sovereign power and bare life. Stanford University Press, Stanford

Agassiz L, Agassiz EC (1868) A journey in Brazil. Ticknor and Fields, Boston

Alves DS (2011) Entrevista com Benedetto Saraceno. Ciên Saúde Colet 16:4695–4700

Amarante P (2007) Saúde Mental e Atenção Psicossocial. Editora Fiocruz, Rio de Janeiro

Bakhtin M (2010) Problemas da Poética de Dostoiévski. Forense Universitária, Rio de Janeiro

Bezerra Júnior B (2011) É preciso repensar o horizonte da reforma psiquiátrica. Ciên Saúde Colet 16:4598–4600

Brink HAT (2007) Grupo poesia: a escrita numa unidade psiquiátrica. Poetry group: writing in a psychiatric unit. Boletim da Saúde 21(2):80–87. http://www.esp.rs.gov.br/img2/GrupoPoesia. 414pdf. Accessed 14 July 2014

Desviat M (2011) Panorama internacional de la reforma psiquiátrica. Ciên Saúde Colet 16:4615–4622

Dumont L (1985) O Individualismo: Uma Perspectiva Antropológica da Ideologia Moderna. Rocco, Rio de Janeiro

Dumont L (1992) Homo Hierarchicus: O Sistema de Castas e Suas Implicações. EDUSP, São Paulo

Faulks S (2010) A week in December. Doubleday, New York

Foucault M (1975) Discipline and punish: the birth of the prison. Random House, New York

Foucault M (1988) Madness and civilization. Vintage Books, New York

Freire P (2005) Pedagogy of the oppressed. Continuum International Publishing Group, New York

Hammell KRW, Miller WC, Forwell SJ, Forman BE, Jacobsen BA (2012) Sharing the agenda: pondering the politics and practices of occupational therapy research. Scand J Occup Ther 19:297–304

Le Breton D (2003) Adeus ao corpo: antropologia e sociedade. Papirus, Campinas

Levav I (2011) Extender la reforma por medio de nuevas acciones de salud mental. Ciên Saúde Colet 16:4592–4593. http://www.scielo.br/scielo.php?pid=S1413-81232011001300004&script=sci_arttext. n. p

Pollard N, Sakellariou D (2012) Politics of occupation-centered practice: Reflections on occupational engagement across cultures. Wiley, Oxford

WHO-AIMS Report on Mental Health System in Brazil (2007) WHO and Ministry of Health, Brasília, Brazil. http://www.who.int/mental_health/evidence/who_aims_report_brazil.pdf. Accessed 25 July 2014

A Situational Analysis of Persons with Disabilities in Jamaica and Trinidad and Tobago: Education and Employment Policy Imperatives

9

Annicia Gayle-Geddes

Abstract

Jamaica and the Republic of Trinidad and Tobago are independent English Speaking Caribbean countries, known as birthplaces for reggae and calypso music, the world's fastest man Usain Bolt, and the Steel Pan. Both are accorded the status of countries of high human development in terms of life expectancy, educational attainment and income by the United Nations Development Program's Human Development Report (2014). The post-independence development strides of both countries however have not equitably improved the socio-economic conditions of persons with disabilities compared to their counterparts without disabilities. Quantitative and qualitative research methods are employed using primary and secondary data analyses to unearth the distinct socio-economic vulnerabilities faced by working-age persons with disability for whom the right to development remains marginally realized. The main barriers that bolster exclusion and cyclical poverty traps for persons with disabilities are distilled through an examination of the socio-cultural environment, education and training, and employment. Recommendations are forwarded to inform practical legislative, policy and program development in the twenty-first century for the Caribbean. The recommendations provide a critical framework to advance the enforcement of the national disability policies in existence and the Convention on the Rights of Persons with Disabilities.

Keywords

Disability • Disabled • Socioeconomic • Public policy • Attitudes • Education and training • Special education • Labor force • Employment • Unemployment • Jamaica • Trinidad and Tobago • Caribbean

A. Gayle-Geddes (✉)
University of the West Indies, Mona, Kingston, Jamaica
e-mail: gannicia@gmail.com

© Springer Science+Business Media Dordrecht 2016   127
P. Block et al. (eds.), *Occupying Disability: Critical Approaches to Community,
Justice, and Decolonizing Disability*, DOI 10.1007/978-94-017-9984-3_9

Acronyms

AEB	Associated Examining Board
CAPE	Caribbean Advanced Proficiency Examination
CXC	Caribbean Examinations Council
CRC	Convention on the Rights of the Child
CRPD	Convention on the Rights of Persons with Disabilities
GCE 'A'	General Certificate of Education Advanced Level
GCE 'O'	General Certificate of Education Ordinary Level
HSC	Higher School Certificate
JSC	Jamaica School Certificate
JSCE	Jamaica School Certificate Examination
JLCL	Jamaica Local Examination
Non-PWDs	Persons Without Disability (ies)
PWDs	Person(s) With Disability (ies)
SSCE	Secondary School Certificate Examination
VREC	Vocational Rehabilitation and Employment (Disabled Persons) Convention, 1983 (No. 159)

9.1   The Development Context and Disability

The socio-cultural environment of Jamaica and the Republic of Trinidad and Tobago reflect an eclectic collage of predominantly African, Indian, Chinese, British, Spanish and French influences resulting from colonization, slavery and indentureship. Jamaica and Trinidad and Tobago gained independence from Britain in 1962 and are ranked as countries of high human development,[1] that is, 96 and 64 respectively of 187 countries assessed (Human Development Report 2014). Both countries became signatories to the Convention on the Rights of the Child (CRC) in 1990 and the Convention on the Rights of Persons with Disabilities (CRPD) in 2007 (Table 9.1). Trinidad and Tobago is also a signatory to the Vocational Rehabilitation and Employment (Disabled Persons) Convention, No. 159 (VREC) since 1999. Further, Jamaica and Trinidad and Tobago have national policies about disability since 2000 and 2005 preceded by the establishment of national disability coordination agencies. The CRC, CRPD, VREC and national policies provide a rights-based framework for the inclusion of persons with disability in the development agenda of both countries.

---

[1]The Human Development Indices for Jamaica and Trinidad and Tobago are 0.715 and 0.766 compared to 0.740 for Latin America and the Caribbean and 0.890 for countries of Very High Human Development (Human Development Report 2014). The Human Development Index (HDI) is a globally comparable composite indicator that combines life expectancy, educational attainment and income data. The HDI serves as a frame of reference for both social and economic development.

Table 9.1   The policy environment of Jamaica and Trinidad and Tobago

Instruments	Jamaica	Trinidad and Tobago
Convention on the Rights of the Child	26 Jan 1990	30 Sep 1990
Convention on the Rights of Persons with Disabilities	30 Mar 2007	27 Sep 2007
Vocational Rehabilitation and Employment (Disabled Persons) Convention, 1983 (No. 159)	Not Applicable	03 Jun 1999
National Disability Policy	2000	2005
State Coordination Agency	Jamaica Council for Persons with Disabilities established 1973	Disability Affairs Unit established 1999

Despite the post-independence development strides of the countries and policy environments, the socio-economic conditions of working age disabled people (15–64 years) compared to their non-disabled counterparts remains unequal. Persons with disability who represent an estimated 15.3 % of the population[2] of 2.7 million persons in Jamaica and 1.3 million persons in Trinidad and Tobago experience similar disability-induced marginalization. This chapter specifically discusses the socio-cultural, education and training, and employment vulnerabilities faced by persons with disability using triangulated quantitative and qualitative research methods based on primary and secondary data. The qualitative primary data includes 10 focus group discussions with individuals with disability and those who are caregivers as well as 10 elite interviews of key disability policy and program officials in Jamaica and Trinidad and Tobago in 2005 and 2013. The quantitative secondary data is sourced from the latest available census data sets of 2001 and 2000 respectively.

The definitions of disability in the national disability policies of both countries are guided by the World Health Organization.[3] Jamaica defines disability as: "…any restriction or lack (resulting from an impairment) of ability to perform an activity in the manner or within the range considered normal for a human being" (National Policy for Persons with Disabilities 2000, 35). For Trinidad and Tobago,

---

[2]The World Disability Report (2011) estimates that 15.3 % of the global population, that is, over a billion people has a disability. Census findings for 2001 and 2000 show that people with disability represent 6.2 and 4.5 % of the population in Jamaica and Trinidad and Tobago. Census findings are associated with underreporting due to disability-related stigma, subjective conceptualizations of defining disability, and limited inclusion of the institutionalized population. Further, the Multiple Indicator Cluster Surveys using the 'ten questions screen' for childhood disability show that 15 % in 2005 and 24 % in 2007 of children 2–9 years had at least one disability in Jamaica (UNICEF 2007, 49 and 2009, 18). The 1984 Marge National Survey "estimates that 16.1 % of children 3–6 years old had at least one category of disability" in Trinidad and Tobago (Cambridge 2009, 3).

[3]Jamaica uses the International Classification of Impairments, Disabilities and Handicaps (1980). Trinidad and Tobago uses the International Classification of Functioning, Disability and Health (2001).

disability is "an umbrella term, covering impairments, activity limitations, and participation restrictions. It denotes the negative aspects of the interaction between an individual (with a health condition) and the individual's contextual factors (environmental and personal factors)" (National Policy on Persons with Disabilities 2005, 2). Despite Trinidad and Tobago's more inclusive and participation-oriented definition of disability compared to Jamaica's more impairment-focused definition, both countries primarily position disability within a traditional medical-oriented model evidenced by the core focus of service provision and lack of legislation to enforce the rights of heterogeneous group of people with all kinds of disability to access key development assets such as education and employment.

Eight main types of disabilities are recorded in census data for both countries (Figs. 9.1 and 9.2). The types of disabilities reported in Jamaica for persons of working age include sight (31 %), physical (20 %), hearing (10 %), mental illness (9 %), multiple (6 %), mental retardation now commonly called intellectual disability (6 %), slowness of learning now commonly called learning disability (4 %), speech (3 %) and other (4 %) (Fig. 9.1). The types of disabilities reported in Trinidad and Tobago for working age persons include seeing (38 %), mobility (23 %), body movements (11 %), gripping (5 %), hearing (9 %), learning (8 %), behavioral (11 %), speaking (9 %), and other (6 %) (Fig. 9.2). While some dissimilarity of disability types exists in both countries,[4] visual and physical disabilities are more prevalent compared to the less visible disabilities (Figs. 9.1 and 9.2). Beyond difference in disability types, international disability severity trends suggest that most individuals have mild or moderate disabilities (Helander 1999; World Report on Disability 2011, 29).[5] While no data exists regarding the severity of disability in Trinidad and Tobago, Jamaican data parallels international findings where 6 and 4 % of children and working age persons with disabilities had severe or profoundly severe disabilities (Paul et al. 1992; Gayle-Geddes 2009).[6] Despite the idiosyncrasies of disability type and severity, which transects with crosscutting issues such as age, gender, and geographic location, disability represents an "identifiable minority group with shared experiences of hardships and discrimination" (Gayle-Geddes 2009).

---

[4]Similar disability types include sight/seeing, physical/mobility/body movements/gripping, hearing, speaking/speech and learning/slowness of learning. However, no clear comparator exists for mental illness, behavioral, mental retardation and multiple disabilities.

[5]Helander (1999) estimates that 58 % of people with disability 15–59 years had mild disabilities and 42 % moderate/severe disabilities. The World Report on Disability (2011) estimates that 15.3 % of the world population had moderate/severe disabilities, while 2.9 % had severe disabilities.

[6]Data for children with disabilities in Jamaica shows 74 % mild, 20 % moderate and 6 % severe (Paul, Desai and Thorburn 1992). Data for working age disabled show 12 % mild, 47 % moderate; 28 % severe and 4 % profoundly severe (Gayle-Geddes 2009).

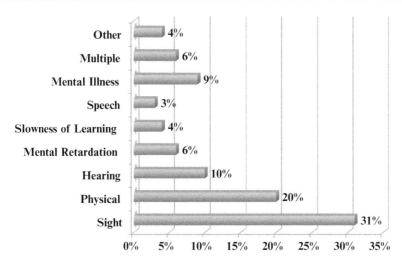

Fig. 9.1   Types of disabilities reported in Jamaica in 2001

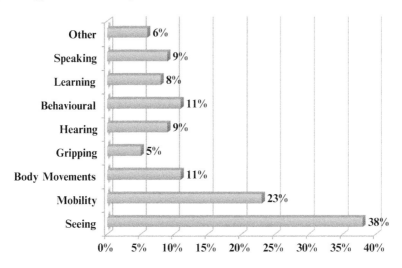

Fig. 9.2   Types of disabilities reported in Trinidad and Tobago in 2000

9.2   The Socio-cultural Environment

The collective disability identity is held robust by the cord of a generally restrictive socio-cultural environment in Jamaica and Trinidad and Tobago. The environment is fused by negative low expectations and limited accommodation amidst an empowered disability identity gaining increased social acceptance. A caregiver from Trinidad and Tobago contends, "nobody knows that a child like mine with many challenges is on the face of this earth ... persons who know me personally ... think it's [disability] a disease and it's stigmatized." Another caregiver from Jamaica asserts: "people who are able-body [non-disabled] discriminate them [disabled] and make them feel that they are less than." The stigmatization and discrimination deny recognition of the humanity of persons with disabilities and thereby stymie, delay and disrupt the desired empowered disability identity on more equal terms with non-disabled counterparts.

A person from Trinidad and Tobago assesses, "It's [having a disability] challenging because at times, I always have to bother somebody . . . it's not a problem for some to help while others might turn up their nose." A disabled person from Jamaica concludes, "society is designed for the accommodation of people without what we call disability and there are more difficulties to overcome for persons with disabilities." Similar to the Jamaican environment, an elite interviewee from Trinidad and Tobago poignantly observes, "many parents still don't understand the sky is the limit or they're scared because they know of the discrimination out there [in society]." The socio-cultural environment therefore inherently sustains voluntary and involuntary exclusion of this minority group through institutional discrimination (e.g. legislation and policies regarding education, employment, healthcare etc.); environmental discrimination (e.g. inaccessible transport and inappropriately designed buildings) and attitudinal discrimination (e.g. low expectations) (Ashton 1999). The debilitating discrimination therefore affects all aspects of the lived experiences of disability.

Much of the limited disability research conducted in the English-speaking Caribbean has focused on children, attitudes and health/rehabilitation-related issues. Elite interviewees in Trinidad and Tobago and Jamaica respectively highlight the pervasive data paucity: "we start off not really knowing accurately what is our disabled population of persons with disabilities in Trinidad and Tobago" and "the census figures aren't right, there are more persons with disabilities in Jamaica." Anderson (2000) and Gayle-Geddes (2009) in Jamaica and Cambridge (2009) and Huggins (2009) in Trinidad and Tobago represent more recent works on the education and/or labor market situation of persons with disabilities. Understanding the education/training and employment situation of persons with varied disabilities represents two core of the socio-economic enablers for independence and sustainable livelihoods which are clearly enshrined in the CRC, the CRPD, the VREC as well as the national disability policies.

9.3   Education and Training Situation

The quantitative data shows that non-disabled persons tend to attain higher education levels in both countries (Table 9.2).[7] Some 10.5 and 5 % of working age disabled persons did not access any education compared to 1.2 and 0.3 % of non-

[7]Chi-square test results show statistically significant associations between highest level of education and disability status with weak relationships for Trinidad and Tobago and Jamaica $(X^2(4) = 21,052.913;$ p = .000; Cramer's V = .172 for Trinidad and Tobago and $X^2(5) = 45,230.683;$ p = .000; Cramer's V = .176 for Jamaica).

Table 9.2 Distribution of working age (15–64 Years) disabled and non-disabled population by highest level of educational attainment (2000 and 2001)

Highest Level of Education	Frequency (%)			
	Trinidad and Tobago (2000)[a]		Jamaica (2001)[b]	
	Non-PWDs (n = 683,891)	PWDs (n = 25,052)	Non-PWDs (n = 1,389,055)	PWDs (n = 69,709)
None	1.2	10.5	.3	5
Pre-primary	0.1	0.4	.3	.8
Primary	33.2	55.6	17.7	30.6
Secondary	60.3	30.6	68.7	51.9
Tertiary	5.2	2.9	12.4	8.3
Special			0.6	3.4

Sources: [a]Census data 2000; [b]Census data 2001
Notes: [1]Secondary (41.1 %) and Vocational (20.1 %); [2]University (7.9 %) and other tertiary (5.4 %); [3]Special educational schools, the level of which was not reported

disabled persons in Trinidad and Tobago and Jamaica. In Trinidad and Tobago, 0.1 % of the non-disabled and 0.4 % of disabled attained pre-primary education; 33.2 % of the non-disabled versus 55.6 % of disabled attained primary; 60.3 % of the non-disabled compared to 30.6 % of disabled attained secondary; and 5.2 % of the non-disabled and 2.9 % of disabled attained tertiary education. For Jamaica, 0.3 % of non-disabled persons and 0.8 % of disabled persons attained pre-primary education; 17.7 %% of the non-disabled versus 30.6 % of disabled attained primary; 68.7 % of the non-disabled compared to 51.9 % of disabled attained secondary; and 12.4 % of the non-disabled and 8.3 % of disabled attained tertiary education.[8]

Non-disabled persons also tend to attain higher certification levels, that is, pass higher level examinations in both countries (Table 9.3).[9] Some 71.5 and 81.1 % of working age disabled lacked any form of certification compared 51.9 and 69.8 % of non-disabled persons in Trinidad and Tobago and Jamaica. In Trinidad and Tobago, 4 % of *PWDs* and 6.1 % of the non-disabled persons possessed Diplomas as well as First and Higher Degrees in 2000. Further, 7.8 % of *PWDs* compared to 6.5 % of the *non-PWDs* had secondary school leaving certificates; 1 % of *PWDs* and 2 % of the *non-PWDs* passed Caribbean Examination Council (CXC) Basic level subjects; while 15.8 % of *PWDs* compared to 33.3 % of the non-*PWDs* passed CXC General Proficiency/General Cambridge Examination (GCE) Advanced level and equivalent

---

[8]A further 0.6 % of the non-disabled compared to 3.4 % of PWDs accessed special education. However, the educational level of the special schools attended was not reported.
[9]In English; 'milk.'
   Chi-square test results show statistically significant associations between highest level of certification attained and disability status with weak relationships for Trinidad and Tobago and Jamaica $(X^2(7) = 4036.146; p = .000;$ Cramer's V = .07 for Trinidad and Tobago and $X^2(6) = 4164.050; p = .000;$ Cramer's V = .054 for Jamaica).

Table 9.3 Distribution of Working Age (15–64 Years) Disabled and Non-Disabled Population by Highest Examination Passed (2000 and 2001)

Highest Examination Passed	Frequency (%)			
	Trinidad and Tobago (2000)[a]		Jamaica (2001)[b]	
	Non-PWDs (n = 661,595)	PWDs (n = 22,759)	Non-PWDs (n = 1,366,459)	PWDs (n = 70,330)
None	51.9	71.5	69.8	81.1
School Leaving Certificate	6.5	7.8	–	–
CXC Basic & Equiv.	2.2[1(a)]	1.0[1(a)]	10.3[1(b)]	7[1(b)]
CXC Gen. & Equiv. 1–3/4	18.5[2(a)]	8.9[2(a)]	7.3[2(b)]	4.2[2(b)]
CXC Gen. & Equiv. 4+/5+	11.6[3(a)]	5.4[3(a)]	3.9[3(b)]	2.1[3(b)]
GCE A, CAPE, HSC 1+	3.2	1.5	.8	.4
College Cert., Dip., Ass. Deg.	2.9[4(a)]	2.1[4(a)]	5.2[4(b)]	3.2[4(b)]
Degree & Prof. Qual.	3.2[5(a)]	1.9[5(a)]	2.8[5(b)]	1.9[5(b)]

Sources: [a]Census data 2000; [b]Census data 2001
Notes: [1(a)] CXC BASIC; [1(b)] CXC BASIC, JSC, JSCE, JLCL and SSCE; [2(a)] GCE 'O'/CXC GEN 1–4 subjects, [2(b)] GCE 'O'/CXC GEN/AEB 1–3 subjects; [3(a)] GCE 'O'/CXC GEN 5+ subjects; [3(b)] GCE 'O'/CXC GEN 4+ subjects +; [4(a)] Diploma or Equivalent Certificate of Achievement; [4(b)] College Certificate, Diploma, and Associate Degree; [5(a)] First and Higher Degree; [5(b)] Degree & Professional Qualification

subjects.[10] For Jamaica, 5.1 % of *PWDs* and 8 % of the non-*PWDs* possessed "College Certificates, Diplomas and Associate Degree" as well as "Degrees and Professional Qualifications" in 2001. Further, 7 % of *PWDs* compared to 10.3 % of the non-*PWDs* passed CXC Basic level & equivalent subjects[11]; while 6.7 % of *PWDs* compared to 12 % of the non-*PWDs* passed CXC General Proficiency/GCE Advanced level and equivalent subjects.[12]

Education and training is highly valued: "If you don't have education, you will not achieve," confirms a Jamaican disabled person. The qualitative discussions with elite interviewees, caregivers and individuals who experience disability in Trinidad and Tobago and Jamaica postulate that access to education and training for persons with disabilities has improved particularly in the last 20 years. However, the quality of education and training accessed is unsatisfactory. An elite interviewee from Trinidad and Tobago contends, "I don't think there is equal opportunity for persons with disabilities in the education system . . . the environment is not accommodating and accessible." An elite interviewee from Jamaica mirrors the assessment, "ignorance is one of the main obstacles, people are not properly sensitized to the abilities of persons with disabilities." Caregivers say:

---

[10]This includes 1–4 subjects in GCE 'O', CXC General; 5+ subjects in GCE 'O', CXC General; and 1+ subjects in GCE 'A', CAPE and HSC examinations.
[11]This includes CXC Basic, JSC, JSCE, JLCL, and SSCE examinations.
[12]This includes 1–3 subjects in GCE 'O', CXC General and AEB; 4+ subjects in GCE 'O', CXC General and AEB; and 1+ subjects in GCE 'A', CAPE and HSC examinations.

The educational system and the way it is designed does not take into account our children. It is left up to the parents to hunt around; many a times to try find some place that these children in their early formative years can be given some help. There is absolutely nothing that is official. It is maybe a little private; some people are trained and in some cases it is not always like that right. So that there is really a great need to address this situation from a governmental level so that it becomes a part of the mainstream. (Caregiver, Trinidad and Tobago)

As long as they don't have any barriers, no one to let them feel like they can't achieve what they set out to do, they function just as well. (Caregiver, Jamaica)

Likewise, elite interviewees conclude that success stories are not the norm, and the environment remains steep with barriers: "even if they break through, it takes a lot of doing...what about the ramps? What about the [sign language] interpreters? What about the e-books? What about these things?" The main barriers identified for programmatic intervention include institutionalized prejudice and stigma; environmental, transportation and other accessibility problems concerning communication and learning aids; limited access to mainstream school offerings buttressed by disparities by type of school and disability type; limited scope of disability specific training programs non-responsive to the modern job market needs; limited enabling support programs to aid with school to work transition; and the cross-cutting issue of financial problems. Such barriers undoubtedly negatively impacts the readiness of persons with disabilities to transition to the labor force.

9.4   Employment Situation

Despite the prevailing attitudes pitted against equal labour force access, persons with disability are resolute self-advocates for workforce inclusion:

...not because he has a physical disability means he cannot [work]...that's depriving him (Disabled Person, Jamaica).
...the only thing I can't do is run and climb, but I can do everything else. (Disabled Person, Trinidad and Tobago).

Like disabled persons and caregivers, an elite interviewee argues, "it is difficult for everybody but more so for persons with disabilities...employers are prejudicial...they assume that you cannot do certain things. So you will be at the bottom of the pile when they are looking to hire." Labor force entry is therefore limited by the low expectations of employers and the low expectations on the part of disabled people themselves regarding anticipated successful employment outcomes. While qualitative findings suggest that labour force participation has increased, the Trinidad and Tobago and Jamaica data show that significantly more non-disabled persons participated in the labour market compared to disabled persons, that is, 31 and 57 % of PWDs versus 62 and 75 % of non-disabled in the respective countries in 2000 and 2001 (Table 9.4).[13] For both countries, disabled and non-disabled

---

[13]The converse is true for the proportion outside the labor force with 69 and 42 % of *PWDs* in Trinidad and Tobago and Jamaica versus 38 and 25 % of non-disabled.

Table 9.4 Labor Force Indicators (2000 and 2001)

	Trinidad and Tobago 15–64 years (2000)[a]		Jamaica 15–64 years (2001)[b]	
	Non-PWDs (n = 714,443)	PWDs (n = 27,097)	Non-PWDs (n = 1,171,430)	PWDs (n = 53,924)
Labor Force Part. Rate (%)	62	31	75	57
Male	78	38	85	65
Female	46	24	65	49
Employment rate (%)	57	28	64	49
Male	73	35	72	54
Female	42	21	56	42
Unemployment rate (%)	5	3	11	9
Male	5	3	13	11
Female	4	3	9	7
Job-Seeking rate (%)	5	3	11	9
Male	5	3	13	11
Female	4	3	9	7
Outside Labor force (%)	38	69	25	42
Male	22	62	15	35
Female	54	76	34	50

Sources: [a]Census data 2000; [b]Census data 2001

males have higher labour force participation than females, with accordingly greater proportions of disabled and non-disabled females being outside the labour force.

Disabled persons experience greater employment disadvantages than non-disabled persons. The employment rate of *PWDs* in Trinidad and Tobago was 28 % compared to 57 % for the *non-PWDs* (Table 9.4). The employment rate of *PWDs* in Jamaica was 49 % compared to 64 % for *non-PWDS*. For both countries, a greater proportion of males accessed employment compared to females for *PWDs* and *non-PWDs* alike. Further, *PWDs* had lower unemployment and job-seeking rates than *non-PWDs* in Trinidad and Tobago & Jamaica; that is, 3 and 9 % for *PWDs* vis-à-vis 5 and 11 % for the *non-PWDs*.

When employed, accessibility and reasonable accommodation challenges may persist. A disabled person says, "sometimes what they say is accessible is not [accessible] when you go there." Other disabled people are at risk for loss of employment upon disability disclosure: "He got a nice job . . . he was honest enough to indicate that he has a disability . . . his supervisor found out and called him in very nicely and indicated, you know, they [employer] really cannot afford to have you working." Further, access to more professional occupations that command higher incomes and related benefits of good working conditions, job security, and promotion opportunities is not generally the norm irrespective of sector or industry of work. Overall, Table 9.5 show generally similar proportions[14] of PWDs and the non-disabled represented in each occupation grouping except for Technicians and Associate Professionals; Clerks; Service & Sales Workers; and Elementary Occupations in Trinidad and Tobago vis-à-vis Clerks; Skilled Agricultural & Fishery Workers; Craft & Related Trades Workers and Elementary Occupations in Jamaica.[15] However, the proportion of disabled persons in elementary occupations[16] in Trinidad and Tobago and Jamaica was sizably higher. Some 29 % of PWDs worked in elementary occupations versus 22 % of the non-disabled people in Trinidad and Tobago. Similarly, 28 % of PWDs worked in elementary occupations versus 22 % of the non-disabled in Jamaica.[17] Qualitative findings suggest that disabled people tend to be restrained to "doing the trades—people making baskets, making chairs" (Caregiver, Trinidad and Tobago). The development of marketable and modern skills is imperative as occupational position often correlates with income potential and related independence, resilience and quality of life. Marketable skills are especially important given the income inequalities which exist[18] as non-disabled persons earn higher income levels than PWDs in both countries

---

[14]Statistically significant associations exist between occupation and disability status for Trinidad and Tobago and Jamaica with very weak relationships ($X^2(8) = 479.138$; p = .000; Cramer's V = .033 for Trinidad and Tobago and $X^2(8) = 1602.861$; p = .000; Cramer's V = .047 for Jamaica).

[15]For Trinidad and Tobago, 17 % of PWDs worked in craft and related trades; 11 % in service and sales; 9 % respectively were clerks and plant and machine operators and assemblers; and 5 % were agricultural workers. Comparatively, 18 % of the non-disabled worked in craft and related trades; 15 % in service and sales; 12 % were clerks; 9 % were plant and machine operators and assemblers; and 3 % were agricultural workers. Cumulatively 20 % of PWDs and 23 % of the non-disabled were legislators, senior officials, managers and professionals; professionals and technicians and associate professionals in Trinidad and Tobago.

For Jamaica, 20 % of PWDs worked in skilled agricultural and fishery work; 15 % in craft and related trades; 12 % in service, shop and market sales; 6 % respectively were clerks and plant and machine operators and assemblers. Comparatively, 15 % of the non-disabled did skilled agricultural and fishery work; 18 % did craft and related trades; and 14 % did service, shop and market sales; 9 % were clerks and 8 % were plant and machine operators and assemblers. Cumulatively 13 % of PWDs and 15 % of the non-disabled were legislators, senior officials, managers and professionals; professionals and technicians and associate professionals in Jamaica.

[16]Elementary occupations are simple and routine tasks which mainly require the use of hand-held tools and often some physical effort.

[17]While 2001 census data is unavailable for Jamaica, Gayle-Geddes (2009, 308) argues, "most PWDs remain in low and semi-skill levels jobs as clerks (26 %), craft and related trade (16 %); elementary occupations (16 %) and service workers and shop and market sales workers (7 %) in 2004."

[18]Measures of central tendency (mean, mode and median) could not be calculated based on the categorical income data available. However, statistically significant associations exist between monthly/annual income earned and disability status for Trinidad and Tobago and Jamaica with weak relationships ($X^2(6) = 3773.424$; p = .000; Cramer's V = .077 for Trinidad and Tobago and $X^2(7) = 1544.167$; p = .000; Cramer's V = .050 for Jamaica).

Table 9.5 Occupation (1991, 2000 and 2004)

	Trinidad and Tobago (2000)[a]		Jamaica (1991)[b]	
	Non-PWDs	PWDs	Non-PWDs	PWDs
Occupation	(n = 435,213)	(n = 8,479)	(n = 692,123)	(n = 31,686)
Legislators, Senior Officials and Managers	7	7	5	5
Professionals	4	4	5	4
Technicians and Associate Professionals	12	9	5	4
Clerks	12	9	9	6
Service Workers & Shop & Market Sales Workers	15[1]	1[1]	14	12
Skilled Agricultural & Fishery Workers	3[2]	5[2]	15	20
Craft & Related Trades Workers	18	17	18	15
Plant and Machine Operators & Assemblers	9	9	8	6
Elementary Occupations	22	29	22	28

Sources: [a]Census data 2000; [b]Census data 1991
Data for 2001 was unavailable
Notes: [1]Service & Sales Workers; and [2]Agriculture

Table 9.6 Monthly income earned by disability status in Trinidad and Tobago (2000)

Income categories ($)	Non-PWDs (n = 607,813)	PWDs (n = 20,665)	Total (n = 628,478)
Less than 500	47.3 %	58.3 %	47.6 %
500–999	7.4 %	15.3 %	7.6 %
1000–1999	18.6 %	12.2 %	18.3 %
2000–2999	11.8 %	6.8 %	11.6 %
3000–3999	4.2 %	2.3 %	4.2 %
4000–4999	4.8 %	2.3 %	4.7 %
5000 and above	5.9 %	2.9 %	5.8 %
Total	100.0 %	100.0 %	100.0 %

Source: Census data 2000

(Tables 9.6 and 9.7).[19] In context of the labor market characteristics, persons with disabilities feel compelled to "work harder" and be "better than the best" to prove themselves and display strong job stick-to-itiveness fearing loss of income and occupational mobility.

---

[19]A greater proportion of PWDs were in the two lowest income groups in Trinidad and Tobago and Jamaica. Some 73.6 % of PWDs compared to 54.7 % of the non-disabled were in the two lowest income groups, earning less than $1000 monthly in Trinidad and Tobago. Approximately a third of *PWDs* compared to a fifth of *non-PWDs* were in the two lowest income groups, earning less than $79,999 annually in Jamaica.

Table 9.7 Annual income earned by disability status in Jamaica (2001)

Income Categories ($)	Non-PWDs (n = 605,189)	PWDs (n = 22,062)	Total (n = 627,251)
Less than 40,000	8.0 %	14.4 %	8.2 %
40,000–79,999	12.9 %	14.8 %	13.0 %
80,000–299,999	52.7 %	50.1 %	52.6 %
300,000–499,999	16.8 %	13.1 %	16.7 %
500,000–999,999	6.7 %	4.6 %	6.6 %
1,000,000–1,499,999	1.7 %	1.8 %	1.7 %
1.5 million–2,999,999	.9 %	.8 %	.9 %
3 million and over	.2 %	.5 %	.2 %
Total	100.0 %	100.0 %	100.0 %

Source: Census data 2001

9.5   Policy Imperatives for the Twenty-First Century

We can do things just the same as the average persons but in different ways so we all would have challenges and it's just being differently able. (Disabled Person, Trinidad and Tobago).
. . . having a disability doesn't say that you are not normal because everybody is normal. (Disabled Person, Jamaica).
At present in Trinidad and Tobago, there are very limited opportunities for persons with disabilities. (Caregiver, Trinidad and Tobago)

The inequalities elucidated through qualitative and quantitative measures require robust legislative, policy and program attention through human rights-based development. Self-advocacy for rights-based provisions is expected to grant such momentum as disabled people are "more aware of their rights and that is what is really driving the thing, in terms of moving them from what I would call the lower class citizens" (Elite Interviewee Trinidad and Tobago). Further, the fact that "disabled persons are achieving more" (Disabled Person and Caregiver, Jamaica) has been a major contributor to changing negative perceptions of disability. Public education is therefore critical to ensure society understands the human rights and abilities of disabled persons as well as the need to create more inclusive institutions and services.

The legislative and policy framework must embrace a twin-track approach that mainstreams disability in all areas of development work and where appropriate, provide program and project support targeted at improving the life chances of persons with disability through identified environmental deficits. Improving both access and quality of education and training and employment provisions as well as transition and supportive services are strategic imperatives needed to improve the long-term development outcomes of disabled people. Thus, the respective national disability policies; the *Draft Special Education Policy* and *Draft Building Codes* (Jamaica); Trinidad and Tobago's *Education Policy Paper 1993–2003* and *Draft Policy on Inclusive Education 2008* and labor rights provisions require legislative enforcement mechanisms to mainstream key development assets for persons with disability and ensure prohibitive consequences for non-compliance. While the development assets of education and employment are emphasized in this paper, other important areas include but are not limited to access to the full range of health services; social protection; early disability identification and diagnosis; and community-based rehabilitation. The crosscutting issue of accessibility of communication methods, the built environment, transportation, assistive aids/technologies; and professional support services require fulsome attention.

"We [PWDs] are same human [beings]. We have the same flesh and the same blood" summarises a disabled person in Jamaica. The policy environment therefore demands a social risk management approach with strategies to prevent, mitigate and cope with disabilities using informal, market-based, public, NGO and private arrangements to address the households and communities of disabled people across the spectrum of disabilities, taking account of severity, gender, overlapping minority identities and urban-rural geographies. The social risk management approach must be evidence-based to replicate best-practices as the findings suggest improvements in the education and labor market situation for persons with disabilities in both countries despite comparatively disproportionate outcomes with non-disabled persons. The research equally must distill contributory factors which result in the comparatively more favorable education and labor force outcomes of disabled persons in Jamaica versus Trinidad and Tobago. Evidence-based policy, program, and project provisions will thereby advance the fulfillment of the national disability policies, the CRC, CRPD and the VREC.

Editors' Postscript If you enjoyed reading Chap. 9 by Gayle-Geddes, and are interested in reading more about postcolonial nation and the state of its disabled citizens, we recommend Chap. 8 "Artistic Therapeutic Treatment, Colonialism & Spectacle: A Brazilian Tale" by Marta Simões Peres, Francine Albiero de Camargo, José Otávio P. e Silva, and Pamela Block, Chap. 19 "Crab and Yoghurt" by Tobias Hecht, and Chap. 20 "Occupying Disability in Brazil" by Anahi Guedes de Mello, Pamela Block, Adriano Henrique Nuernberg. Or if you would like to read more about intersection of socio-economic injustices and ableism, we recommend Chap. 21 "Black & Blue: Policing Disability & Poverty Beyond Occupy" by Leroy Franklin Moore Jr., Lisa 'Tiny' Garcia, and Emmitt Thrower.

References

Anderson S (2000) In pursuit of excellence: educational barriers, opportunities and experiences of Jamaican students with disabilities. Ph.D. dissertation, University of the West Indies, Mona

Ashton B (1999) A rights based approach to disability, development and the intergenerational bargain. Paper presented at the development studies association annual general meeting, Bath, 13th September 1999

Cambridge I (2009) Why social disability studies at the University of the West Indies, St. Augustine? Caribbean Dialogue 14(1 & 2):1–12

Gayle-Geddes A (2009) A marginalized people: the state of the attitudinal environment, education and employment of persons with disabilities in Jamaica. Ph.D. dissertation, University of the West Indies, Mona

Helander E (1999) Prejudice and dignity: an introduction to community based rehabilitation, 2nd edn. UNDP Interregional Program for Disabled People, New York

Huggins J (2009) The disabled in the Caribbean. Caribbean Dialogue 14(1 & 2):13–24
Ministry of Labor and Social Security (2000) National policy for persons with disabilities. Ministry of Labor and Social Security, Kingston
Ministry of the People and Social Development (2005) National policy on persons with disabilities. Trinidad and Tobago, Port of Spain
Paul TJ, Desai P, Thorburn MJ (1992) The prevalence of childhood disability and related medical diagnoses in Clarendon, Jamaica. West Indian Med J 41:8–11
UNICEF (2007) Progress for children: a world fit for children. Statistical review number 6. UNICEF, NewYork. http://www.unicef.org/publications/files/Progress_for_Children_No_6_revised.pdf. Accessed 12 Aug 2013
UNICEF (2009) Progress for Children: a report card on child protections http://www.unicef.org/protection/files/Progress_for_Children-No.8_EN_081309(1).pdf. Accessed 12 Aug 2013
United Nations Development Program (2014) The human development report 2014. United Nations Development Program, New York
World Health Organization (2011) World report on disability 2011. World Health Organization, Geneva. http://whqlibdoc.who.int/publications/2011/9789240685215_eng.pdf. Accessed 12 Aug 2013

Part II
Disability and Community

Editors' Note: For an introduction to Part II see Sect 25.2

Akemi Nishida

Abstract

This chapter addresses debilitating impacts of neoliberal academia and ways to resist it; and it does so through critical analysis of disability studies. With insights of disability studies, it pushes the conversations not to stop at how oppressed academics are under the neoliberal regime, but to ask what it means to participate in higher education which is traditionally contested for its ablism and saneism. As neoliberalism came to corporatize education, academics' are evaluated based on financial value of their work and their capacities to fulfill its expectation. Through a concept of hyper-productivity—one of the key characteristics of neoliberal academia—this chapter describes how expectation of neoliberal academia comes to be internalized as desire or a standard to measure one's value as academics. Using the social model of disability, this chapter untangles how the expectation for hyper-productivity is constructed as well as how such neoliberalization amplifies ableism and sanism in academia. Finally, examples of disability-centered activism organizing are shared to provide ways to improve mainstream education justice movements to be more accessible and inclusive. Significance of collective care is reviewed as a way to sustain academics as they fight for education justice and to actualize democratic ways of living.

Keywords

Neoliberalism • Higher education • Collective care

A. Nishida (✉)
Disability and Human Development, Gender and Women's Studies, University of Illinois at Chicago, Chicago, IL, USA
e-mail: anishida922@gmail.com

© Springer Science+Business Media Dordrecht 2016
P. Block et al. (eds.), *Occupying Disability: Critical Approaches to Community, Justice, and Decolonizing Disability*, DOI 10.1007/978-94-017-9984-3_10

Persistently to critique a structure that one cannot not (wish to) inhabit is the deconstructive stance. (Spivak 1993, p. 284, cited in Landry and Maclean 1996) ... This is why it is especially important to choose as an object of critique something which we love, or which we cannot not desire, cannot not wish to inhabit, however much we wish also to change it (ibid, p. 7)

Academia provides its participants tremendous privilege. The correlation between one's educational background and income level has long been a topic of scrutiny (Levine 2001). The relationship between power and knowledge production is an intimate one and has been theorized heavily within academia itself (Foucault 1990, for example). Academic privilege affects those who participate in academia (in this case, higher education) differently, though, based on each individual's status within academia: tenured professor, adjunct professor, graduate student, undergraduate student, and more. The addition of intersecting identities (e.g., race, gender, disability, class, and more) and social injustice makes even sharper distinctions of how the privilege and power distributed across academia is experienced differently; how some individuals are marginalized within spheres of academia, while others accumulate their privilege as so-called 'experts'. Just as more degrees after last names are said to bring more income, the current rise in education debt complicates such a notion. This chapter examines the experiences of academics within neoliberal academia while paying close attention to the ways academic demands and expectations are distributed differently along lines of able-body/sane-mind privilege. Disability studies and its analysis of how academic privilege works through ableism and saneism inform and guide this chapter as such analysis provides critical insights into the ways academia is built on ableist and saneist foundation and practices. It thus deepens our understanding of disabling effects of neoliberal academia. This chapter poses a series of questions: how are contemporary academics' lives and wellbeing shaped and/or disabled by the neoliberal academia?; inasmuch as individuals are oppressed and victimized by the neoliberal academy, what does it mean for them to also participate in and perpetuate such ideologies un/intentionally?; how can the analytical lens of disability studies be applied to further understand mechanisms of neoliberal academia?; and what are the ways to resist the neoliberalization of academia in sustainable way?

This chapter first addresses the questions above by briefly explaining neoliberal-ism and neoliberal academia. Secondly, it lays out impacts of neoliberal academia experienced by those who are part of higher education; third, it looks at the intersection of neoliberal academia, ableism, and saneism; fourth and finally, this paper explores the ways individuals working in academia can resist such neoliberal academic ideologies through accessible and sustainable activism and the practice of collective care. The following arguments are supplemented by surveys of individuals working in higher education, mostly in nations of the Global North.[1] This chapter

---

[1] I do not mean to say that neoliberal academia and its impact are unique to these nations. It is definitely affecting academia of different nations; while degree and nature of such impact varies depending on the nation (please see Naidoo 2008, for example).

was initially written for a lecture at a U.S. university; and, as I am part of the U.S. higher education system, parts of this piece have been written as a first-person account. Finally, while this chapter focuses on neoliberal academia, many of the concepts discussed here are relevant to other spheres of society due to neoliberalism's managerial relationship to every aspect of society.

> The mantras of neoliberalism are now well known: Government is the problem; Society is a fiction; Sovereignty is market-driven; Deregulation and commodification are vehicles for freedom; and Higher education should serve corporate interests rather than the public good (Giroux 2013, October).

As Giroux eloquently summarizes above, neoliberalism is often illustrated as a political theory that pushes certain liberal economic policies such as free trade and open markets, as well as the privatization and deregulation of various sectors of the society (Harvey 2005). Harvey (2005, p. 2) argues that such theory is built on the belief that "[H]uman well-being can best be advanced by liberating individual entrepreneurial freedoms and skills within an institutional framework characterized by strong private property rights, free markers, and free trade." These theories thus privilege those who are rational, logical, and autonomous enough to successfully participate in competitive business markets. It has come to economize (and make profits out of) every aspects of our lives (Brown 2014). As much as neoliberalism shapes political and economic structures of our society, including social virtues, it also affects and forms our beliefs, desires, behaviors, and our bodyminds.[2] As the role of the state shifts from provision of safety nets for its citizens to the creation of a "good business or investment climate," people are put in competition with one another and are made increasingly responsible for their individual roles and productivities (Harvey 2005, p. 70). Education is one of the public sectors that continues to lose its public funding. Spaces of education are aggressively privatized, and have come to be part of the neoliberal machine shaping rational, logical, autonomous social capitals (Barkawi 2013; Davies and Bansel 2010; Fabricant and Fine 2013; Giroux 2013, for example). It is now an individual's responsibility to achieve their own quality education; thus education is geared towards shaping individuals to be citizens who are good consumers and can enter and successfully compete in the market-driven world.

Many scholars describe the neoliberalization of academia as a synonym for aggressive privatization (Barkawi 2013; Brown 2009; Davies and Bansel 2010; Fabricant and Fine 2013; Giroux 2014). Del Gandio (2010, para. 7) describes how "[Academia's] primary function is to serve the neoliberal enterprise." The characteristics of neoliberal academia, particularly within higher education, include:

---

[2]A concept of "bodymind" is used throughout the chapter, instead of separating body from mind, in order to emphasize the deeply intertwined nature of body and mind. Please refer to Price (2011), for example, for a further conceptualization of "bodymind".

- Research and education are no longer considered public goods, but as business investments. Schools, and in this case universities, are run by nonacademic corporate figures;
- academic work is valued based on its financial value;
- thus, departments and individuals are evaluated based on the market value of their work which is expected to reflect individuals within the department and the department budget at large;
- such evaluation fuels competition among universities, departments, and individuals; thus undermining collegiality;
- research is heavily influenced by corporate funders and their business interests;
- instead of educating students to be critical thinkers and encouraging them to do more imaginative and innovative work, academia increasingly implements standardized delivery systems to efficiently increase human capital for financial profits;
- students are treated more as customers and the roles of professors are centered around customer satisfaction;
- an increase in adjunct and short-term contract jobs that rarely provide full benefits;
- exploitation of faculties and administrative staff as common practice;
- the expansion of inequality between those who can afford quality education and those who cannot;
- A decrease in the amount of resources spent on working to make academia more accessibility and inclusive for diverse student and faculty bodies.

(Barkawi 2013; Bowley 2010; Brown 2009; Canaan and Shumar 2008; Davies and Bansel 2010; Fabricant and Fine 2013; Giroux 2014).

While the neoliberalization of academia manifests in a wide range of practices, this chapter focuses on one of neoliberalism's main characteristics: hyper-productivity. Davies and Bansel (2010) discuss that the neoliberal moment in which we live depends on and generates a complex enmeshment in linear time—an end-product driven time. Indeed, academics are embedded in the era of a knowledge economy that treats knowledge as a commodity. In such contexts we often tend to focus exclusively on, or have an access only to, *products* or *outcomes* rather than *processes*. By looking closely at the process of academia-in-the-making, this chapter untangles how productivity, or *hyper*-productivity, is an expectation and desire within academia under neoliberalism. Productivity is often identified as a key factor or virtue for anyone seeking legitimization as a valuable citizen, worker, or individual. More specifically, "publish or perish" is a common phrase used in academia and sums up a valuing of certain kinds of products and productivity. Within the current state of neoliberalism, academics are pressured to be not only productive but to be *hyper*-productive.

As the discourse of "funding scarcity" circulates and comes to shape the reality of academia, academics are forced to enter the competition (against other schools, departments, or colleagues) for what some call "economic survival" (Barkawi 2013; Davies and Bansel 2010). To survive, academics experience a demand to produce un-achievable amounts of publications and grant proposals for funding while, at the same time, balancing these duties with other responsibilities such as teaching. These products are by-and-large assessed according to their financial value and are used to assess one's capacity for efficiency. Further, valuing and demanding hyper-productivity from academics also leaks into their private time when they are supposedly away from work obligations. For example, the development of the internet and related technology means that the speed of academic life has become exceptionally fast, with speedy communication as the norm. These technologies' mobile status creates environments as if there are no time restrictions on work, with the expectation that academics be held accountable to being on-call e-mails 24/7. The physical and emotional impact of these demands accumulates in their bodyminds, including an evacuation of energy and time when engaging daily chores or when attending to relationships with others. Such conditions have prolonged, and at a time disabling, impacts on academics.

> I work roughly 100 hours a week and am getting more and more behind as the years go by. I am simply unable to keep up with demands on my time let alone handle more requests. I feel extremely guilty about this, but it's important that I push folks away so that I can continue to produce research and do the work that I do. (An anonymous academic quoted in Rosin 2014, March 23)

This quote demonstrates how academics' priorities are set up based on academic agendas. The never-ending list of to do's demands hyper-productivity and a shameful and hopeless relationship to one's ability to fulfill these expectations of hyper-productivity. My own relationships with other academics mean that I routinely hear how there is no imaginable outside to academia, with little self-value or worth found in anything not geared towards academic success or legitimation. Academics are both managed and surveilled by neoliberal academia. This means academics and academics-in-training often internalize neoliberalism's ideologies. It is getting harder to separate academic life from private life; academic values and customs now dominate the everyday life and self-worth of academics. Because success in academia *is* their desire, academics are disciplined by neoliberal expectations of success. Such internalization of hyper-productivity has its cost: sometimes debilitating costs. A recent survey of over 14,000 academics in the UK describes that nearly half of the survey participants answered that "[T]heir general or average level of stress was high or very high," and close to one-third of them responded that "[T]hey often experienced levels of stress they found unacceptable" (Court and Kinman 2008, p. 3). This study further shows a slight uplift in stress levels among participants of the same 2008 survey, as compared to earlier studies done in 1998 and 2004. These numbers are attributed to ever-increasing workloads, extended work hours, and difficulty managing academic as well as nonacademic life demands (Court and Kinman 2008). Similarly, a study done by the Higher Education Research Institution at the University of California at Los Angeles (Hurtado et al. 2012) shows a large number of faculty members experience work-life stress caused by self-imposed high expectations (84.4 %), lack of personal time (82.2 %), or managing household responsibilities (74.7 %) Among the various sources of stress these full time faculty members mentioned, it is notable that significantly larger numbers of public university and college faculty members are stressed out by reasons such as "institutional budget cuts" or "institutional procedures and "red tape," especially when compared with private university and college counterparts (p. 4). When the "managing of household responsibilities" as well as a "lack of personal time" rank higher on the list of stress sources, it is easy to imagine how academic demands affect academics' private, personal, or family time, and vice versa. One of the reviewers of this chapter shares their personal account of the debilitating impacts of neoliberal academia:

> As I read this section I kept thinking to myself, yes this happened to me, this happened to my colleague recently, this grad student dropped out, this one got into a car and randomly drove until they ended up in the Midwest (from a state of the East Coast), that one had to be picked up by their parents and that one had to be driven to the hospital. I'm not entirely sure how many times this year my colleague, who is a director of graduate studies in [an academic department], had to look after students suspected of serious depression, but I know they took least one to the ER. This problem is very real to me. And it is an occupational issue—neoliberalism encourages occupational imbalance that is unhealthy. There is tremendous occupational injustice in academia.

Survey results and this personal narrative beg further reflexive questioning of *what* is lost as academics are put under the demands to perform the *good* and *reliable* faculty members or graduate students. As everyday lives are consumed extensively by the demands of the workplace, academics' bodyminds (as well as the bodyminds of those they love) are neglected and ignored.

Another point from Rosin's earlier quote painfully represents how, under neoliberal academic conditions, academics come to internalize that it is an individual responsibility to fulfill unachievable amounts of work at un-sustainable hyper-productive levels. Thus, when they fail to be able to take on more work or work harder, shame and guilt appear and spread. In other words, people's productivity is understood within the framework of individual capability, ability, and competency. Failure to keep up with such demands becomes an individual's responsibility to fix in private in order to keep working as an academic. This is where disability studies' conceptualization of the medical and social models provides an analytic lens. In general, the medical model of disability understands disability as a biomedical impairment which resides in an individual's bodymind. Thus, such impairments or disabilities are expected to be cured and fixed in order to rehabilitate the disable person into a productive citizen. When the disability is not curable, disabled people are segregated and regulated in institutions such as nursing homes and prisons. Against this pervasive medical understanding of disability, disability rights activists in the 1970s and 1980s formulated the social model, which argues that an analysis of disability should shift from understanding disability as an individual bodymind problem to be fixed, towards understanding that one's difficulty in participating in society comes from an ableist society. Environmental inaccessibility and exclusionary social norms allow only certain behaviors, cognitive and mental processes, emotions, and physiques to exist in public, thereby preventing disabled people from participating in the society.[3] In resisting this and fighting back,

---

[3]Recently, in the realms of disability studies and activism, many people are working to extend the analysis outlined above by improving the social model through critique (please see Kafer 2013, for example).

disability communities work to remove stigma from disabled people's bodymind by placing the cause of disablement or exclusion of disabled people on the role of society. Disability activists continue to demand that society, *not* the bodyminds or behaviors of disabled people, needs to be fixed and changed. Shifting the blame to society by articulating systematic ableism allows disability to emerge and coalesce as an identity around which people can come together to fight ableism.

Similarly, the capacity to fulfill demands of hyper-productivity within academia has been made into an individual issue and personal responsibility. This means that any obstacle for an individual's productivity is expected to be dealt with privately and by oneself. As described later in this section, such individual responsibility and labor is often subcontracted to others: often women who engage in paid or unpaid reproductive labor (e.g., care and other domestic work). The subcontracting of labors in order to redeem and support a working academic's productivity can include finding and hiring of babysitters for their children or care providers for aging parents, finding editors to edit their work, Thus, any disruption to a hyper-productive frequency of work is expected to be immediately resolved, even if it means sacrificing time for self-care (e.g., sleeping, eating, or bathing) or time with loved ones (Gill 2009; Hurtado et al. 2012). Though these processes towards becoming hyper-productive in academia are to some extent common, they are often made invisible, ignored, and unquestioned. Public expressions of concern or skepticism are often seen as whining or a sign as an individual is unfit to succeed within the academy. Since these stories fade to the background of individual responsibility, we often fail to recognize these experiences as a collective phenomenon and as a reason for political action.

Within the social model of disability, disability studies and communities shifted the burden previously attributed to individual bodyminds (as disability or incapacity to participate in the society was solely attributed to an individual's bodymind). Instead, social conditions began to be understood as barriers for disabled people's engagement of society. Following this line of thinking, how can such a shift be made in order to understand academia's demands for hyper-productivity as a socio-politically constructed? To begin with, the expectation for such hyper-productivity—publishing a number of quality works, getting funding, teaching, and other services—is constructed in profit-centered ways that are not necessarily in alignment with human-centered ways or ways that facilitate collaborative works. Fish (2009, para. 13) reports a trend within neoliberal academia where "[A] state's contribution to a college's operating expenses falls … demand for the 'product' of higher education rises and the cost of delivering that product (the cost of supplies, personnel, information systems, maintenance, construction, insurance, security) skyrockets." This illustration of ever-decreasing budgets, and the increasing bureaucratic costs and demands for more productivity makes it easy to imagine worn-out academics bearing these burdens on their shoulders. In other words, creation of demands and expectation for hyper-productivity barely takes into account people's wellbeing, limited capacities, or their responsibilities outside of academia (such as their relationships with families and friends and community activities they may otherwise engage). Demands for productivity are deeply intertwined with various types of social injustices and unequal distribution of resources. For example, those with class and institutional privileges use such wealth and privilege to outsource their everyday chores and responsibility to free up their time to do more work and appear as productive as possible. This leads to a further accumulation of privilege. As discussed elsewhere, particularly in feminist studies, the outsourcing of labor is distributed unequally along gender, race, class, immigration-status lines. Thus, society is constructed to favor those who can fit into the social norm of certain physical, mental, emotional, and/or cognitive capacities, with the assumption that people can function as such. If one's physical make up fits within the social norm, such as having arms and fingers that function to type on a keyboard, the person's body is suited to the form in which the computer is constructed.[4] In this way and others the production of knowledge is standardized. One's physical make-up is not the only social norm that affects one's productivity in academia. Others include the virtues placed on being present, on the ability to participate, to engage in collegiality that exclude those who cannot or have a hard time figuring out and adapting to unspoken social norms, to interact with each other face-to-face, or express what are considered as appropriate emotions at appropriate timing (Price 2011; Wolframe 2013).

Academia has both historically and contemporarily excluded disabled people while privileging those who can fit in the academic norm (please see Wolanin and Steele 2004, for example). The neoliberal academy amplifies the difficulties disabled people face in relation to academia: both entering and participating in it successfully. The academies have a set of fundamental prerequisites in order to enter it: being a productive, rational, logical and autonomous individual (Price 2011). Such prerequisites exclude many disabled people due to the exclusiveness of such prerequisites in general, and due to the inaccessibility of university spaces and other inaccessible social conditions (e.g., the lack of accessible transportation or care providers for those who attend school). Disabled people's journeys in maneuvering and negotiating ableist/saneist space continue even when they enter higher education. For example, as discussed previously, academics are expected to perform as productive and capable faculty members or students in such public space. This can mean that for many disabled individuals, coordination with disability service office (in private) is the only way to receive the accommodation services necessary to continuing their lives on campus. As much as it is understood that individuals should take care of their own access needs, the process of advocating for one's own needs simultaneously compensates for the ableist and saneist shortcoming of universities that determine and gate-keep who is allowed to inhabit the university space. The process of accommodation can be largely avoided if a school utilizes universal design and universal learning design. Price (2011) complicates the business of accommodation.

---

[4]Or if one uses dictation software to write paper vocally, one is required to be able to clearly speak what s/he intends to write down.

We are accustomed to thinking of classroom accommodations in terms of measurable steps that help "level the playing field": note-takers; extra time on exams; captions on videos; lecture slides posted online; Braille and large-print handouts; the presence of a sign interpreter. But what accommodations can be offered for the student who is earnestly participating, but in ways that do not fall into the (usually rationalist) pattern of classroom discussions and activities? Although the notion of a classroom "discussion" implies that it is open to all perspectives, this setting is in fact controlled by rigid expectations: students taking part in a "discussion" are expected to demonstrate their knowledge of the topic at hand, raise relevant questions, and establish themselves as significant, but not overly dominant, voices in crowd of at least fifteen—and usually many more—other persons. (p. 59–60)

Indeed, our society, including academia, is filled with unwritten and subtle rules. Violations of these unwritten social rules are rarely tolerated.

This set of disability studies and community analyses of academia beg for reflexive questions, such as: as much as academics are victimized, oppressed, and exploited by the academy under neoliberalism, what are the impacts or implications of their participation in such an academy, particularly knowing that the academic structure excludes many? Participation in academia means that academics are holders of educational privilege which consequently ties them to specific social responsibilities. Such privilege and responsibility beg further questions: what should be done with such privilege and responsibilities? As people continue to participate within academia, what are the ways these individuals can collectively practice resistance against neoliberal academia?

The following section focuses on ways to resist and transform the conditions of ableist, neoliberal academia. With the rise of the Occupy Movements in the last several years in the U.S., student-led activism has encouraged those within academia to resist the neoliberalization of education such as the privatization of public education, tuition fee hikes, and an increase in part-time teaching positions. As such activism has been documented already (for example, please see McCathy 2012), the rest of this chapter is spent exploring ideas that make such *macro* activism more accessible and inclusive, while foregrounding the possibility and importance of practicing *micro* resistance within our everyday lives. The first point to be discussed is on how to make activism accessible and more inclusive. This requires the rearrangement of a liberatory education movement's agenda to prioritize accessibility and inclusion. It can entail increasing and diversifying entry points for participation such as through the internet and social media (and making it more than just a subsidiary space), rather than relying solely on and prioritizing direct physical actions. People's needs, desires, and availabilities vary, making their capacity for activism different. The second point highlighted here is the practice of community care as a crucial form of micro-resistance: actualizing democratic practices and sustaining ourselves both in activism and academia. These two points underscore differences between mainstream movements and disability-centered movements.

Within disability-centered organizing for social justice it is common practice for participants to spend time acknowledging each other's accessibility needs and desires prior to the initial meeting so that plans can be made to collectively actualize everyone's full participation. For example, people take time discussing through email, phone, face-to-face, or Facebook messaging about the physical, emotional, and cognitive support they need and can offer. This mutual support seeks to expand and transgress traditional care provider and recipient roles. Participants make sure the meeting is accessible through long-distance participation such as by phone and internet for those for whom the city pollution is too intense, for whom face-to-face meetings are too overwhelming, or for those whose care providers' schedules remain in conflict with the meeting's time. Participants pair up in order to reach the meeting spot together when geographical navigation is a challenge. Other considerations for accessibility include: identifying desirable working styles; collectively agreeing to work-speed; how future meetings impact and interact with care provider's schedules and general energy levels.

Even such well-prepared plans have unexpected changes: acute health issues arise, personal energy levels drop, and complications with a care provider's schedules occur. This is what disability community calls Crip Time.[5] Crip Time reflects the fact that people require double or triple amounts of time to travel across the often inaccessible city of New York, for example. Crip Time reminds us the importance of patience and flexibility as we work with each other. Part of the meeting's time is dedicated to checking in with participants to ensure everyone's comfort and participation is maximized. These meetings are not only a space for task-based conversations but are also a space of social support. It is always collective, creative, and imaginative work to move and organize collectively with disability community: this is the only way for us to have sustainable activism.[6]

These strategies are brought up here not to present them solely as disability community-specific tactics, but to say that these tactics have a lot to do beyond disability centered organizing. Here, they are shared as ways to transform the ableist, saneist, and neoliberal academic (or activism) practices we often engage in and in order to work collectively for more genuinely beneficial and sustainable ways. Feminists of color, womanists, and transnational feminists all speak and write about the importance of acknowledging the differences we embody and the different standpoint within which each of us is situated (Lorde 1984; Mohanty 2003; Smith 1998, for example). Only with such recognition can we figure out ways to unite and share an agenda together. Here, I am adding different working styles we embody (e.g., speed of processing information or preferable ways of communicating with each other), in addition to the different standpoints. Taking the time to get to know each other, connect with each other, learn from each other's work ethics and styles is crucial in figuring out ways to collaborate and build something bigger than any of us individually. People become part of activist movements in order to resist and change

---

[5] Please see Kafer (2013) for more reference to the concept of 'crip time.'
[6] Mingus' article on INCITE Women of Color Against Violence Blog (2010, August 23) also provides an example of how disability communities move together to attend a conference as a collective.

the status quo—in order to build a better society. It is critical, then, to reflect on what kind of society we want to create (e.g., an accessible and inclusive society) through the specific forms of resistance and protest we engage (e.g., accessible and inclusive activist strategies). The process of how people carry on transformative activist movements is telling of what kind of society can be built. A fully inclusive and accessible society will not be borne out of exclusive and inaccessible movements.

In addition to this activism and organizing, I want to touch on community or collective- care, which I understand to be a fundamental component of micro-resistance. As much as it is crucial to work for radical and fundamental transformation, I do not want to dismiss the realities of people's everyday lives and how do they treat themselves and others while they work to change neoliberal academia. As academics (and others) are exploited by the academy, our mindbodies are exhausted, injured, and they retain a lot of trauma as well as stress. When we are busy and exhausted from our work as academics, not only does care for ourselves fall by the wayside, but so too does our capacity to care for others who are important to us. Community and collective care are ways for academics to keep ourselves sustainable physically and emotionally. In particular, community care is critical not only for our wellbeing, but also because it is a tangible way to resist the neoliberal academy's compulsion for individualization by nurturing our capacities for democracy.

Scholars as well as activist movements (e.g., disability justice) have started to embrace a practice of interdependence: where there is an acknowledgement that none of us are truly independent and that we depend and need each other to heal ourselves and resist the oppressive conditions we live under today. The practice of interdependence is definitely not a new concept as it has been practiced in many cultures. Yet increasing attention to the practice of interdependence signifies the needs and yearnings for such fundamentally collective and democratic modes of living in our everyday lives. It is a journey and constant trial-and-error practice to interdependently meet everyone's needs without making anyone feel like their labor is exploited or being burned out. It is a journey and practice I believe that we need to keep trying, and we need to do it carefully. Healing justice activist, Padamsee (2011, June 19, para. 15) notes, "If your liberation is wrapped up with mine- for me that means that it matters how you *feel* and what you are *feeling*. Your well-being is our liberation, and I would hope that you would say the same" (emphasis original). Indeed, such recognition of dependency and practices of interdependence are the first step towards breaking neoliberal demands for individual responsibility towards hyper-productivity. Thus, it is crucial to integrate inclusivity and accessibility as well as interdependent measurement in the larger education justice movements.

10.1 Conclusion

Throughout this chapter, I trace neoliberal conditions and trends (such as hyper-productivity) within academia, as well as the ways these conditions impact all academics, but academics with disabilities in particular. Part of this tracing involves identifying the characteristics of professional academic life under neoliberalism as well as the forms of resistance academics can take when confronting higher education's many constraints and expectations. Oppression and stress for those who participate in neoliberal academia are real. These realities impact the bodyminds of academics as well as their loved ones—their mental and physical wellbeing are at stake. Such academic demands for hyper-productivity are often turned into individual responsibility and capacity; thus any obstacles towards achieving hyper-productivity are expected to be dealt with individually and privately. While such struggle is true, it is also true that participation in such institutions is intricately tied to educational privilege and exclusivity (based upon metrics where not everyone is admitted). Such privilege and its accompanying responsibility urge the matter not to be stopped at the point of discussing how oppressed academics are, but to be pushed to explore ways to unlearn, give back, or dismantle such privilege. It is a balancing act of liberation to heal from the oppression experienced by academics within neoliberal academia as much as to engage with and be aware of their privilege and responsibility in a society which favors a hierarchy of knowledge and people with higher education degrees. One key to sustaining such a balancing act is collectivity: to collectively refuse the demands placed on academics as individuals and build solidarity and care is to actualize democratic strategies for creating a more inclusive academy.

Editors' Postscript If you liked reading Chap. 10 by Nishida and are interesting more on how neoliberal social structure plays out in disabled people's everyday lives, we recommend Chap. 14 "Occupying Seats, Occupying Space, Occupying Time: Deaf Young Adults in Vocational Training Centers in Bangalore, India" by Michele Friedner. Or Chap. 21 "Black & Blue: Policing Disability & Poverty Beyond Occupy" by Leroy Franklin Moore Jr., Lisa 'Tiny' Garcia, and Emmitt Thrower and Chap. 2 "Krips, Cops and Occupy: Reflections from Oscar Grant Plaza" by Sunaura Taylor with Marg Hall, Jessica Lehman, Rachel Liebert, Akemi Nishida, and Jean Stewart address accounts on larger Occupy Wall Street Movement and responses from disability communities.

References

Barkawi T (2013, April 25) The neoliberal assault on academia. Aljazeera. http://www.aljazeera.com/indepth/opinion/2013/04/20134238284530760.html#.U2-gQSGaZX1.facebook. Accessed 25 July 2014
Bowley G (2010, July 31) The academic-industrial complex. The New York Times. http://www.nytimes.com/2010/08/01/business/01prez.html?pagewanted=all&action=click&module=Search&region=searchResults&mabReward=relbias%3As&url=http%3A%2F%2Fquery.nytimes.com%2Fsearch%2Fsitesearch%2F%3Faction%3Dclick%26region%3DMasthead%26pgtype%3DHomepage%26module%3DSearchSubmit%26contentCollection%3DHomepage%26t%3Dqry106%23%2Facademic+industrial+complex. Accessed 25th July 2014
Brown W (2014) Sacrificial citizenship: neoliberal austerity politics. Speech presented at the Graduate Center, The City University of New York, New York
Brown W (2009) Save the University: a teach-in on the UC crisis [Video file]. http://www.youtube.com/watch?v=aR4xYBGdQgw. Accessed 25 July 2014
Canaan JE, Shumar W (eds) (2008) Structure and agency in the neoliberal university. Routledge, New York

Court S, Kinman G (2008) Tracking stress in higher education. University and College Union, London

Davies B, Bansel P (2010) Governmentality and academic work: shaping the hearts and minds of academic workers. J Curric Theor 26(3):5–20

Del Gandio J (2010, August 12) Neoliberal and the academic-industrial complex. Truthout. http://truth-out.org/archive/component/k2/item/91200:neoliberalism-and-the-academicindustrial-complex. Accessed 25 July 2014

Fabricant M, Fine M (2013) The changing politics of education: privatization and the dispossessed lives left behind. Paradigm Publication, Boulder

Fish S. (2009, March 8). Neoliberalism and higher education. The New York Times. http://opinionator.blogs.nytimes.com/2009/03/08/neoliberalism-and-higher-education/?_php=true&_type=blogs&_r=0. Accessed 25 July 2014

Foucault M (1990) The history of sexuality. Volume 1: An introduction (trans: Hurley R). Vintage Books, New York. (Original work published 1976, Paris: Editions Gallimard)

Gill R (2009) Breaking the silence: the hidden injuries of neo-liberal academia. In: Flood R, Gill R (eds) Secrecy and silence in the research process: feminist reflections. Routledge, London

Giroux HA (2013, October 29) Public intellectuals against the neoliberal university. Truthout. http://www.truth-out.org/opinion/item/19654-public-intellectuals-against-the-neoliberal-university. Accessed 25 July 2014

Giroux HA (2014) Neoliberalism's war on higher education. Haymarket Books, Chicago

Harvey D (2005) A brief history of neoliberalism. Oxford University Press, Oxford

Hurtado S, Eagan K, Pryor JH, Whang H, Tran S (2012) Undergraduate teaching faculty: the 2010–2011 HERI faculty survey. University of California, Los Angeles

Kafer A (2013) Feminist, queer, crip. Indiana University Press, Bloomington

Landry D, Maclean G (eds) (1996) The Spivak reader. Routledge, New York

Levine A (2001) The remaking of the American university. Innov High Educ 25(4):253–267

Lorde A (1984) Sister outsider. Crossing Press, Berkeley

McCathy MA (2012) Occupying higher education: the revival of the student movement. New Labor Forum 21(2):50–55

Mingus M (2010, August 23) Reflections on an opening: disability justice and creating collective access in Detroit. On INCITE women of color against eiolence blog [Web log post]. http://inciteblog.wordpress.com/2010/08/23/reflections-from-detroit-reflections-on-an-opening-disability-justice-and-creating-collective-access-in-detroit/. Accessed 25 July 2014

Mohanty CT (2003) Feminist across boarders: decolonizing theory, practicing solidarity. Duke University Press, Durham

Naidoo R (2008) Entrenching international inequality: the impact of the global commodification of higher education on developing countries. In: Canaan JE, Shumar W (eds) Structure and agency in the neoliberal university. Routledge, New York

Padamsee YM (2011, June 19). Communities of care, organizations for liberation. On naya maya [Web log post]. http://nayamaya.wordpress.com/category/liberation/. Accessed 25 July 2014

Price M (2011) Mad at school: rhetorics of mental disability and academic life. The University of Michigan Press, Ann Arbor

Rosin H (2014, March 23) You're not as busy as you say you are. Slate. http://www.slate.com/articles/double_x/doublex/2014/03/brigid_schulte_s_overwhelmed_and_our_epidemic_of_busyness.html. Accessed 25 July 2014

Smith B (1998) Writing on race, gender and freedom: the truth that never hurts. Rutgers University Press, New Brunswick

Spivak GC (1993) Outside in the teaching machine. Routledge, New York

Wolanin TR, Steele PE (2004) Higher education opportunities for students with disabilities: a primer for policymakers. The Institute for Higher Education Policy, Washington, DC

Wolframe PM (2013) The madwoman in the academy, or, revealing the invisible straightjacket: Theorizing and teaching saneism and same privilege. Disabil Stud Q 33(1). Retrieved from http://dsq-sds.org/article/view/3425

Soul Searching Occupations: Critical Reflections on Occupational Therapy's Commitment to Social Justice, Disability Rights, and Participation

11

Mansha Mirza, Susan Magasi, and Joy Hammel

Abstract

In this chapter we analyze the construct of participation and the reality of participation disparities for people with disabilities. We also critically reflect on the professed role of occupational therapy (OT) in advancing social justice by facilitating disabled people's participation in society. We begin the chapter by debating the construct of participation as a nuanced, individually-determined phenomenon. We also highlight the futility of attempts to capture this construct through a single magical number or normative comparisons. Taking a more critical perspective, we draw attention to the heterogeneity of participation experiences even among people with disabilities. We follow this with a pitch for pluralized notions of disability participation to include diverse expressions of individually, contextually and culturally-defined interests.

In the second half of this chapter we highlight social, economic, and political conditions that marginalize people with disabilities thereby limiting their participation opportunities. Drawing upon contemporary disability studies literature we argue the need for a materialist understanding of participation that foregrounds the role of societal inequities. A materialist understanding of participation also calls for restructuring rehabilitation practice and power imbalances within traditional rehabilitation settings in the interest of a more just society that facilitates individually-determined expressions of participation. We conclude the chapter by offering ideas for 'occupying' OT practice, teaching, and research, and reorienting these to the profession's social justice beginnings.

Keywords

Disability • Participation disparities • Occupational therapy

M. Mirza (✉) • S. Magasi • J. Hammel
University of Illinois at Chicago, Chicago, IL, USA
e-mail: mmirza2@uic.edu

© Springer Science+Business Media Dordrecht 2016
P. Block et al. (eds.), *Occupying Disability: Critical Approaches to Community,
Justice, and Decolonizing Disability*, DOI 10.1007/978-94-017-9984-3_11

11.1   Introduction

Despite the lack of a singular purpose, or perhaps because of it, the Occupy Movement(s) that began in September 2011 came to represent a collective call for a more egalitarian society. Some commentators, both supporters and skeptics, used the catchphrase 'Occupational Therapy' to characterize the movement(s) (e.g. Chicago Tribune 2011; Dauphenee 2011; Spurr 2011; Surpin 2012). This curious choice of words was likely a play upon the Movement's title, its bid to 'rehabilitate' unjust social and economic structures, and its own need for 'rehabilitation' after flagging interests. The commentators who coined the phrase were arguably unaware of the history of OT or that the field traces its roots to the urban social reforms of the U.S. Progressive Era (Frank et al. 2008). Yet the catchphrase unwittingly gives pause to those of us who identify professionally, academically, or personally with the field.

The history of OT in the U.S. is closely tied to social justice and activism. The field's early founders were dedicated to reforming treatment of people with mental illness and improving impoverished urban communities, which were considered a hotbed for physical and mental ailments. As the field became more established, its activist roots gave way to an ever increasing alliance with clinical medicine, which has continued to dominate the field (Frank and Zemke 2009). It was not until 2010 that social justice was added (and later retained) as a guiding principle in the field's influential ethics code, but after much debate and resistance (ADVANCE March 31 2011; Brown 2011).

The field has witnessed a recent revival, albeit a modest one, in its social justice thrust. Occupational therapy scholars have noted a growing interest in societal inequalities and a practice trend toward political engagement and social transformation (Braveman and Bass-Haugen 2009; Frank and Zemke 2009). The pervasiveness of this trend and the extent to which it has penetrated clinical practice is debatable. Yet, for at least two decades, prominent voices in OT have argued for a greater focus on marginalized populations and for interventions to be guided by a social justice framework (Townsend 1993; Townsend and Wilcock 2004; Thibeault 2002, 2006).

In this chapter we reflect on the social justice ideals of OT[1] and the pursuit of these ideals in dialectical collaboration with disability studies and the disability rights community. We do so by foregrounding 'participation', a construct that has become the holy grail of practice in OT and other rehabilitation fields (Hemmingsson and Jonsson 2005), and has also emerged as a key theme in disability rights discourse (Boyce and Lysack 2000; Galheigo et al. 2012). We argue that this seemingly simple term is in fact a complex, multilayered construct that lends itself to

---

[1]The OT Code of Ethics and Ethics Standards (Reed et al. 2010) describes seven principles that OT personnel are accountable for. Justice is the fourth principle described in the document, which asserts that "While opinions differ … the issue of justice continues to focus on limiting the impact of social inequality on health outcomes." (p. S22). In the newest version of the code of ethics, 'social justice' has been replaced with the more generic 'justice'.

myriad and sometimes divergent interpretations. Therefore, without deconstructing participation and clarifying its usage in our practice and scholarship we run the risk of misappropriating the term and turning it into a weak stand-in for social justice. We propose a materialist reframing of participation and argue that such a reframing is necessary if participation is to become, as Townsend and Wilcock (2004) suggest, a benchmark for advancing justice for the people we serve. Finally we consider some ways in which such a reframing can be incorporated in OT practice, pedagogy, and research.

11.2 Participation and Its Discontents

Participation has emerged as a key outcome in rehabilitation interventions for persons with disabilities, mainly because of its central place in the International Classification of Functioning, Disability, and Health (ICF), the WHO's influential disability framework (Heinemann 2010). Within OT, the concept of participation has been incorporated in practice, theory, and in the professional lexicon (Hemmingsson and Jonsson 2005). Prominent journals in the field have embraced participation as their central focus (e.g. OTJR: Occupation, Participation, and Health) or dedicated whole sections to participation outcomes (e.g. American Journal of OT). Professional bodies have also endorsed the centrality of participation to OT practice (e.g. the American Occupational Therapy Association [AOTA] 2008; World Federation of Occupational Therapists [WFOT] 2004).

Yet we have done little to elaborate how we conceptualize participation and its linkages with the social justice ideals of the field. If we claim our primary professional role as facilitators of participation (AOTA 2008) for persons with disabilities we owe it to ourselves and the people we work with to critically discuss and debate just what we mean by participation. Not doing so would render participation a mere buzzword, or worse still, a cover up for perpetuation of old practices in the garb of contemporary and progressive jargon (Maskos and Siebert 2006).

There is risk of participation being defined and used in ways that are incongruent with the experiences and goals of persons with disabilities. For example, the ICF conceptualizes participation as functional performance in context (WHO 2001). Contrary to this notion of participation qua performance, people with disabilities conceive participation as being actively engaged in self-chosen activities and communities *and* having the freedom, opportunities, and supports to do so (Hammel et al. 2008; Milner and Kelly 2009). Yet instruments and assessments continue to be developed in the field using functional performance as a proxy to operationalize and measure participation (Dijkers 2010). The express purpose of such instruments is to build evidence for the effectiveness of our interventions. However such developments pander to a 'politics of evidence' (Morse 2006; Denzin 2009), the irony of demonstrating putative benefits of our services in ways that are in line with funders' or insurers' expectations but completely at odds with the values of service recipients.

Another misstep is defining participation outcomes and interventions based on normative standards for the 'general', non-disabled population (Dijkers 2010). This often entails foisting on disabled people an obligation to participate, to ascribe to expected modes of participation, and to assimilate within mainstream society, its flaws and shortcomings notwithstanding (Maskos and Siebert 2006). Whereas disabled people often desire alternative modes of participation, some of which are not only outside of mainstream society but also subversive of conventional expectations. Even when 'equal' participation is desired, equality is not a stand-in for sameness but rather fairness in access to rights, opportunities, and resources.

For example disability activist and artist Sunaura Taylor staunchly asserts her right to *not* participate in paid employment. She argues that in the resolutely capitalist and corporate American economy even her most ardent contributions are likely to be undesirable. Rather than participating at the fringes of the employment sector (in sheltered workshops, for example), she chooses to participate at the heart and center of disability rights rallies and protests. While affirming her right to participate on her own terms, Taylor also laments that her chosen path is often unrecognized or undervalued as true participation (Taylor 2004).

Consideration must also be given to the heterogeneity of participation among people with disabilities. Disabled people vary in their participation preferences, and also in the material and social contexts that condition their participation experiences (Brown 2010). For example, Kasnitz and Block (2012) remind us that the North American and Western European disability communities are steeped in the independent living paradigm, a paradigm that espouses individual choice and control and exalts the autonomous and independent subject (Kelly 2010; Smith and Routel 2010). One of the authors, who self-identifies as a 'crip American woman', recalls an incident in Guatemala, and her own misplaced, 'gringa' sense of outrage when a Guatemalan disability rights activist thought nothing of being manually carried up a flight of stairs to participate in a meeting with the local mayor. Such examples underscore the wide variations in culturally-accepted ways of achieving participation and the pitfalls of imposing one cultural view on another (Kasnitz and Block 2012).

Similarly, research with disabled North Americans from ethnic minority backgrounds shows that their participation narratives do not conform to participation values commonly extolled in mainstream disability discourse (Mirza and Hammel 2011). Values such as decisional autonomy, self-determination, and individualism are derivatives of Western thinking and culture (Kelly 2010; Smith and Routel 2010). Disabled people from diverse cultural backgrounds might disavow these values in favor of shared, interdependent, and more communal forms of participation (Mirza and Hammel 2011). Similar arguments have been made regarding the participation of persons with severe cognitive disabilities. Recognizing and celebrating only autonomous expressions of participation limits participation possibilities for people with cognitive disabilities and perpetuates their disenfranchisement (Erevelles 2002). Therefore a more inclusive conceptualization of participation ought to be rooted not in the autonomous individual, but instead in the possibilities of interdependence and community supports (Erevelles 2011).

The above arguments call for more pluralistic notions of disability participation achieved independently or interdependently and including diverse expressions of individually, contextually and culturally-defined interests and values (Kasnitz and Block 2012). Thus for occupational therapists pursuing participation goals, it is important to recognize that meaningful and satisfactory participation likely varies from one disabled individual to the next and from one environment to another, even for the same person (Heinemann et al. 2010). That is not to say there are no universal commonalities across individual experiences. Instead, and taking a cue from transnational feminism (Mohanty 2003; Milevska 2011), we argue that the individual and the universal are dialectically related. In other words, individual experiences of participation, distinct as they may be, are deeply conditioned by material realities and structural barriers that are common across large numbers of people with disabilities. Thus participation goals differ starkly from clinical goals. The latter tend to be uniform across people with disabilities, and in their uniformity they render invisible material and structural disparities. In contrast, experiences of participation and participation disparities, while uniquely individual, illuminate common conditions of deprivation and oppression, a topic that we turn to in the next section.

11.3 Contours of Participation Disparities

Participation disparities occur when barriers to participation are rooted in structural inequalities. Completely satisfactory participation across desired venues and at all times is well-nigh impossible for anyone regardless of disability. For example, non-participation in the workforce (when this is a desired goal) is not a disparity if reasons for non-participation include taking time off volitionally to attend graduate school or raise one's children. However, this becomes a disparity when participation in the workforce is hindered by lack of disability-related accommodations, discriminatory hiring policies, and the possibility of losing one's public health insurance. Thus disparities in participation do not stem from life situations that happen to all of us and impose competing demands on our time and resources. Disparities arise when societal discrimination, inadequate social policies, and economic inequalities constrain participation opportunities for specific groups of people.

As a social group, disabled people experience inequalities across various domains. At the heart of these inequalities is the disproportionate poverty experienced by people with disabilities. Of the 36 million disabled people in the U.S., about 12 % of the total U.S. population, 21 % (aged 16 and older) live below the poverty level compared with 11 % of their nondisabled counterparts (Disabled World News 2011). Families raising disabled children are more likely to live in poverty and face greater financial hardship compared with other families (Fujiura and Yamaki 2000; Wang 2005; Parish 2008). The situation is also getting progressively worse. According to the Current Population Survey, the income gap among households with and without a person with a work limitation (the survey's definition of "disability") has grown steadily, from a difference of about $19,000 in 1980 (in 2008 dollars) to nearly $28,000 in 2008 (U.S. Census Bureau, Current Population Survey as cited in National Council on Disability 2011). Educational disparities and pervasive unemployment are believed to be contributors to high poverty levels among people with disabilities. For example, 72 % of disabled people in the U.S. aged 16 and older are not in the labor force compared to 27 % of non-disabled people (Disabled World News 2011). Some disabled people might find employment opportunities in the informal economy. However informal employment is frequently characterized by high-risk jobs, little or no job security, and absence of non-wage compensation or fringe benefits (Burton Blatt Institute 2011). Employment disparities are related to disparities in educational attainment. Only 13 % of people with a disability aged 25 and older have a bachelor's degree or higher compared with 31 % for those with no disability. Furthermore, the proportion of disabled people with less than a high school graduate education (28 %) is more than double that of nondisabled persons (12 %) (Disabled World News 2011).

People with disabilities also experience inequalities in other important areas such as transportation, housing and healthcare. According to a recent survey conducted in the U.S., 34 % of people with disabilities reported having inadequate transportation compared with 16 % of people without disabilities (Kessler Foundation and National Organization on Disability 2010). Finding appropriate housing is also a constant challenge. The National Council on Disability (NCD) reports that disability-related discrimination is the most frequent type of housing discrimination, 30 % higher than discrimination based on race. Housing discrimination complaints based on disability also increased by more than 20 % between 2005 and 2009 (NCD 2011). In addition, it is nearly impossible for the large number of people with disabilities living on fixed Supplemental Security Income (SSI) to find safe, accessible and affordable housing without receiving housing subsidies, which typically tend to be in short supply. According to one stipulation, people receiving SSI would need to triple their income to rent a one-bedroom apartment at the national average (NCD 2011). It is not surprising then that large numbers of homeless adults living in shelters identify as persons with disabilities (U.S. Department of Housing and Urban Development 2009).

People with disabilities also experience disadvantages in access to healthcare. In the U.S., disabled people are disproportionally affected by draconian insurance policies that deny healthcare coverage because of preexisting health conditions and impose annual and lifetime caps on benefits (National Council on Disability 2011). Lack of adequate insurance coverage renders even basic healthcare unaffordable. According to a 2009 survey, people with disabilities in all U.S. states were more likely to report cost as a barrier to healthcare compared to people without disabilities (Centers for Disease Control and Prevention 2011). Other barriers such as physically inaccessible facilities and diagnostic equipment, lack of sign language interpreters, and insensitive health professionals further hinder healthcare access for people with disabilities (Sinai Health System and Advocate Health Care 2004; Wheeler 2013; Yee 2013).[2]

---

[2]This chapter was written before implementation of the Affordable Care Act, which was intended to mitigate some of these barriers.

In addition to barriers in the real world people with disabilities also experience barriers in accessing the virtual world. The digital divide disproportionately affects disabled people whose access to the Internet and other information technologies is significantly hindered by financial constraints, inaccessible websites, and dearth of adaptive hardware equipment and software programs (Mirza et al. 2006; National Council on Disability 2011). This places disabled people at a major disadvantage in a world where the Internet has become the mainstay for information dissemination and social networking.

Taken together, the above inequalities constitute an overall environment replete with challenges for the vast majority of people with disabilities. An environment where disabled people must negotiate daily barriers to ensure basic survival is hardly conducive for meaningful participation. Thus *individual* quests for participation do not occur in a vacuum but in a *universal* environment of inequitable social and economic conditions. Participation experiences of people with disabilities, regardless of how uniquely individual they may be, are similarly constrained by shared conditions of chronic poverty, pervasive unemployment, unstable and unaffordable housing, discriminatory workplace policies, lack of educational opportunities, substandard healthcare, and inaccessible transportation and information technologies. The latter conditions are pervasive enough to disadvantage even middle-class and affluent people with disabilities, thereby lending credence to the notion that second-class citizenship and participation disparities among disabled people are often socially engineered (Wendell 1996). In the next section we propose a reconceptualization of participation that foregrounds the role of these social and economic conditions.

11.4 Toward a Materialist Understanding of Participation

Noted disability studies scholar Nirmala Erevelles theorizes disability as a materialist construct. In this theorization, disability is inextricably linked with structural inequalities. First, structural inequalities engender conditions of war and poverty, which play a role in the creation and proliferation of disability. Second, structural inequalities are manifestations of transnational capitalism, which in its relentless pursuit of profits and productivity, casts disability as an immanent disadvantage. Finally, structural inequalities are synonymous with material conditions that hinder basic survival of and life opportunities for people with disabilities (Erevelles 2011).

The above argument underscores the role of political economy in conditioning disability experiences. In the U.S. and much of the rest of the world, political and economic resources are organized in the service of transnational capital. This creates a political economy where profiteering, consumerism, and staying competitive in the global economy are of paramount importance. Consequently, public welfare is offloaded to the private sector and subject to market solutions. Economists, disability studies scholars, and political theorists (Amin 1977; Eisenstein 1998; Mohanty 2003) have long argued that there is another dimension to this political economy, a dark underbelly characterized by underdevelopment and widespread inequalities. People with disabilities occupy a near permanent yet hidden presence in this underbelly. Deemed unfit to contribute to competitive labor markets, their only way to contribute to a profit-oriented economy is as clients of various service industries (Albrecht 1992). Their biggest value derives from their commodification as beds in institutions (Russell 2000).

In the U.S. there exists a long-standing bias toward institutional placement of people with disabilities versus their integration in communities of choice (Shirk 2006). Medicaid, the largest publicly-funded healthcare program for low-income people in the U.S., requires coverage of institutional care for persons with disabilities whereas home and community-based services are optional (NCD 2011). According to recent reports, 57 % of Medicaid long-term care dollars was directed toward institutional care. The few recent gains in home and community-based care are at risk of being reversed as states attempt to balance their budgets (NCD 2011). In times of economic crises, public programs for people with disabilities are among the first to be eliminated, a further testament to the fact that the welfare of citizens with disabilities is not a primary goal of market-driven economies.

Within this political economy, people with disabilities are often assigned to spaces that are marginal at best, such as inner cities, nursing homes, sheltered workshops and special education classes. Some scholars characterize these spaces as a 'Third World' that thrives in the backyard of the 'First World'; a world whose existence is seldom acknowledged and whose denizens are consequently rendered invisible (Watts and Erevelles 2004; Erevelles 2011). We believe that this 'Third World' should be foregrounded in any critical discussion about participation of people with disabilities. Thus participation is a materialist construct; its expression (or lack thereof) reflects broader structural inequalities. Without acknowledging these structural inequalities what we have is a vapid 'First World' construction of participation that ignores 'Third World' realities.

Drawing upon the arguments of other scholars (e.g. Amin 1977; Dhaliwal 1996; Farmer et al. 2006; Erevelles 2011), we posit that OT interventions based on "deso-cialized" notions of participation are likely to be ineffective in challenging existing inequalities. Instead we propose a materialist understanding of participation where participation is not a stand-alone end goal but rather a *process* of striving toward *individual goals* whilst pushing back against *universally inequitable conditions*. In the next section we offer examples of how this can be attempted in OT practice, research, and education.

11.5   Where Do We Go from Here?

We believe that the way forward is to align ourselves with the disability rights community in a shared pursuit of social justice. Instead of framing a separate, professionally-delimited version of justice, we suggest the pathway of 'reflective solidarity' (Mohanty 2003), enacted through democratic dialogue and a praxis-oriented shared struggle. The collective struggle we envision is distinct from professional advocacy in that it is not framed to serve professional self-interests or to preserve the relevance of OT vis-à-vis other rehabilitation professions. Rather we envision a politically active struggle launched shoulder-to-shoulder with diverse communities of people with disabilities and grounded in the principles of mutual understanding and accountability where common interests are foregrounded while differences are also acknowledged and discussed (Mohanty 2003).

We acknowledge that the above vision is not the undertaking of individual occupational therapists. Having been practitioners ourselves and in constant dialogue with our colleagues in practice we understand that translating lofty ideals into reality is a daunting enterprise. Therapists feel disempowered to engender radical change in traditional practice settings where restrictive healthcare policies and misguided funding priorities favor biologically-based, short-term, and expert-driven interventions (Townsend et al. 2003). What we propose here is as much about individual actions as it is about change in the overall tenor of OT practice, and healthcare practice in general. What we need is a collective consciousness raising that inspires us to reflect critically on where we have fallen short of our discipline's ideals and to galvanize change in our practice, research, and education. Examples where this has been attempted in our own work and in the work of others follow.

In the practice arena, a fitting example comes from the work of Galheigo and colleagues (2012) at the University of Sao Paulo, Brazil. This enterprising group of occupational therapists, used a 'territorial' approach to facilitate the social participation of people with disabilities living in impoverished urban areas in Sao Paulo. Their approach involved mapping the terrain of material and subjective conditions of disabled people including the local economy of their neighborhood, housing conditions, availability of resources, social networks, and prevailing cultural attitudes about disability. Their interventions ranged from individual clinical care and assistive technology to group and sociocultural activities and human rights forums involving local churches, community centers, volunteers, and community leaders. These interventions were evaluated through personal trajectories and life story narratives of the people served.

The above example might be difficult to replicate in the U.S. given restrictive healthcare policies and the clinical/institutional bias of public health insurance programs. As a result, employment opportunities for occupational therapists are largely restricted to traditional clinical settings. However, even in this constrained environment there are examples of therapists who buck the trend. Some therapists have found a home in non-traditional settings. For example, Barbara Kornblau, a licensed occupational therapist and educator, serves as Executive Director of the Society for Participatory Medicine. She is also the founder and CEO of Disability Health Equity, an organization that strives to eliminate healthcare disparities faced by people with disabilities (Kornblau 2013). The work of Maggie Heyman is another example. Kronenberg and Pollard (2006) describe her approach of blending OT principles with Native American spiritual beliefs while working in a Native American boarding school in the U.S. northwest. The school's mission, endorsed by the Affiliated Northwest Tribes, focused on enrichment and future prosperity of Native American peoples while preserving their cultural heritage (Ojibwa 2011). Heyman's work at the school involved supporting students to transition to higher education and return to serve their tribes and communities.

Aside from a few exceptions, the vast majority of occupational therapists are employed in traditional settings. Even in such settings, however, there are examples of therapists who subvert professional norms. For example, Mattingly (1998) describes an 'underground practice' among therapists who furtively orchestrate clinical sessions around activities that, while central to a patient's well-being, might not be reimbursable under health insurance policies. These activities remain hidden because they are either redefined in biomedical terms or not reported in clinical documentation. Similarly Dhillon and colleagues (2010) report that therapists routinely engage in advocacy during their clinical work but refrain from discussing or documenting these activities to avoid pushback from employers. There are also examples of therapists who have colluded with disabled nursing home residents to get them out into their communities in defiance of administrative authorities (Gossett Zakrajsek et al. 2014, see Vic's case study). In addition, the Affordable Care Act might open up opportunities to locally implement similar community-focused interventions as the previously described program implemented in Sao Paulo. New assessments to identify environmental factors that influence participation (Heinemann et al. 2011) are also being developed and can be potentially helpful in guiding such interventions.

In the research arena there are several examples of projects driven by the collective vision we described at the beginning of this section. Hammel, in partnership with two Centers for Independent Living, developed and evaluated a community living program to support the transition of disabled people from institutional to community settings (Minkler et al. 2008). This is a trailblazing example of using traditional clinical research methodology to build evidence for a non-traditional social justice intervention. Paul-Ward's (2009) qualitative research serves as another example. Her study highlights inadequacies within the U.S. foster care system with a goal to improve the life opportunities of children in foster care. Similarly Magasi and colleagues' recent research focuses on investigating healthcare disparities among low-income disabled people in the U.S. Their project is in response to nation-wide shifts in healthcare delivery from the traditional, state run fee-for-service model to privately-administered managed care. Magasi and colleagues' work focuses on investigating healthcare disparities among disabled Medicaid beneficiaries as a result of these shifts (Magasi et al. 2013). Finally, Mirza is working in partnership with disability activists and immigrant communities to address service disparities and social isolation of new immigrants and refugees with disabilities settling in the U.S. (Mirza et al. 2014).

A final arena where we need to foster change is OT education so that lessons from the above endeavors are carried forward by the next generation of OT researchers and clinicians. There have been long-standing calls to make OT training curricula more dynamic and socially relevant. Some have noted that educational institutions privilege first-world and middle-class norms which are then translated into OT tools, assessments, and interventions. Therapists trained in the 'vacuum of the rich' are unlikely to understand or effectively address the needs of socially and economically marginalized groups (Thibeault 2006; Beagan 2007). Others have argued that freshly-minted occupational therapists are often well-versed with the microlevel interplay between individual functioning, occupational goals, and the local environment. However they lack knowledge of political, economic, and social processes that constrain disabled people's participation (Grady 1995; Frank and Zemke 2009).

Thus there is a need to revitalize OT curricula by introducing interdisciplinary coursework in areas that are currently lacking. We acknowledge that this is an uphill task especially in an environment where academic institutions are succumbing to economic pressures and aligning educational offerings with industry-driven interests (Thibault 2006). However opportunities exist to transform educational curricula within the constraints of contemporary economic realities.

For example, in the U.S., educational standards established by the national accrediting agency for OT education offer several possibilities for introducing new coursework or adding new content to existing courses. A core educational standard calls for knowledge and understanding of the history and philosophy of the OT profession (ACOTE 2011). As Kronenberg and Pollard (2006) argue, the philosophical base of OT is far broader that biomedical understandings of health and disability. Other educational standards require knowledge and understanding of societal factors that affect the health and wellness of populations (including people with disabilities) who are at risk of social injustice, occupational deprivation, and service disparities (ACOTE 2011). These standards can be met by infusing disability studies and social justice training throughout OT curricula and fieldwork experiences (Block et al. 2005; Cottrell 2005). Indeed there are examples of accredited institutions offering masters and doctoral level educational opportunities corresponding to these standards. These opportunities entwine OT education with political and social engagement with underserved populations (Kronenberg and Pollard 2006; Suarez-Balcazar et al. 2013).

What we are calling for here is an activist praxis and pedagogy of OT enacted in solidarity with people with disabilities. This endeavor is vital for personal, professional, and political reasons. On the personal front, disability touches all our lives, either directly or through family members. Therefore it is in our personal interests to advocate for disability justice. More importantly, we need to remember that as OT professionals we make a living from serving people with disabilities. It is therefore imperative that we fulfill this responsibility in ways that are not just evidence-based but also socially responsible (Kronenberg and Pollard 2006). If not, then we risk becoming entrenched in the 'disability business' that thrives off the oppression of people with disabilities (Albrecht 1992). On the professional front we also need to be cognizant of the fact that the same political economy forces that constrain the lives of people with disabilities – market-driven economies, profit-oriented healthcare systems, and restrictive insurance policies – also thwart our professional goals and ideals. Finally, on a broader political level we need to acknowledge that our fates are bound with those of the most marginalized in our society. Participation disparities experienced by people with disabilities reflect a more pronounced manifestation of degraded social conditions that affect us all such as shrinking public services, unaffordable health insurance, lack of secure employment, impoverished neighborhoods, and growing income gaps (Taylor

2004). Shared conditions of degradation warrant a shared resistance struggle of the kind we described at the beginning of this section.

11.6 Conclusion

At the 2006 World Federation of Occupational Therapy Conference, key note speaker Sohail Inayatullah, debated alternative futures for OT. He cogently argued that hopeful alternative futures often stem from acceptance of voices from the margins. He labeled these marginal voices as 'the Bedouins in OT', those who envision a different future and challenge the status quo (Inayatullah 2007).

In this chapter we have amplified some of these marginal voices, our own as well those of clinician and scholars. Our collective endeavors move away from reductionist, biomedically-focused clinical goals toward broader social justice pursuits specifically addressing participation disparities for people with disabilities. Our work is guided by a nuanced and critical conceptualization of disability participation, which includes diverse expressions of individually, contextually and culturally-defined interests. Our work also underscores the need for a materialist understanding of participation in light of social, economic, and political conditions that marginalize people with disabilities thereby limiting their participation opportunities. A materialist understanding of participation calls for restructuring rehabilitation practice and power imbalances in the interest of a more just society that facilitates individually-determined expressions of participation. Such a restructuring is only possible by embracing a political practice of OT where we reacquaint ourselves with the profession's social justice roots (Frank and Zemke 2009). If we endeavor to address existing inequalities we must first acknowledge and confront societal factors that feed these inequalities. Failing to do so is tantamount to silent compliance with existing injustices (Townsend and Wilcock 2004). May the tribe of 'the Bedouins in OT' grow.

Editors' Postscript If you liked Chap. 11 by Mirza et al. and you are interested in how occupational therapists have engaged with disability studies across the lifespan, we recommend Chap. 12: "Refusing to Go Away: The Ida Benderson Seniors Action Group" by Denise M. Nepveux and Chap. 17: "Self Advocacy and Self Determination for Youth with Disability and their Parents during School Transition Planning" by Eva Rodriguez. If you are interested in creative interplay between disability and occupational therapy, see Chap. 24 "If Disability is a dance, who is the choreographer?" by Neil Marcus, Pamela Block and Devva Kasnitz.

References

Accreditation Council for OT Education (2011) 2011 accreditation council for occupational therapy education standards and interpretive guide. http://www.aota.org/Educate/Accredit/Draft-Standards/50146.aspx?FT=.pdf. Accessed 9 July 2013
ADVANCE for Occupational Therapy Practitioners (2011) Social justice: to be or not to be? AOTA members debate one of the hottest issues expected to come before the 2011 Represen-

tative Assembly. Adv Occup Ther Pract 27(7):8. http://occupational-therapy.advanceweb.com/Archives/Article-Archives/Social-Justice-To-Be-or-Not-to-Be-2.aspx. Accessed 9 July 2013

Albrecht GL (1992) The *disability business*: rehabilitation in America. Sage, Newbury Park

American Occupational Therapy Association (2008) Occupational therapy practice framework: domain and process (2nd ed.). Am J Occup Ther 62(6):625–683

Amin S (1977) Imperialism and unequal development. Monthly Review Press, New York

Beagan B (2007) Experiences of social class: learning from occupational therapy students. Can J Occup Ther 74(2):125–133

Block P, Ricafrente-Biazon M, Russo A, Chu KY, Sud S, Koerner L, Vittoria K, Landgrover A, Olowu T (2005) Introducing disability studies to occupational therapy students. Am J Occup Ther 59(5):554–560

Boyce W, Lysack C (2000) Community participation: uncovering its meaning in CBR. In: Thomas M, Thomas MJ (eds) Selected readings in community-based rehabilitation, CBR in translation (series 1). Asia Pacific Disability Rehabilitation Journal, Bangalore, pp 42–58

Braveman B, Bass-Haugen JD (2009) Social justice and health disparities: an evolving discourse in occupational therapy research and intervention. Am J Occup Ther 63(1):7–12

Brown M (2010) Participation: the insider's perspective. Arch Phys Med Rehabil 91(9 suppl. 1):S34–S37

Brown EJ (2011) 'Social justice' stays in ethics code. Adv Occup Ther Pract 27(9):7. http://occupational-therapy.advanceweb.com/Archives/Article-Archives/Social-Justice-Stays-in-Ethics-Code.aspx0. Accessed 9 July 2013

Burton Blatt Institute (2011) Disability and economics: the nexus between disability, education, and employment. Briefing seminar series. Department of Economic and Social Affairs, United Nations, New York. http://www.un.org/disabilities/docu,ents/events/1July2011_economics_panel_nexus.pdf. Accessed 9 July 2013

Centers for Disease Control and Prevention (2011) Cost as a barrier to care for people with disabilities: a tip sheet for public health professionals. http://www.cdc.gov/ncbddd/documents/Cost_barrier%20Tip%20sheet%20%20_PHPa_1.pdf. Accessed 10 Sept 2012

Chicago Tribune (2011, October 9). Occupational therapy: making sense of the Wall Street protests. http://articles.chicagotribune.com/2011-10-09/news/ct-edit-occupy-20111009_1_protests-occupational-therapy-financial-crisis. Accessed 1 Sept 2012

Cottrell RPF (2005) The Olmstead decision: landmark opportunity or platform for rhetoric? Our collective responsibility for full community participation. Am J Occup Ther 59(5):561–568

Dauphenee B (2011, November 19) N.S. Movement requires a little occupational therapy. The Chronicle Herald. http://thechronicleherald.ca/opinion/34456-ns-movement-requires-little-occupational-therapy. Accessed 1 Sept 2012

Denzin NK (2009) The elephant in the living room: or extending the conversation about the politics of evidence. Qual Res 9(2):139–160

Dhaliwal A (1996) Can the subaltern vote? Radical democracy, discourses of representation and rights, and questions of race. In: Trend D (ed) Radical democracy: identity, citizenship, and the state. New York, Routledge, pp 442–461

Dhillon SK, Wilkins S, Law MC, Stewart DA, Tremblay M (2010) Advocacy in occupational therapy: exploring clinicians' reasons and experiences of advocacy. Can J Occup Ther 7(4):241–248

Dijkers MP (2010) Issues in the conceptualization and measurement of participation: an overview. Arch Phys Med Rehabil 91(9 suppl. 1):S5–S16

Disabled World News (2011, July 27) Figures facts and statistics relating to disability in America today supplied by the U.S. Census Bureau. http://www.disabled-world.com/disability/statistics/census-figures.php#ixzz25Z6VzlHT. Accessed 15 Sept 2012

Eisenstein Z (1998) Global obscenities: patriarchy, capitalism, and the lure of cyberfantasy. New York University Press, New York

Erevelles N (2002) (Im)material citizens: cognitive disability, race and the politics of citizenship. Disabil Cult Educ 1(1):5–25

Erevelles N (2011) Disability and difference in global contexts: enabling a transformative body politic. Palgrave Macmillan, New York

Farmer PE, Nizeye B, Stulac S, Keshavjee S (2006) Structural violence and clinical medicine. PloS Med 3(10):e449. 1686–1691. doi:10.1371/journal.pmed.0030449

Frank G, Zemke R (2009) Occupational therapy foundations for political engagement and social transformation. In: Pollard N, Sakellariou D, Kronenberg F (eds) A political practice of occupational therapy. Elsevier, New York, pp 111–136

Frank G, Block P, Zemke R (2008) Introduction to special theme issue anthropology, occupational therapy, disability studies: collaborations and prospects. Pract Anthropol 30(3):2–5

Fujiura GT, Yamaki K (2000) Trends in demography of childhood poverty and disability. Except Child 66(2):187–199

Galheigo SM, Oliver FC, Ferreira TG, Aoki M (2012) People with disabilities and participation: experiences and challenges of an occupational therapy practice in the city of Sao Paulo, brazil. In: Pollard N, Sakellariou D (eds) Politics of occupation-centered practice. Reflections on occupational engagement across cultures. Wiley-Blackwell, Chichester, pp 128–145

Gossett Zakrajsek A, Mirza M, Chan N, Wilson T, Karner M, Hammel J (2014) Supporting institution-to-community transitions for people with psychiatric disabilities: findings and implications from a participatory action research project. Disability Studies Quarterly 34(4)

Grady A (1995) 1994 Eleanor Clarke Slagle lecture—building inclusive communities: a challenge for occupational therapy. Am J Occup Ther 49(4):300–310

Hammel J, Magasi S, Heinemann A, Whiteneck G, Bogner J, Rodriguez E (2008) What does participation mean? An insider perspective from people with disabilities. Disabil Rehabil 30(19):1445–1460

Heinemann AW (2010) Measurement of participation in rehabilitation research. Arch Phys Med Rehabil 91(9 suppl. 1):S1–S4

Heinemann AW, Tulsky D, Dijkers M, Brown M, Magasi S, Gordon W, DeMark H (2010) Issues in participation measurement in research and clinical applications. Arch Phys Med Rehabil 91(9 suppl. 1):S72–S76

Heinemann AW, Coster W, Hammel J (2011) Measuring environmental factors that influence community participation. Paper presented at 2011 NARRTC (National Association of Rehabilitation Research and Training Centers) annual conference, Bethesda, MD, 27–28 April 2011. http://www.ric.org/app/files/public/1663/pdf-NARRTC-Heinemann-Coster-Hammel-25-Apr-2011.pdf. Accessed 9 July 2013

Hemmingsson H, Jonsson H (2005) An occupational perspective on the concept of participation in the international classification of functioning, disability and health—some critical remarks. Am J Occup Ther 59(5):569–576

Inayatullah S (2007) Alternative futures of occupational therapy and therapists. J Futur Stud 11(4):41–58

Kasnitz D, Block P (2012) Participation, time, effort and speech disability justice. In: Pollard N, Sakellariou D (eds) Politics of occupation-centered practice. Reflections on occupational engagement across cultures. Wiley-Blackwell, Chichester, pp 197–216

Kelly C (2010) Wrestling with group identity: disability activism and direct funding. Disabil Stud Q 30(3/4). http://www.dsq-sds.org/article/view/1279. Accessed 21 Sept 2012

Kessler Foundation and National Organization on Disability (2010) Survey of Americans with disabilities. http://www.2010disabilitysurveys.org/pdfs/surveyresults.pdf. Accessed 17 Sept 2012

Kornblau B (2013) Policy implications at the intersection of race, ethnicity. and disability: where are we & where can we go? Paper presented at health disparities research at the intersection of race, ethnicity, and disability: a national conference, Washington, DC, 25–26 April 2013. http://www.ohsu.edu/xd/research/centers-institutes/institute-on-development-and-disability/public-health-programs/project-intersect/upload/BKornblau.pdf. Accessed 10 July 2013

Kronenberg F, Pollard N (2006) Political dimensions of occupation and the roles of occupational therapy. Am J Occup Ther 60(6):617–626

Magasi S, Reis JP, Martin M, Wilson T (2013) "There ain't no care in it!" – an examination of medicaid beneficiaries with disabilities' healthcare experiences. Paper presented at the second OT summit of scholars, Chicago, IL, 10–11 May 2013

Maskos R, Siebert B (2006) Self-determination: the other side of the coin: reflections on a central but ambiguous term of the German Disability Rights Movement. Disabil Stud Q 26(2). http://dsq-sds.org/article/view/693/870. Accessed 17 Sept 2012

Mattingly C (1998) Healing dramas and clinical plots: the narrative structure of experience. Cambridge University Press, Cambridge

Milevska S (2011) Solidarity and intersectionality: what can transnational feminist theory learn from regional feminist activism. In: Feminist review conference proceedings, e52–e61. http://www.palgrave-journals.com/fr/conf-proceedings/n1s/full/fr201129a.html Accessed 25 July 2014

Milner P, Kelly B (2009) Community participation and inclusion: people with disabilities defining their place. Disabil Soc 24(1):47–62

Minkler M, Hammel J, Gill C, Magasi S, Breckwich Vásquez V, Bristo M, Coleman D (2008) Community-based participatory research in disability and long-term are policy: a case study. J Disabil Pol Stud 19(2):114–126

Mirza M, Hammel J (2011) Crossing borders, pushing boundaries: disabled refugees' experiences of community and community participation in the US. Res Soc Sci Disabil Spec Issue Disabil Commun 6:157–186

Mirza M, Anandan N, Hammel J, Madnick F (2006) A participatory program evaluation of a systems change program to improve access to information technology by people with disabilities. Disabil Rehabil 28(19):1185–1199

Mirza M, Luna R, Mathews B, Hasnain R, Hebert E, Niebauer A, Mishra UD (2014) Barriers to healthcare access among refugees with disabilities and chronic health conditions resettled in the US Midwest. J Immigr Minor Health 16:733–742

Mohanty CT (2003) Feminism without borders. Duke University Press, Durham

Morse JM (2006) The politics of evidence. Qual Health Res 16(3):395–404

National Council on Disability (2011) National disability policy: a progress report – October 2011, Washington DC. http://www.ncd.gov/progress_reports/Oct312011. Accessed 25 July 2014

Ojibwa (2011, November 13) The Chemawa Indian school. Native American Netroots: a forum for American Indian issues. http://www.nativeamericannetroots.net/diary/1171/the-chemawa-indian-school. Accessed 9 July 2013

Parish SL (2008) Material hardship in U.S. families raising children with disabilities. Except Child 75(1):71–92

Paul-Ward A (2009) Social and occupational justice barriers in the transition from foster care to independent adulthood. Am J Occup Ther 63(1):81–88

Reed K, Hemphill B, Ashe AM, Brandt LC, Estes J, Foster LJ, Homenro DF, Jackson CR (2010) Occupational therapy code of ethics and ethics standards. Am J Occup Ther 64(6 Suppl.):S17–S26

Russell M (2000, January/February) Stuck at the nursing home door: organized labor can't seem to get beyond the institutional model. Ragged Edge Magazine. http://www.raggededgemagazine.com/0100/a0100ft1.htm. Accessed 11 Sept 2012

Shirk C (2006) Rebalancing long-term care: the role of the medicaid HCBS waiver program (trans: N. H. P. Forum). The George Washington University, Washington, DC

Sinai Health System & Advocate Health Care (2004) Improving access to health and mental health for Chicago's deaf community: a survey of deaf adults. Final survey report. The Urban Institute, Chicago. http://www.healthtrust.net/sites/default/files/publications/improvingaccess.pdf. Accessed 25 July 2014

Smith P, Routel C (2010) Transition failure: the cultural bias of self-determination and the journey to adulthood for people with disabilities. Disabil Stud Q 30(1). http://dsq-sds.org/article/view/1012/1224. Accessed 1 Sept 2012

Spurr B (2011, October 13–20). Occupational therapy: occupy T.O. movement struggles to squeeze consensus out of confusion. NOW Mag 31(7). http://www.nowtoronto.com/news/story.cfm? content=183157. Accessed 1 Sept 2012

Suarez-Balcazar Y, Hammel J, Mayo L, Inwald S, Sen S (2013) Innovation in global collaborations: from student placement to mutually beneficial exchanges. Occup Ther Int 20:97–104

Surpin J (2012, March 27) Occupational therapy. Occidental Weekly. http://occidentalweekly.com/uncategorized/2012/03/27/occupational-therapybr/. Accessed 1 Sept 2012.

Taylor S (2004, March) The right not to work: power and disability. Mon Rev 55(10). http://monthlyreview.org/2004/03/01/the-right-not-to-work-power-and-disability. Accessed 15 Sept 2012

Thibeault R (2002) In praise of dissidence: Anne Lang-Étienne 1932–91. Can J Occup Ther 69(4):3–10

Thibeault R (2006) Globalization, universities and the future of occupational therapy: dispatches for the majority world. Aust Occup Ther J 53:159–165

Townsend E (1993) Muriel driver lecture: occupational therapy's social vision. Can J Occup Ther 60(4):174–184

Townsend EA, Wilcock AA (2004) Occupational justice and client-centered practice: a dialogue in progress. Can J Occup Ther 71(2):75–87

Townsend E, Galipeault JP, Gliddon K, Little S, Moore C, Klein BS (2003) Reflections on power and justice in enabling occupation. Can J Occup Ther 70(2):74–87

U.S. Department of Housing and Urban Development (2009) The 2008 annual homeless assessment report. Office of Community Planning and Development, U.S. Department of Housing and Urban Development, Washington, DC

Wang, Q. (2005). Disability and American families (2000) Census 2000 special reports. United States Census Bureau, Washington, DC

Watts IE, Erevelles N (2004) These deadly times: reconceptualizing school violence by using critical race theory and disability studies. Am Educ Res J 41(2):271–299

Wendell S (1996) The rejected body. Routledge, New York

Wheeler B (2013) Project intersect focus groups preliminary findings. Paper presented at health disparities research at the intersection of race, ethnicity, and disability: a national conference, Washington, DC, 25–26 April 2013. http://www.ohsu.edu/xd/research/centers-institutes/institute-on-development-and-disability/public-health-programs/project-intersect/project-intersect-conference.cfm. Accessed 9 July 2013

World Federation of Occupational Therapists (2004) Position paper on community-based rehabilitation. http://www.wfot.org/ResourceCentre.aspx#. Accessed 15 Sept 2012

World Health Organization (2001) International classification of functioning, disability and health (ICF), Geneva. http://www.who.int/classifications/icf/en/. Accessed 25 July 2014

Yee S (2013) Health disparities for people with disabilities. Paper presented at health disparities research at the intersection of race, ethnicity, and disability: a national conference, Washington, DC, 25–26 April 2013. http://www.ohsu.edu/xd/research/centers-institutes/institute-on-development-and-disability/public-health-programs/project-intersect/project-intersect-conference.cfm. Accessed 9 July 2013

Refusing to Go Away: The Ida Benderson Seniors Action Group

12

Denise M. Nepveux

Occupying means refusing to go away.
—Dana Spiotta, 2012

Abstract
This chapter draws upon critical gerontology, urban studies, and occupational justice to analyze rhetoric and activism surrounding the closure of a popular senior center in downtown Syracuse, New York. In a context of downtown gentrification and entrepreneurial governance, city administration employed logics of ageism and austerity to justify the closure. Although elder participants could not block the closure, they steadfastly refused to permit pejorative framings of their largely low-income elder community as passive, frail and burdensome. They used street theater and marches to resist their invisibility. They formed an action group and persisted in maintaining community ties and a presence in the city while pursuing their long-term vision of an accessible, centrally located, and senior-controlled community center.

Keywords
Senior center • Community • City • Older adults • Gentrification • Activism • Protest • Austerity • Procedural justice

D.M. Nepveux (✉)
Program in Occupational Therapy, School of Health Professions and Education, Utica College, Utica, NY, USA
e-mail: dmnepveu@utica.edu

© Springer Science+Business Media Dordrecht 2016
P. Block et al. (eds.), *Occupying Disability: Critical Approaches to Community, Justice, and Decolonizing Disability*, DOI 10.1007/978-94-017-9984-3_12

12.1 Introduction

The Ida Benderson Senior Citizens Center closed its doors on September 30, 2011. It had been a well-attended place of leisure and socializing in downtown Syracuse, New York since 1975, serving lunches daily to dozens of older city residents. Popular among low-income elders and those who used public transportation, it was perhaps "the most integrated place" in this racially and economically divided city (Lloyd September 28, 2011, quoting Howie Hawkins). Its participants represented a wide spectrum in terms of age, education level, housing status, disability status, family status, neighborhood of residence, and even gender expression. Word of its impending closure mobilized to action residents who rarely have had a visible presence or voice in city affairs.

In this chapter, I draw upon critical gerontology (Holstein and Minkler 2003; Katz 2000; Martinson and Minkler 2006; Minkler and Estes 1991; Phillipson 2011), urban studies (Hall and Hubbard 1996; Lepofsky and Fraser 2003; Attoh 2011) and occupational justice (Kronenberg and Pollard 2005; Stadnyk 2008) to interrogate the rhetoric, activism and organizing that surrounded the Center's closure and to reflect upon their implications for city governance and urban citizenship with respect to low income elder residents. I do not write from a distant or disinterested position, but as a scholar-activist who helped organize older city residents in resisting the Center's closure and who has participated in activism, arts production and community projects with the Ida Benderson Seniors Action Group on a weekly basis since October, 2011.[1] Rather than objectivity, I strive for transparency, veracity and rigor in my observations and analysis. My methods are performance ethnography and discourse analysis.[2] Before I proceed to describe events and analyze rhetoric surrounding the closure of the Ida Benderson Center, I introduce three crucial and interrelated contextual aspects.

---

[1] I learned of the Ida Benderson Center in August, 2011, when I read in the Syracuse Post-Standard (Knauss August 19, 2011a) that the center was threatened with closure. I attended a pair of lively hearings at City Hall and then collaborated with Syracuse University Assistant Professor of Religion Vincent Lloyd to assist senior participants in getting their voices heard by decision makers and the media. I have met weekly with the Ida Benderson Seniors Action Group (IBSAG) since the Center closed. Using transcripts I made from Syracuse Common Council Hearings of September 2011, I wrote the original text and music of a musical melodrama, the *Ida Benderson Blues*, in order to dramatize, preserve, and mobilize discussion around this and similar issues affecting elders. Members of IBSAG reviewed and revised the text. Tim Eatman assisted the group in revising the melody and Susan Schoonmaker arranged the piece. A local political musical theater troupe, D.R.E.A.M. Freedom Revival, worked with the Action Group to arrange this piece for band, choir, and soloists and to stage a free performance and community dialogue featuring Action Group members entitled "Snow on the Rooftop, Fire in the Furnace" in Syracuse in February 16, 2013 (Caceres February 20, 2013).

[2] Performance ethnography uses intensive participant observation and other participatory methods to generate artistic representations of lived experience in context. Discourse analysis is a research tradition that seeks to uncover how power functions in a given setting by deconstructing speech and other forms of expression.

12.2   Globalization, Entrepreneurial Cities, and Urban Aging

City governments today must address the realities that their "economic fortunes are increasingly tied to global economic trends" (Hall and Hubbard 1996, p. 159; also see Hyra 2012; Lepofsky and Fraser 2003, p. 128). This is due both to federal government devolution and globalization. Although globalization of capital and communications transformed some major cities into "world" cities, many formerly prosperous industrial cities such as Syracuse, New York experienced significant economic downturns, layoffs, and decades of insecurity as industrial sectors moved overseas. Thousands of Syracuse residents were laid off from industrial jobs in the 1970s and 1980s as long-established manufacturing operations of Carrier, General Electric, General Motors and Chrysler moved out of state or overseas. Between 1950 and 2000, the city gradually lost 36 % of its population, largely to surrounding suburbs (Spirou 2011, p. 185). Once a thriving industrial city, Syracuse is now an economically struggling center of regional governance, civil society and service industries. As discussed below, it is seeking to reimagine and revitalize itself in ways that respond to these economic and demographic changes.

Globalization has been characterized by rising inequality within and between nations and within cities. Like other postindustrial upstate New York cities such as Rochester, Utica and Buffalo, Syracuse is now a racially, ethnically and economically diverse but deeply segregated city surrounded by largely white and middle class suburbs. Although the financial services, advanced manufacturing, and higher education sectors offer some mid-level and elite salaried jobs, the local service and tourism economy emphasizes casualization of labor and minimum-wage service jobs.

Phillipson (2011) suggests that effects of globalization and deindustrialization have "fragmented and distorted the experience of community and place for older people and other social groups" (p. 283) in cities such as Syracuse. Indeed, most elders in Syracuse were at the heights of their working careers (i.e., 30s 40s or 50s) at the time of massive industrial lay-offs. They have thus witnessed, and in many cases directly experienced deep changes in Syracuse generally and their own neighborhoods. Because of their (or their spouse's) abridged working life, many—particularly women—are left without significant pensions or Social Security benefits. In this context, governmental devolution of social services and social welfare (Lepofsky and Fraser 2003, pp. 129–130) creates precarity among large numbers of lower income elders in Syracuse.

Older people who live in urban neighborhoods segregated by age and class suffer disproportionate effects of economic insecurity and geographic inequality that are heightened under globalization. While old age is often stereotyped as a period of "inevitable spatial withdrawal" (Rowles 1978, cited in Phillipson 2011), much evidence points to the strong influence of environmental conditions that restrict the mobility and well-being of urban elders, particularly those who live on limited incomes, in deteriorating and neglected neighborhoods, and those with disabilities. Mobility restrictions are imposed by inaccessible housing, fear of crime and limited public transportation. Other effects on seniors of neighborhood conditions include mental health problems and decreased social and practical support as neighbors and family members move away seeking work and the neighborhood fabric of trust wears thin (Klinenberg 2002, cited in Phillipson 2011, pp. 285–286).

Cities' efforts to respond to globalization's opportunities and pressures occur in both political-economic and symbolic spheres. Researchers in urban studies have noted that cities are reimagined as economic "growth machines" (Lepofsky and Fraser 2003, p. 157) and mayors as creative, entrepreneurial minds behind these machines. Mayors and their administrations track both federal government programs and global business and communication trends for relevant threats and opportunities. Further, they engage in creative rebranding of their cities in an effort to attract people and investment.

Syracuse has engaged in "place marketing" (Hall and Hubbard 1996, p. 150)— an effort to redevelop and reimage the city as a center of consumerism, culture and entertainment in order to attract prospective residents, tourists and businesses (Spirou 2011). This first was manifested in the redevelopment of an industrial area north of downtown into Carousel Mall, now known as Destiny. The Destiny development has been strongly criticized locally as a "sweetheart deal" favoring the developer over the interests of the city, offering insecure and low-waged jobs, and bringing little benefit overall to the local economy. More recent, and ongoing, is the revival of several sections of the downtown business district into shopping and entertainment districts featuring commercial storefronts with market-rate rental housing above the street level. These private developments are subsidized by federal historical preservation funds as well as multi-year property tax break deals with the city of Syracuse. They actively court young urban professionals and "empty nesters" as prospective residents and consumers.

As contemporary cities strive to reinvent themselves for economies of consumption rather than production, questions arise from an occupational justice perspective as to whether new development processes and outcomes promote inclusion, equity and empowerment for all, or whether they further inequality and entrench poverty for some groups. We may ask: to what extent do these processes of urban revitalization and rebranding result in social exclusion for elders, particularly low-income elders? (Phillipson 2011, p. 285)

Other key points of contestation involve the purpose and focus of city governance, the meaning and purpose of cities themselves, and the question of "the right to the city" (Attoh 2011): who has the right to participate in shaping the city?

Older people are often virtually absent from, or not taken seriously within decision-making processes about city revitalization. Elders may be cast solely as "victims" of change rather than as citizens with input rights or agents of change (Phillipson 2011, p. 288, citing Riseborough and Sribjilanin 2000). Thus one may ask: to what extent are elders included as a constituency in decision-making; and when they are, which sub-groups of elders have a voice?

12.3 False Positive: Disability Shaming and Neoliberal 'Responsibilization'

In addition to recognizing the political economic context in which cities emphasize attracting residents and investment capital over deliberative justice, it is important to understand ideological trends currently shaping aging policy and programs, how they intersect with globalization and neoliberal governance, and how they foster marginalization of certain elders.

In an effort to counteract the portrayal of old age as a time of decline and withdrawal from life roles and activities, gerontologists over the past several decades have introduced new frameworks that promote active and participatory living in latter decades of life. These include "successful aging," "positive aging," "productive aging" and "civic engagement." All are both descriptive and prescriptive, in the sense that their lines of research document practices that correlate with health and wellbeing in later life. This work has been influential in popular media, across health and social service professions and in policy.

Critical gerontologists have cautioned that these discourses, when used prescriptively rather than descriptively, carry paradoxical risks. By creating narrow ideals of wellness and productivity that few elders will achieve and fewer will be able to sustain, these frameworks risk reinforcing images of most elders as burdens upon family members and the state (Holstein and Minkler 2003). By doing so, they may heighten, rather than alleviate fears and shame that people experience in relation to aging.[3] For example, Katz (2000) has shown that elders both internalize and resist pressures to be visibly active, recognizing such pressures as intrusions into their autonomy and sense of self-worth. Katz refers to activity regimes imposed on elders as a "managerial" approach to aging, i.e., a form of disciplinary surveillance closely linked to governance.

As taken up in policy, programs and popular media, these discourses thus tend to promote particular behavioral scripts and images that hold individual elders largely, if not solely, responsible for how they have aged, and how they will now live out their years. They tend to disregard the roles of gender, race, working conditions, poverty and other forms of social inequality in the production of

---

[3]Gerontological frameworks are often simplified and essentialized in popular discourse and policy. "Successful aging" is ostensibly intended by its creators simply to describe a set of health practices, such as regular exercise, that stave off ill health and impairment in old age (Holstein and Minkler 2003). But the label "successful aging," and the way in which it is taken up in popular discourse, tends to shame and devalue those of us who do live with disabilities or illnesses. It emphasizes individual effort over societal responsibility to accommodate diverse and aging bodies (Holstein and Minkler 2003). "Productive aging," which honors and seeks to facilitate a wide array of contributions elders make to their families and communities, including self-care and caring for others, tends to be operationalized for research in terms of measurable economic contributions. And "civic engagement," which originators of the term define broadly to include voting, neighborhood participation, mutually supportive relationships, and activism, is commonly operationalized in research only as formal volunteerism (Martinson and Minkler 2006).

health and disability (Thomas 1999). Further by favoring the healthy, vigorous, and economically productive, they risk deepening existing social hierarchies among and toward elders.

Such discourses also place little weight on the intrinsic worth, dignity and individual experience of aging. In doing so, they risk devaluing and neglecting to support many elders, including those who live with chronic conditions, those who contribute primarily to their families and friends, those who rely upon supportive services for their survival and well-being, and those nearing the end of life.

Discourses of positive, active, productive, and engaged aging, and programs and policies inspired by them, thus participate in what Butler and Anathanasiou (2013) describe as the neoliberal governance process of "responsibilization": in a context of a postindustrial service economy and a declining state role in social welfare and community infrastructure, elders are not only made responsible their own health, but must also fill in growing gaps of service and support for their communities and nation. As "productive aging" and "civic engagement" rise to prominence over earlier discourses, it is likely that those elders who prefer relatively passive recreation and socializing will be seen as less than contributing citizens and thus unworthy of either voice in decision making or investments in their wellbeing.

12.4   Elder Activism

Few studies of grassroots, issue-based elder activism have been published. Martinson and Minkler (2006) cite several examples of senior activism at the national level, such as the Grey Panthers and Older Women's League. In several recent instances, elders have initiated or joined in activism at the local level to contest service cuts. Older adults in New York City organized in 2011–2012 to successfully resist the closure of dozens of senior centers. The Jane Addams Senior Caucus in Chicago has collaborated on several campaigns with disability activists and with Occupy Chicago activists. They have taken up cross-cutting matters of rights and freedoms for disabled people and elders and thus resisted neoliberal measures of human value. Such actions unapologetically confront ideals of "successful," nondisabled and independent elders who rely only upon their personal resources for survival and wellbeing.

It bears noting that elder activism differs markedly from the image broadly promoted of elder civic engagement, which as noted above, tends to be operationalized as volunteerism that supports established organizations and institutions (Martinson and Minkler 2006). Rather than simply filling the lacunae left by government retrenchment, elder activists in New York City, San Francisco, and Chicago, have called attention to ill effects of austerity upon marginalized groups in the community.

What follows illustrates another example of elder activism that resists compliance with neoliberal activity regimes, but expresses a demand for dignity and the right to participate in city life and decisions affecting one's community. In the following sections, I recount events leading up to the closure of the Ida Benderson

Center, and interrogate the ways in which the slated closure was framed and understood by different parties. Each of these sections opens with a stanza from the *Ida Benderson Blues*, a brief operatic piece I co-created and performed with the Action Group and other community artists to memorialize and retell the debate around the closure and the resistance enacted by Center participants.

12.5 The Ida Benderson Senior Citizens Center

It's been our home, our family,
and we have all we need
because we meet each other's needs.
Together we are strong and free.
                    —From The Ida Benderson Blues

"See you at Ida," was once a common farewell on the sidewalks of downtown Syracuse. The Center gave elders a centrally located, easily accessible and free daytime space in which to socialize and meet new friends. Like other senior centers across the United States, the Ida Benderson Center utilized a community center model. City residents above age 60 were free to participate on a drop-in basis. Its modest storefront space included several distinct areas: a kitchen, a billiard room with three tables; a computer nook; a general area with a number of eight-seat and four-seat tables and a piano. The Center was city-funded at about $300,000 per year, largely through Federal Community Development Block Grants. Meals were provided by Catholic Charities through a federal contract administered by Onondaga County. City parks employees managed the Center. Older adults, paid minimum wage through the federal Experience Works program, served meals and staffed the shop and front desk (Jackson June 7, 2010).

One key to the Ida Benderson Center's popularity was its location at the city's Common Center, just north of the Fayette and Salina intersection where buses from all corners of Greater Syracuse dropped off passengers. From this home base, elders could venture out to stroll or to visit downtown shops, the post office, and other services. On warm afternoons, a few participants would gather on the sidewalk bench in front of the Center to smoke, converse, and observe street life. The Center's neighbors on the block included a deli, a family owned jewelry store, and a donut shop to the south, and a gym and a comedy club to the north. Above the Center's storefront space was commercial space including a Merrill Lynch office. Across the street stood Perseverance Park, essentially a landscaped seating area, which later became the site of Occupy Syracuse (Ramsey-Lefevre and Kuebrich 2011; Hannigan 2012). Just south of Perseverance Park stood the city bus terminal, a roofed waiting area with benches along South Salina Street. Behind the bus terminal towered the Chase Bank building.

Another key to the Center's popularity was its diverse, tight-knit community (Jackson, June 7, 2010). Participants at the Center largely—although not solely—occupied "the lower rungs on the socioeconomic scale" (Patrick Hogan, quoted in Knauss August 19, 2011a). Two other city-sponsored senior centers in Syracuse were located in city park clubhouses difficult to reach by bus. Unlike the Ida Benderson Center, these centers attracted predominately white participants who either lived in nearby senior buildings or owned cars and could drive themselves. The Ida Benderson Center was frequented by large numbers of African American "regulars," particularly those from the Near West and South Sides of the city, as well as people of diverse ethnicities and national origins, largely from the North Side. Regular attendees included one transgendered participant, a number of deaf elders, and several insecurely housed or homeless elders. Many participants needed housing assistance or other social service supports, and staff considered social service advocacy to be part of their jobs (Jackson June 7, 2010). Long-time participants recalled that Ida Benderson had advocated for the Center to be located at the Common Center in order to be accessible to all, including impoverished city residents. Former staff recalled that, despite her elevated social station, Benderson readily danced with everyone at occasions, regardless of their gender, dress, or degree of cleanliness or grooming.

As is evident from photo documentation in the Syracuse Post-Standard, the Ida Benderson Center's heyday occurred under the Driscoll Administration (2001– 2009), when an ambitious director, the late Deborah "Debbie" Bova, solicited volunteers, grants and in-kind donations to supplement city allocations. Participants happily remember outings, holiday dinners, and dance parties of this era. Such events were memorialized in large murals in the Center. By the time of its closure under the Miner administration in 2011, however, the Ida Benderson Center offered few scheduled activities beyond the meals it served and occasional outings. Still, it remained popular, attracting dozens of regulars daily for lunch, leisure activities and socializing. A number of people told me stories of how losses of home (e.g., via a fire) or the death of a spouse precipitated their visiting the center for the first time. They found support there, established friendships and had oppertunities to help others as well.

12.6   Desperate Times, Prudent Measures: The City Administration Perspective

These are trying times.
Cities have to count our dimes.
We find we must collaborate
in order to increase (not to cut!) your services.
Outsourcing is what we need.
—From The Ida Benderson Blues

Although rumors circulated among regulars prior to the announcement, some first became aware of the City's plan to close the Center when Parks Commissioner Baye Muhammad visited on August 18, 2011 (Knauss August 19, 2011a). He announced to those present the city's plan to partner with the local Salvation Army. The Salvation Army, he said, intended to expand its Adult Day Care Program in order to substitute for and improve upon the Ida Benderson Center's offerings. This location, he added, would be closing soon, but the Ida Benderson Center (including the name) would continue at the Salvation Army site.

About 50 Center participants, along with staff and some family members, filled half the Council chambers at a Common Council Parks and Recreation Committee meeting on September 6, 2011. Muhammad clarified that his department was requesting $120,000 over two fiscal years to support the integration of the Ida Benderson Center's 300 registered participants into the Salvation Army's Day Program. Funds would go directly to the Salvation Army. After two years, the city would cease involvement in this program. Muhammad emphasized that in these "trying times," with further cuts anticipated in Federal Community Development Block Grants to cities, partnership and collaboration with the private sector were the only avenues to improving city services. As he responded to pointed questions from Councilors, Muhammad repeatedly redirected them from the language of "closing" the Center or "cutting" a valued program, asserting instead that the city's proposed engagement with the Salvation Army represented a promising public-private partnership. "We're not closing the center," Muhammad insisted, "we're just shifting it down the street," (Shepperd September 15, 2011).

The Center, he said, occupied rented space, and was simply too costly to maintain at that location. Foreseeing the approaching end of an overpriced ten year lease agreement, the City had prudently entered discussions a year earlier with the Salvation Army. The City saw the Salvation Army's program as duplicating and improving upon the Center's offerings; thus, a consolidation of the programs seemed wise and fiscally responsible.

Mayor Miner later issued a statement affirming that, "[t]he agreement with the Salvation Army provides expanded and better services for our seniors while ultimately saving the city money" (Kenyon September 19, 2011).

12.7 Older Adults Need Care: The Salvation Army Perspective

We seek to increase—not to cut—your services
We've heard that you need nursing care
So come on down the street
All your needs we're sure to meet
We'll assign you your own seat.
                            —From The Ida Benderson Blues

Parks Commissioner Muhammad made a second argument: Parks department workers were not trained to provide medical care for what he described as this "frail population." Ambulance calls to the Center had been frequent, he said. "Six to eight calls per month" was the only data the Miner Administration offered to justify their assessment of medical need. According to Muhammad, the City's partnership with the Salvation Army would enable "better care," with more staff and a registered nurse present at all times, and at a much lower cost.

It went unstated that the "better care" available at a lesser cost from the Salvation Army was possible through a different model and funding structure. Older adult day care programs, which in New York State are licensed as Social Day Programs, differ from senior centers. Whereas senior centers are characterized by free-flowing, voluntary participation on a drop-in basis, Social Day Programs are structured, professionally driven, medical-model programs. These programs charge participants a daily rate, which depending upon an individual assessment of need, may be reimbursable as a community-based long term care benefit under Medicaid and some private medical insurance programs (Nepveux 2011).

The Common Council invited the local Salvation Army (SA) executive director, Linda Wright, to speak at a Council meeting later that week. Center participants filled half the chamber once again. In a brief statement, Wright emphasized the broad range and flexibility of social, recreational and rehabilitative services available at the SA senior program, as well as its ratio of one staff to five clients.[4] Some seniors called out from their seats in the Council chambers that they were not frail and did not need nursing care. When Wright was asked by a Councilor how she would feel in the elders' position, being forced to leave a cherished place behind and given no choice but to join another program, she responded that she believed that the Ida Benderson seniors were an intelligent group, and as such she was hopeful that they would recognize that this move was indeed in their best interests. Speaking with a television reporter following one of the Common Council hearings, Mayoral Chief of Staff Bill Ryan shrugged off the elders' resistance as rigidity and reluctance to accept change, which he said were characteristics of older adults.

12.8 Procedural Injustice: The Common Council Perspective

What is this charade?
Quite a backroom deal you've made
You act without consulting us
Or giving them a voice
And do you think it's fair
And do you even care?
You say they have no choice
And you know what's best for them?
—From The Ida Benderson Blues

In each hearing, several Councilors accused the Administration of having blindsided them, the Center participants, and the community with a decision that clearly had long been in the works. Councilor Nader Maroun derided the hearings as a "charade," in the sense that the Center's closure was already a forgone conclusion (Shepperd September 15, 2011). Although Commissioner Muhammad and Chief of Staff Bill Ryan asserted that Councilors should have noticed line item changes in the FY 2011–2012 budget months earlier, Councilor Patrick Hogan, himself a former

---

[4]Such a ratio is required under New York State Medicaid policies for Social Day Programs; it is not characteristic of senior centers.

Parks and Recreation Commissioner, contested what he framed as a paternalistic and undemocratic approach taken by the City. Why, he and other councilors wondered aloud, should the Salvation Army have been consulted so long before the Council? Why was no needs assessment performed? Why was there no discussion with the Center participants about which options might be palatable to them? Why were no other locations considered? Why no public consultation? Few answers were forthcoming from Muhammad or Ryan, except to reaffirm the appropriateness and inevitability of the closure from a fiscal standpoint.

Hogan had asserted to the Post Standard two weeks earlier that he was "not prepared in these fiscal times to turn our backs on these seniors, who are probably some of the neediest folks we have in the community." He was not alone in this sentiment. Council President Van Robinson, with full backing of the Council, refused to bring the proposed Salvation Army funding initiative to a vote. The Council could not prevent the closure, but they could refuse to fund a program that seemed unlikely to find many former Ida Benderson participants at its doors. Allocating city funds to a Christian nonprofit Social Day Program at the edge of downtown could not mitigate or justify the closure of what for decades had been a public, nonsectarian, drop-in recreation center at the Common Center, or the "heart of Syracuse," named in honor of a Jewish community leader.

12.9   Losing Home, Family, and City: Center Participants' Perspectives

You don't seem to know
What this place has meant to us
It's been our home, our family
And is this how you see fit to treat the elderly?
They're changing the downtown
Rich folks don't want us around
Reminding them of poverty, vulnerability, mortality . . .
—From The Ida Benderson Blues

At each of the hearings, Center participants stepped or rolled to the microphone one by one. Several insisted that the Center had met their needs by simply providing a space in which they had formed a unique community and looked after one another. The words "family" and "home" were invoked several times, as they had been in previous coverage of the Center (Knauss August 19, 2011a; Jackson 2010) and in their letter to the Mayor. Speakers emphasized the freedom and camaraderie of the Center, and feared that they would lose both in the highly structured Salvation Army Day Program. They also spoke of the paid and unpaid work they had enjoyed at the Center, and the sense of contribution this gave them. They spoke of how the Center enabled them to spend time downtown, and thus to remain part of the city that they had helped to build. Other community members testified to the Center's place in the city's history and changing fabric; they suggested that the administration should have sought another location within a downtown full of empty storefronts, rather than eliminating the Center altogether and effectively driving seniors out of the downtown core. Retired Councilor John Murray pointed out the relative thrift of a senior center in its contribution to keeping seniors out of "assisted living, nursing homes or hospitals." Senior Sue Hollister, a North Side resident who traveled by electric scooter, presented a petition she had initiated with 249 signatures to keep the center open. She asserted that "it ain't over until the fat lady sings, and I ain't sung yet."

On the Friday following the second hearing, Vincent Lloyd and Green party candidate Howie Hawkins visited the Center to hear seniors' views and ask what they wished to do. Hollister and other seniors handwrote a letter to the Mayor, requesting that she "come to listen to the Ida Benderson Center family in person" and hear their concerns. Twenty five participants signed the letter.[5] Hollister and a few others delivered it in person to her office that afternoon.[6]

Mayor Miner accepted their invitation and visited the following Tuesday, September 12. Mayoral staff kept the gathered press and a few protesters outside on the sidewalk while Miner circulated, declining to address the group as a whole but instead speaking with seniors one table at a time. This blocked participants' intention to speak with a strong and unified voice. Hollister and others later told me that the Mayor appeared to listen to their concerns but was unyielding in her stance that the "move" to the Salvation Army site was definite. Speaking with the press afterward, Miner asserted: "This is a decision that is going to go forward" (Knauss September 13, 2011b). She emphasized the fiscal necessity, and framed the closure of the first of many painful decisions the city would need to tolerate to prevent bankruptcy.

Not all seniors were convinced by the Mayor's rhetoric of austerity, however. Center participant Mary Lawler, speaking with a reporter (Knauss September 13, 2011b) on the sidewalk after the Mayor's visit, commented "[t]hey have a vision for the city of making this into upper-class apartments . . . That's the basic reason for closing this center, to make preparations for that." Indeed, the closure coincided with development of market-rate housing in a number of nearby buildings and moving the bus hub south, out of the Common Center. From Lawler's perspective, it was gentrification—not the Center's cost, and not medical concerns—that motivated the city's plan.

The protests escalated and broadened after the Mayor's visit. Democrats, Republicans, and Green Party candidates assembled on the sidewalk outside the Center on Friday, September 16 to declare their unity in opposition to the Mayor on this matter. Although this was to be a press conference by candidates and office-holders, seniors claimed turns at the microphone and their comments were aired on the evening news. James Shields, a senior who worked in the kitchen and rode his bicycle to the Center every day, garnered laughter when he quipped, "The Mayor says we are frail.

---

[5]Handwritten letter available at: http://solidaritycny.files.wordpress.com/2011/09/ib-invitation.pdf
[6]Image of the group that delivered the letter: http://solidaritycny.wordpress.com/2011/09/12/mayor-miner-agrees-to-visit-ida-benderson/

Do I look frail?" This comment was characteristic of some other assertions I heard seniors make, asserting that their (claimed) nondisabled status made them not only free of care needs, but significantly different from the population attending the Day Program at the Salvation Army.

Following this event, Center staff members were instructed by the Parks and Recreation Commissioner not to allow community organizers (such as Vincent Lloyd or me), protest-related activities or materials to enter the Center. Prior to this, we had freely interacted with staff and participants both inside and outside on the sidewalk. This made organizing across groups more difficult, as communications had been largely by word of mouth, and through flyers photocopied by organizers. A number of the Center participants had mobile phones, however, and word could also be sent through seniors to others inside the center.

Organizers made sign-making materials available in Perseverance Park across from the Center early on the morning of Monday, September 19th. A few seniors crossed the street to make signs, and a few passers-by also joined in. Later that morning, about 50 disability, peace and labor activists, Center participants, Common Councilors, other local politicians gathered and community members gathered at Plymouth Congregational UCC Church, historically a center of progressive resistance on the south end of downtown. They marched up Salina Street banging pots and pans and chanting slogans opposing the closure. More seniors joined in with handmade signs—some written on pieces of cardboard boxes—when the rally paused in front of the Center around noon. The group continued to the front steps of City Hall, where it rallied with songs and speeches (Kenyon September 19, 2011). Council Chair Van Robinson, an African American who had worked in the Civil Rights Movement, cited continuity with the Civil Rights history and tradition and vowed to see this issue through.

Ten days later, Center participants Sue Hollister, Mary Carr and Virginia Dolin assembled in front of the Center, and before television cameras, to have their heads shaved in a mock barber shop scene (Knauss September 28, 2011c). James Shields wielded the clippers. "They can take my hair, but they can't take my spirit," Hollister said (Donaldson September 29, 2011). Carr commented that they had contemplated a sit-in in the Mayor's office, but felt that their "old bones wouldn't be able to take sitting that long" (ibid). About ten of their peers gathered around the women, holding signs. One poked fun at the Mayor's claim that the impending closure was simply a move: "Miner's Cuts: We don't cut hair, we just relocate it." Another read, "Seniors, are you ready for back-to-the-streets?" Carr led the group in singing and inventing new verses to "This Little Light of Mine" and "We Shall Not Be Moved,[7]" both anthems of empowerment in the Civil Rights Movement.[8]

Instead, it was the Mayor and her administration who remained unmoved. The Center's last day, September 30th, was met with goodbye rituals inside the Center,

---

[7]Video footage available at: http://videos.syracuse.com/post-standard/2011/09/ida_benderson_protest.html
[8]http://folkmusic.about.com/od/toptens/tp/CivilRightsSong.htm

and more protests outside the Center and in front of City Hall. Lois Dwyer, a retired nurse, was the last participant to leave the Center, departing with her rolling walker through the alley doors. Protesters also used chanting, noisemaking and signage to unsettle a late afternoon Mayoral celebration in the glass-enclosed City Hall Commons marking the conclusion of Syracuse's participation in IBM's Smarter Cities Challenge.[9]

12.10 Don't Stop: The Ida Benderson Seniors Action Group

> *When somebody takes something from you, don't stop. Because if we stop, they're gonna keep taking.*
> —Mary Carr, speaking to WAER News

One week after the Center closed, a small group of former Center participants met at Plymouth Church in downtown Syracuse. After meeting every Friday for a few weeks, they named themselves the Ida Benderson Seniors Action Group.

The Ida Benderson "family community," as they called themselves in their letter to the Mayor, had no known (to this writer) history of collective self-advocacy or activism. The center itself had no mechanism for internal democracy, thus had not afforded seniors opportunities to learn self-governance or advocacy. Individuals among them, however, had a wide array of experience and knowledge. One gentleman had worked for a number of years in community organizing and voter education on the city's predominately Black south side. One was an ordained minister. Others—both men and women—had been involved in the civil rights movement, or more recently in groups such as Public Citizen. A number of early participants, including Mary Carr, were African American South Side residents who had experienced not only job loss from deindustrialization, but neighborhood destruction at the hands of government when Highway 81 was built through their neighborhood; these experiences seemed to make these elders more skeptical of the group's prospects in fighting overwhelming power, but also gave them a moral indignation that inspired self-advocacy.

Mary Lawler—a white Catholic nun and former school teacher—explained to a reporter,

All we need money for is a small, warm, comfortable, safe place where we could gather around the table and talk to each other, and listen to each other, and help each other to cope with the struggles that we face as we age . . . We have to start small, but we'll stick together and we'll be a support to one another. (Mary Lawler, quoted in Clark 2011)

---

[9]The IBM Smarter Cities Challenge helps cities use data to "make smarter, more strategic investments in their communities, maximizing value in the long term." Syracuse's participation was concerned with collecting and using data concerning vacant and blighted housing. http://smartercitieschallenge.org/about.html

12.11 Discussion: Ageism, Austerity and Entrepreneurial Governance

In this chapter, I have sought to unpack the rhetorical strategies and tactics of resistance employed by various parties in the weeks leading up to the closure of the Ida Benderson Center and by the Action Group that formed in its wake. Ageism, entrepreneurial governance and fiscal crisis made powerful partners in the rhetoric legitimizing the closing of the Ida Benderson Center. Although privatizing and eventually offloading[10] a heavily utilized senior center constituted a significant cutback of city efforts for elder residents, the Miner administration sought to portray this act as a responsible and beneficent act. In order to convince the public, it called upon ageist stereotypes, the logic of neoliberal austerity, and a vision of managerial governance necessary to the entrepreneurial city. I consider each of these in turn here.

In discussions around the closing, the seniors who attended the Ida Benderson Center were "othered" in multiple ways, in keeping with critiques of discourses of positive aging. These elders, a large number of whom were elders of color, were portrayed as those who had aged unsuccessfully and whose days were spent in unproductive pursuits. They were depicted as incapable of contribution, interdependence, genuine community, or even generating their own fun, but instead as a population of individual service recipients in need of structured activity, professional care, protection and direction. They were described as uniformly rigid, passive and frail. When the SA director asserted that she believed these seniors were "intelligent," this assertion was a thin one, borne of persuasive flattery rather than genuine confidence in seniors' judgment. This fits with what Katz (2000) describes as a managerial approach to elders, in which they should comply with regimes of activity regardless of what the activity itself, the group of people, and the context mean to them. Activity is presented as an inherent good that will stave off dependency, which in this logic entails loss of personhood. Yet elders experience a loss of autonomy when others choose for them.

The administration described Center participants as medically frail and implied that they were unable—implying cognitive decline—to make good decisions for themselves. They were also portrayed as rigid, i.e., arbitrarily resistant to change, even when change was objectively in their best interests. Such portrayals, which are deeply rooted in ageist stereotypes (Gullette 2011), helped to protect the administration from seeming callous in its coercive handling of elders.

---

[10]The Mayor was requesting $60,000 per year for two fiscal years to fund the "transition" to the Salvation Army, after which, financial responsibility for the relocated/consolidated program would be entirely on the Salvation Army. The SA, however, would of course be able to fundraise from private donors or foundations for the program, and also bill the federal government's Medicaid program whenever services to individual participants could be justified as community-based long term care. Presumably over passing years, former Ida Benderson Center participants would develop specific support needs that would justify Medicaid billing.

By portraying elders as not knowing what was best for them, the administration sought to silence or delegitimize elders' claims that closing the center would harm them as individuals and destroy what Center participants described as their newfound "family." The mayor took a paternalistic but arguably compelling stance of having acted responsibly not only for the welfare of Center participants, and also for the fiscal good of the whole city.

Bolstered by the authoritative location of the mayor's office, austerity-based arguments functioned to diminish any claims by elders and allies on the council. As Goodley et al. (2014) point out, the discourse of neoliberal austerity succeeds rhetorically by creating a crisis that justifies sidelining other concerns and principles of democratic governance. It calls upon all citizens—in a way that creates a false equality of effects—to "make do and mend" (Goodley et al. 2014, p. 1). In the Ida Benderson Center closing, concerns regarding procedural and distributive justice, community preservation and human flourishing were made to seem frivolous in light of impending bankruptcy. Yet, in the background remained the mayor's overall policy emphasis on not only averting fiscal disaster but taking bold and innovative steps to foster economic growth (as exemplified in the city's participation in IBM's Smarter Cities initiative), which, in one activist's words, entailed "cleaning up downtown" of bus commuters, loiterers, and elders.

12.12 Seniors Talk Back: Voice, Embodied Activism, and Occupation

In efforts to counteract this powerful trifecta, and—I believe—in expressions of genuine indignation and distress, seniors contested the ways in which they as individuals and their senior center were portrayed. Against a powerful backdrop of ageist and paternal rhetoric, they presented themselves as diverse, assertive, knowledgeable and creative individuals united across race and gender to save their senior center and its community. They did so via written and spoken speech acts, gathering support via a petition and collaboration with other groups, collective visibility at marches, demonstrations and other gatherings on the sidewalk in front of the center, and head shaving: a stark embodied demonstration of elder women's commitment and sense of urgency.

As they were combating ageist stereotypes and paternalistic threats to their autonomy, seniors and their allies also called city administration to moral and civic responsibility. They confronted, on a moral basis, city government retrenchment and entrepreneurial preoccupations at the expense of a vulnerable group. Closing a busy and readily accessible center was irresponsible in a context of scarce and peripherally located recreational offerings for an aging and isolated population.

Finally, elders and allies called out the Miner administration for colluding with business interests to "clean up downtown" of elders and other low-income city residents in an effort to draw young middle class renters downtown and thus to court business and real estate development interests. In doing so, they asserted their dignity and their right to the city. Perhaps they also set an example that other marginalized communities could follow.

12.13 Conclusion: Senior Resistance, Occupation and a Broader Vision

"We are not gone, and we are still looking for a place to go."
–Mary Carr, speaking to WAER News

Thanks in part to a city constitution that empowered the mayor to close city services without Council consent, the prerogatives of downtown gentrification ultimately overwhelmed the efforts of low-income elders and allies to demand procedural justice. Although city administrators framed this act as both fiscally responsible and in these elders' best interests, Center participants maintain that the Mayor misrepresented their needs, steamrolled their resistance and thus failed in her responsibility to them. Closing the center saved the city $120,000 a year for rent and enabled the fitness center next door to expand into part of the former Center space. It also greatly reduced the presence of elders along the sidewalks near the Common Center.

The Ida Benderson seniors did manage to claim a voice in this decision, and to communicate clearly how the closure would affect them. They were denied the opportunity to influence the decision, but the media did respond by airing their views and actions on several occasions in September, 2011. Whenever the Mayor's performance was discussed in the following years, this closure was brought up. Further, in key interviews and debates prior to election 2012, candidates for Common Council were asked their views on the Center's closure. The Center's closure came to be emblematic of either a disciplined Mayor who made the "tough choices" under conditions of austerity, or a city prioritizing business interests and gentrification over the welfare needs of its majority population.

At the time of this writing, market rate apartments continue to be developed and leased along S. Salina and adjacent streets, such that despite rapid growth of housing stock, downtown occupancy remains at 99 % (Delaney February 15, 2012). Federal grants and municipal multi-year tax breaks support investments in downtown properties. The block just south of the Center is a major area of residential and commercial redevelopment. The rented storefront space that the Center had occupied for decades remained empty for two and a half years after the Center was closed, until the fitness center next door expanded in what was interpreted by the press to be "another sign of growth and resurgence in downtown Syracuse" (Web Staff April 9 2014). Another part of the space has recently become occupied by Federal Citizenship and Immigration Services—hardly the lively commercial storefront envisioned by the Downtown Committee and other entities interested in downtown gentrification, but perhaps emblematic of federal government shifts in funding priorities away from urban low-income community programs, which since the Nixon administration were supported by Community Development Block Grants.

Action Group members praise some aspects of downtown growth—particularly prospects for a downtown grocery—but feel pushed aside by what they perceive as its sole focus upon priorities of youth and those who can afford to pay. They now face a downtown with few public restrooms, few places to rest, a bus terminal distant from most of their destinations downtown, and no place to meet up informally as city residents and community members. Members of the Ida Benderson Center community, however dislocated and dispersed, did not allow the mayor's abrupt action to dissolve them entirely. They persist at the time of this writing in the form of an Action Group. As of May 2014, members of this community—not bound by neighborhood of residence but by intentionality and mutual recognition—continue determinedly to gather weekly and to make their presence known at every opportunity. The majority of Center alumni have, understandably, grieved their loss and moved on to socialize in other settings. But a core group has persisted and has come to enjoy and value the group itself. The group has developed ground rules and a shared set of rituals. Collective singing has been part of pre-meeting activities. Members bring food to share, open meetings with a social check-in, and close with "appreciations" of each person in attendance. The group functions without a constitution or elected officers, but with flexibly established roles. Decisions are made and meeting agendas are set by consensus. Members strategize about how to keep their community together, raise awareness, and work toward establishing a new senior center downtown. The Action Group has spoken publicly, organized social gatherings and forums, created and performed musical theater and collaborative dance to convey their story and its relevance to Syracuse, and sponsored booths at community fairs that encourage dialogue about the city. They also have created and continue to maintain a perennial flower and herb garden to beautify a busy but neglected corner downtown and thus to concretely demonstrate their ongoing presence and contributions.

The Action group has developed a shared vision of a cooperative community center run by seniors, for seniors. It would continue in the inclusive tradition of Ida Benderson by encouraging diverse participation, "proactive behavior and community-mindedness" (Lisa Bogin, personal communication May 2014). Members would work with other groups and agencies to promote a larger vision for Syracuse than an entrepreneurial city administration and development interests have considered: a positive and unified community identity that pursues equity and embraces and accommodates difference. The group faces many hurdles in achieving this vision, but persisting and refusing to go away are achievements in and of themselves. In the words of Action Group member Dorothy H.,[11] "We were kicked and we're still kickin'."

Editors' Postscript If you enjoyed reading this chapter, we would like to recommend that you also look at Chap. 11 "Soul searching occupations: Critical reflections on Occupational Therapy's Commitment to Social Justice, Disability Rights, and Participation" by Mansha Mirza, Susan Magasi and Joy Hammel. These authors are all occupational therapists who describe how they do collaborative research. Chapter 16 "6: Beyond Policy—A Real Life Journey of Engagement

---

[11]Last name withheld at Dorothy H.'s request.

and Involvement" by Stephanie de la Haye covers some of this ground as does Chap. 17, also by an occupational therapist, Eva Rodrigues "Self Advocacy and Self Determination for Youth with Disability and their Parents during School Transition Planning." These chapters really explore community.

Acknowledgements I would like to express my thanks and appreciation to members of the Ida Benderson Seniors Action Group and its larger community, without whom this work would not be possible. Thanks to Lisa Bogin and Dorothy H. of the Ida Benderson Seniors Action Group and to David Hill for reviewing and offering suggestions on this chapter.

References

Attoh KA (2011) What kind of right is the right to the city? Prog Hum Geogr 35(5):669–685
Butler J, Anathanasiou A (2013) Dispossession: the performative in the political. Polity Press, Cambridge
Caceres N (2013, February 20) Don't close the doors on them just yet. South Side Stand.http://mysouthsidestand.com/events/don%E2%80%99t-close-the-doors-on-them-just-yet/. Accessed 25 July 2014
Clark A (2011, November–December) Ida Benderson and the war economy. Syracuse Peace Council Peace Newsletter 809. Retrieved from http://www.peacecouncil.net/pnl/november-december-2011-pnl-809/ida-benderson-and-the-war-economy. Accessed 25 July 2014
Delaney R (2012, February 15). Walkability, new apartments draw residents to downtown Syracuse. WRVO News. http://wrvo.org/post/walkability-new-apartments-draw-residents-downtown-syracuse. Accessed 25 July 2014
Donaldson T (2011, September 29) Three senior women shave heads in protest. South Side Stand.http://mysouthsidestand.com/voices/three-senior-women-shave-heads-in-protest. Accessed 25 July 2014
Goodley D, Lawthom R, Runswick-Cole K (2014) Dis/ability and austerity: beyond work and slow death. Disabil Soc 29(6):980–984
Gullette M (2011) Agewise: fighting the new ageism in America. University of Chicago Press, Chicago
Hall T, Hubbard P (1996) The entrepreneurial city: new urban politics, new urban geographies? Prog Hum Geogr 20(2):153–174
Hannigan C (2012, September 14). A year later, where's Occupy Syracuse now? The Syracuse Post-Standard. Retrieved from http://www.syracuse.com/news/index.ssf/2012/09/a_year_later_wheres_occupy_syr.html. Accessed 25 July 2014
Holstein MB, Minkler M (2003) Self, society and the "new gerontology". The Gerontologist 43(6):787–796
Hyra DS (2012) Conceptualizing the new urban renewal: comparing the past to the present. Urban Aff Rev 48(4):498–527
Jackson K (2010, June 7) Ida Benderson senior center 'a warm and comfortable place to be." The Constitution/Urban CNY News Online Edition. http://www.urbancny.com/ida-benderson-senior-center-a-warm-comfortable-place-to-be/. Accessed 25 July 2014
Katz S (2000) Busy bodies: activity, aging, and the management of everyday life. J Aging Stud 14(2):135–153
Kenyon J (2011, September 19) Seniors fight for Ida Benderson Senior Center. CNY Central News. http://www.cnycentral.com/news/story.aspx?list=190258&id=664818. Accessed 25 July 2014
Knauss T (2011a, August 19). Strapped for cash, Syracuse plans to close Ida Benderson Senior Center. The Syracuse Post-Standard. http://www.syracuse.com/news/index.ssf/2011/08/strapped_for_cash_syracuse_pla.html. Accessed 25 July 2014

Knauss T (2011b, September 13) Syracuse mayor meets with seniors unhappy about Ida Benderson center's closing. The Syracuse Post-Standard. www.syracuse.com. Accessed 25 July 2014

Knauss T (2011c, September 28) Syracuse seniors shave heads to protest closing of Ida Benderson center. The Syracuse Post-Standard. http://www.syracuse.com/news/index.ssf/2011/09/syracuse_seniors_shave_heads_t.html. Accessed 25 July 2014

Kronenberg F, Pollard N (2005) Introduction: a beginning... In: Kronenberg F, Simo Algado S, Pollard N (eds) Occupational therapy without borders: learning from the spirit of survivors. Elsevier/Churchill Livingstone, Edinburgh, pp 1–13

Lepofsky J, Fraser JC (2003) Building community citizens: claiming the right to place-making in the city. Urban Stud 40(1):127–142

Lloyd V (2011, September 28) Letter to the editor: campus should rally to preserve vital center for elderly. The Daily Orange. http://www.dailyorange.com/2011/09/letter-to-the-editor-campus-should-rally-to-preserve-vital-center-for-elderly/. Accessed 25 July 2014

Martinson M, Minkler M (2006) Civic engagement and older adults: a critical perspective. The Gerontologist 46(3):318–324

Minkler M, Estes CL (1991) Critical perspectives on aging: the political and moral economy of growing old. Baywood, Amityville

Nepveux D (2011, September 28) Include seniors in city's recreation plan. The Syracuse Post-Standard (Syracuse, NY). http://blog.syracuse.com/opinion/2011/09/include_seniors_in_citys_recre.html. Accessed 25 July 2014

Phillipson C (2011) Developing age-friendly communities: new approaches to growing old in urban environments. In: Handbook of sociology of aging. Springer, New York, pp 279–293

Ramsey-Lefevre A, Kuebrich B (2011, November-December) A day in the life of Occupy Syracuse. http://www.peacecouncil.net/pnl/november-december-2011-pnl-809/a-day-in-the-life-of-occupy-syracuse. Accessed 25 July 2014

Shepperd W (2011, September 15) Benderson center: safe! caring! clean! closing? The Eagle CNY News. http://www.theeaglecny.com/news/2011/sep/15/benderson-center-safe-caring-clean-closing/. Accessed 25 July 2014

Spiotta D (2012) Untitled. In: Lang AS, Lang/Levitsky D (eds) Dreaming in public: the building of the occupy movement. World Changing, New York. http://occupywriters.com/works/by-dana-spiotta. Accessed 25 July 2014

Spirou C (2011) Urban tourism and urban change: cities in a global economy. Routledge, London

Stadnyk R (2008) Occupational justice for older adults. In: Coppola S, Elliott SJ, Toto PE (eds) Strategies to advance gerontology excellence: promoting best practice in occupational therapy. American Occupational Therapy Association, Bethesda, pp 445–460

Thomas C (1999) Female forms: experiencing and understanding disability. Open University Press, Buckingham

Web Staff (2014, April 9) Fitness club expands as resurgence of downtown Syracuse grows. Time Warner Cable News. http://centralny.twcnews.com/content/search/723883/fitness-club-expands-as-resurgence-of-downtown-syracuse-grows/#sthash.5fFBp4aO.dpuf. Accessed 25 July 2014

Why Bother Talking? On Having Cerebral Palsy and Speech Impairment: Preserving and Promoting Oral Communication Through Occupational Community and Communities of Practice

13

Rick Stoddart and David Turnbull

Abstract

A technique for facilitating oral communication with a person with speech impairment, based on time spent in communication regarding that person's life story and his everyday activities, is placed within the framework of enabling an occupational community. The goal is to develop ongoing resources for instructing therapists, other health professionals and human service providers, whose communities of practice and agendas of which, are not necessarily congruent with those so engaged.

Keywords

Disability • Speech impairment • Occupational community • Communities of practice • Oral communication • Ethics

13.1 Introduction

My name is Rick and I have a condition named cerebral palsy. People who do not know me may find it hard to understand what I say. However I'm very patient and am always willing to teach.

My name is David and I have a communication disability. My ears are culturally attuned to normal speech. When I first heard Rick speak a few years ago I couldn't understand him. I thought back then, this guy has something he really wants to say. So I went around to his place and Rick taught me how to understand. Now we get together in various locations and teach others to listen and understand. That's what we do together.

R. Stoddart (✉) • D. Turnbull
James Cook University, Queensland, Australia
e-mail: ricki.stoddart7@bigpond.com; davidturnbull4886@gmail.com

© Springer Science+Business Media Dordrecht 2016
P. Block et al. (eds.), *Occupying Disability: Critical Approaches to Community, Justice, and Decolonizing Disability*, DOI 10.1007/978-94-017-9984-3_13

Rick doesn't write much. He has a computer and a keyboard with a perspex cover with holes in it so his fingers can touch one key at a time. That isn't Rick's preferred mode of communication. Rick would rather spend an hour talking than spend that amount of time typing.

David writes a great deal. In this chapter David gets to do the writing. To back up what is written here, we have (are producing) videos in which Rick does quite a bit of talking (see to begin with, http://www.youtube.com/watch?v=BFObghvzVZU). This form of text production has the advantage that people who prefer not to read can get to view it and listen and learn what Rick has to say.

Rick has a large number of life experiences in which he has learned firsthand what it is like to be discriminated against on the basis of his impairments. David only knows about these second hand. The first goal of this chapter is to tell parts of Rick's story. The reason for telling the story is that it enables us to justify our claim that there is an ethical imperative for an engagement in an occupational community and communities of practice in relation to people with speech impairments.

Neither of us are therapists or health workers. Rick has always wanted to be a worker of some sort, but somehow this goal has mostly eluded him. He just wants to do what any other bloke does, have a proper job, do a full day's work, go home and relax. He wants his work to be fulfilling. David has always wanted to be part of a community. Not just any kind of community, but rather a community based on meaningful occupational engagements. David writes, lives in a house he has built for himself, is married and has a family, gardens, does photography and filmmaking with his son Robin, teaches ethics and philosophy. David is unashamedly fulfilled occupationally speaking whereas Rick is not so much so, even though Rick has a place he calls home that shows his fine taste in art, and into which he invites people with pride. Rick lives alone and for the most part the people in his life are human service workers who come and go at regular intervals. Sometimes Rick feels so occupationally deprived and alienated from the wider community it breaks his heart and undermines his will to live.

There is an imbalance between us from the beginning. But this lack of occupational symmetry is somewhat overcome by understanding ourselves as part of each other's community. In a community at least some of what is good for one person gets shared with others. These benefits do not automatically flow unless there are deliberate acts in which they are shared. The reason why Rick and David got together to teach has to do with sharing in the occupation of storytelling. The best stories originate from within someone's lived experience. David has spent many years advocating for people with disability albeit from an outsider perspective. What David lacks is insider experiential knowledge, and he does not have any legitimacy to speak about disability on his own accord. Rick imparts his knowledge to David and Rick also legitimizes every aspect of our mutual engagement through his own participation and enthusiasm. The reason we are writing this chapter and making a video is to invite others into the same sort of sharing that goes on between us.

The video will show clearly how we teach communication. The technique is simple and can be learned in under half an hour in a group setting. It is worth individually practicing the technique with someone in real life as it cuts across conventions that are deeply ingrained into us from childhood. The process involves breaking accepted rules of allowing a speaker to continue uninterrupted, and because it is widely considered 'rude to interrupt', trainees may have to overcome certain internal inhibitions in doing so. Consent from the speaker with the speech impairment must be sought to do so. Interruption is vital, because if a listener misses crucial words and phrases, the whole meaning of a speech act is immediately distorted, with potentially disastrous consequences, for example in a healthcare setting. Interruption by consent presents an opportunity for the listener to repeat back the speaker's speech as it unfolds, and for the speaker to correct it phrase by phrase, or if need be, word by word or letter by letter. Doing this places the listener immediately in a questioner role, and the initial disadvantage of being the listener gives way to the advantage gained by being in a position to readily clarify intended meaning. The emphasis shifts from "have I heard you?" to "have I understood what you are saying?" From the speaker's perspective there is an added advantage of being able to repeat sentences, phrases, words and letters until such time as the listener has understood them, and this provides an opportunity for making an additional emphasis on crucial aspects of the message, or clarifying further and drawing out implications of what has been said initially. The result is enhanced communication and enables greater depth of comprehension between speaker and listener. An exact description of the technique would require an entire book chapter, which is why we have elected to model it by the use of video.

The big goal we have for this chapter is to discuss the ethics of what we are doing. The ethics requires us to give a justification for creating such an emphasis on Rick's bothering to talk, when others would prefer him to adopt another method or have someone else do it for him. Some people point to the advantages of assistive communication technology. Time is short, they say. We do not have the time it takes to understand Rick orally. Some would like to make the use of such technology a condition for Rick engaging with professional people particularly if he has a teaching role. They would also like Rick to have some teaching qualifications of the sort they recognize as valid. Knowledge is what we have, they say. What Rick has is a need for expert supervision.

Challenging these views sets up a requirement for engaging with communities of practice. We use the term 'community of practice' to mean a community in which professional or academic elites are in a position of power and authority. We wish to engage such elites in reflection on the ethics of their practice in relation to other communities. Practitioners are invited into a dialogue about the boundary conditions that exist between their professional lives and the lives of people who do ordinary things in the wider community. We wish to draw a distinction between occupational communities and communities of practice to highlight the power imbalances between someone like Rick and, say, a health services provider.

We also wish to challenge those communities of practice, in advocacy circles, or in community development circles and the like, that insist on drawing a clear cut distinction between disabled and non-disabled people. We wish especially to avoid the notion that there is a disability community to which all people with disability belong. When Rick was asked if he regards himself as disabled he asserted categorically: "Not now, not ever." From his own perspective Rick does not wish to be associated with people with disability. He regards himself as a unique human being with individual desires and goals like anyone else. It follows directly from this that Rick would take offense if he was to be regarded as a disabled research subject in matters of academic research. David has honored this stance by regarding Rick as his colleague in all matters of intellectual inquiry, and does not make any differentiations over matters of formal academic qualification. We each have a unique set of skills to offer, and we have found them to be highly complementary.

13.2   Rick's Story

According to Rick's own account his mother died before he was born and that is how he acquired cerebral palsy. Rick's grandmother was the influence that made a lasting impression on his life. His grandmother brought Rick up entirely on her own without any external assistance. She taught him to put the maximum amount of effort and concentration into everything he did. He never missed a day of school and after he finished school he went on to learn data entry on computers. Rick also learned from his grandmother to stick up for his dignity and rights, and not to let other people's impressions of him dictate terms. In Rick's mind he is mentally normal; he becomes annoyed when people judge him to be less intelligent than he actually is through their superficial impressions.

When Rick's grandmother died, in his early 30s, he went into group home accommodation with a large disability service. This event followed a big disappointment when in 1984 he was asked if he wanted a job with the disability service agency doing what amounted to secretarial work for the social worker. This job did not materialize, even though Rick had moved to a completely different city specifically in order to fill it, and he was relegated to the ranks of helplessly unemployed service recipients. In 1991 he was the first person from that service to go into so called 'independent living,' Whilst Rick was enabled to have occupancy of a dwelling space he could call his own home, he nevertheless experienced what occupational therapists have come to term occupational deprivation (Townsend and Whiteford 2005). Rick has support workers coming into his home three times a day for daily care, who had no further input into his daily activities. Even though occupancy of his own home gave Rick the right to organize and decorate it the way he wanted, his situation was such that he had many hours each day with nothing meaningful to do. Then employment and community development agencies became involved and these had modest degrees of success. For about 5 years he had about 10 h a week doing data entry for a wild life rescue organization, until that paid work finished. A community development agency enabled him to get into various volunteering capacities. Beyond that Rick's time was spent watching television or on the computer performing tasks such as organizing his budget.

Occupational deprivation was only one aspect of the humiliating way Rick was being forced to live. In order to move about Rick is obliged to take wheelchair taxis. He is frequently abused by taxi drivers who make no effort to understand his speech, and accuse him of having no money to pay for the trip. And that is only at the beginning of a journey. When he had to go to the hospital during bouts of sickness, interactions with hospital staff soured his view of the medical system. On one occasion a doctor asked: "why aren't you in a nursing home?" On other occasions nursing staff talked with each other in a demeaning way about him whilst in his earshot. A typical hospital response was to demand that he be accompanied by a carer, even though the service he received had no provision for carers to accompany clients to hospital. Rick formed a personal vision in which he would do something about showing the transport and medical systems a better way to treat people: with respect and dignity.

13.3 Working Together Within Occupational Communities and Communities of Practice

The specific notion of occupational community has not been fully articulated in community development circles, and not even in occupational therapy and occupational science, even though these disciplines acknowledge the life-encompassing community based dimensions of occupation (Christiansen and Townsend 2010; Curtin et al. 2010; Pollard et al. 2010; Townsend and Whiteford 2005; Townsend and Poltajko 2007). The notion of communities of practice is gaining wider currency based on the work of Wenger (1998, 2010; Snyder and Wenger 2010) and Blackmore (2010), utilizing research into organization dynamics and group learning. In this chapter we discuss the conceptual difference between the two types of community and give examples of how they are related. Conceptually, occupational communities are grounded in everyday activities, whereas communities of practice are grounded in professional and organizational roles. The distinction is not absolute, and is only useful when we come to discuss the boundary conditions that occur when people with everyday concerns find themselves confronted with professional and organizational practices and values.

One community development agency worked with Rick looking for opportunities for Rick to have a valued social role (Wolfensberger 1991). The worker helped Rick become a member of a consumer advisory board at the local hospital. The worker evidently thought this fitted the goal of finding Rick a meaningful occupational outlet. For Rick it only meant more frustration sitting in meetings that did not present him a way to address his personal burning issues.

As David's background includes business and life coaching (which he now terms occupational coaching) we together devised a scheme whereby Rick would start up his own communications coaching business. Working together we negotiated paid teaching commitments with the university, conducting communications lectures for therapy and medical students. We also conducted a pilot program for nurses at the local hospital, and demonstrated an effective capacity to deliver oral communications training in a timely and cost efficient manner. As we write, the work is ongoing at the university and we are in our seventh consecutive year of delivering lectures.

Even though this has been an exciting journey for Rick, demonstrating the ability Rick has to engage students and professionals alike and show how communication

is possible using simple techniques that require no specialist training, we have to
admit that Rick's vision is far from being fulfilled.

Rick's vision is to conduct oral communications training to health and human
service professionals, transport and other workers and their managers. Our experience shows that this training is most effective in face-to-face encounters where
members from the training group can experience firsthand what it is like to engage
with a person with cerebral palsy and with severe speech impairment. Invariably we
find that when this occurs, people report that the experience is both challenging
and rewarding. They discover they are learning new skills that are relevant to
their work. We are continually provided with first hand evidence that training
in oral communication immediately breaks down some of the prejudice amongst
professionals and students towards the person with the speech impairment.

We have found that we can conduct effective basic training in groups of up to
20, even for durations of only half an hour. During that time trainees self-assess
their comprehension of Rick's speech. We have devised a 7-point scale, and find
that trainees generally improve at least a couple of points on that scale within half
an hour of engagement with the program. In lecture scenarios, the situation is more
limiting as lectures generally are to audiences of over 100 students; however the
lectures are immensely popular, as Rick has a strong and engaging presence in front
of an audience. In one lecture to medical students we had about 10 students come
up afterwards to volunteer to learn more, and we started up a focus group with them
that lasted throughout the year. A similar event occurred with a combined class of
therapy students.

Along the journey we realized that achieving the goal of Rick becoming more
extensively involved in training and teaching oral communication depends on more
people being involved, in order for Rick to not depend on David doing the liaison
and facilitation role. This has led us to develop a vision to enable an occupational
community for Rick that will link specifically to a wider array of organizational
settings and communities of practice.

Some health professionals however see no point in undergoing the training that
Rick offers on the grounds that Rick ought to be first prepared to use assistive
communication technologies, and until he does so, attempts at oral communication
are a waste of their professional time and resources. The tension between these
perspectives creates an ethical problematic, that we wish to address.

We take a scholarly view of occupational community as it is articulated in the
anthropological literature, and what comes to the fore is the political aspect of such
communities. Inevitably, by invoking this notion, we are committing ourselves to
some form of political action, and we wish to highlight the salient features of this.

The term 'occupational community' has been current in the anthropological
literature since the mid twentieth century when Lipset (1956) applied the concept in
his study of the printer's union in the United States. Initially the concept related to
work-based situations where there is a flow-over amongst workers from shared work
to shared leisure, enhancing a sense of solidarity that provided a platform for more
radicalized political activity. This concept was expanded by Blauner (1960) and
Lockwood (1966). Blauner, in studies of remote fishing and farming communities,

emphasized social isolation of the workers from mainstream society, accompanied by a high job satisfaction: factors that combined to enhance the likelihood of leisure associations with workmates. Blauner also noted the development of a distinctive worldview in which values derived from the occupational setting provided the standards for workers' evaluations of the world around them. Lockwood added to these criteria a sense of autonomy from supervisory constraints and a distinct occupational subculture that created a sense of belonging and the 'us versus them' political outlook.

The 'us versus them' criterion and the latent political impact of such a form of community identification came to dominate scholarly discussion of the concept in the 1970s and 1980s (see Bulmer 1975 for an overview of the issues). Lockwood (cited in Davis 1986, pp. 129–130) regarded occupational communities to be of anthropological interest only where workers were characterized by a strong proletarian 'us versus them' attitude, and where the identity of 'us' (the workers) is associated with a strong negative occupational imagery associated with 'them' (the bosses). Salaman (cited in Davis 1986, pp. 129–130) by contrast, emphasized positive occupational self-imagery as the criterion of most importance in occupational community formation. This imagery comes through in the sense of group solidarity, high value associated with the occupational role, and a positive self-image associated with the occupation. Dona Lee Davis in her 1986 study of a Newfoundland fishing village explored this further, going well beyond previous emphases on male worker roles, highlighting the roles of women, and in particular emphasizing spirituality and caring. Lee-Ross (2008) discussed how problematic an occupational community can be from a management perspective, and the distinction he draws nicely fits with our differentiation of such a community from an organizational community of practice.

The salient point for us is that identification with an occupational community ideally comes from a positive identification with an occupation (Salaman's emphasis), rather than merely an identification with a state of disqualification or marginalization, which expresses a sense of personal or group injustice (Lockwood's emphasis). In following through the implications of these differences, we place a great deal of emphasis on Salaman's position in describing the sort of working and wider living engagements we envisage for Rick, despite his having to deal with issues of disqualification.

This emphasis places us both in a position of disagreement with various strands of disability activism (under the slogan of "nothing about us without us") whereby the relevant community is regarded as a "disability community" (or "community of disabled people") organized by disabled people themselves opposing issues of injustice and oppression (Oliver 1996a, b). In agreement with the stance taken by disability researcher Tom Shakespeare (2006), we strongly support the notion of collaboration between disabled and non-disabled people, as is evidenced by the partnership we have formed. This partnership serves the purpose of breaking down barriers for Rick into such workplaces as the academic environments, overcoming at least for a time the position whereby he is regarded as intrinsically a recipient of services, not a provider of them. In these episodic encounters Rick provides David and our audience with an essential link to the world of lived experience of people with speech impairments and other forms of disability. Our claim is that Rick's own testimony is an example of a boundary condition between the lived world of people with speech impairments and professional and service providers. Rick is the boundary condition in his own person because he inhabits both worlds, as a service recipient and as a communications teacher and instructor.

13.4 Occupational Community and Communities of Practice: Exploring Boundary Interactions

Before exploring the importance of boundary interactions we must pause to consider the barriers faced by people with speech impairments. In human service situations there typically is a disjunction between the emphasis on work on the part of carers and the emphasis on leisure on the part of people being cared-for. The predominant service expectation is that people with disability will find leisure-based relationships with people like themselves, for example from going to a weekly indoor bowls outing. Rick personally finds this expectation unacceptable, particularly when having personally trained care workers in communication, they then "try to take over and tell me what to do, like going to bowls." (Rick's words)

In light of the anthropological literature, the blurring of boundaries of work, leisure and care provides scope for the formation of occupational communities. The issue is not that the occupational community supports someone's work. It is that whatever occupation it is being engaged in, such occupation signifies a distinctive form of community life. In Rick's situation, an occupational community can be regarded as being formed from his insistent use of oral communication, and occurs when people come into his home, and are required to act according to standards placed on them by Rick as a homeowner. In Rick's case such requirements include care workers being trained in oral communication. Rick extends this training beyond his home to include drivers of wheelchair accessible taxis, shopkeepers, bank tellers, medical personnel and such people as he meets on a day-to-day basis. These are all part of Rick's occupational community, as he meets the same people on a regular and repeated basis. Rick only interacts with people who also willingly enter into a communicative relationship with him on his own terms. However sometimes Rick is forced by various exigencies to interact with people who treat him with disrespect, and refuse to acknowledge him as a communicating person.

If we take Salaman's lead in emphasizing positive identifications as part of the basis for the formation of an occupational community, we must also recognize the problem posed by the issue of disqualification. Despite Rick being able to make choices as to who comes into his home regularly as a carer and who he shops with, and so forth, he also has to contend with the continual reminder that he is the object of other people's work, and not an equal partner in reciprocal social relations. These situations of experienced inequality are the precise point at which boundary interactions occur. Rick's social status as object of care, originates in the communities of practice that inform those who impose this identity on him.

Rick is thereby faced with the following problem. From his perspective an occupational community extends around him on all sides where people are linked through their interactions with him through oral communication. On the other hand, from various organizational perspectives Rick is a client, and has to be made subject to the limitations placed on clients. The disjunction between perspectives is what is at issue.

As important is it is for carers to be familiarized to impaired speech, Rick's vision is to familiarize the wider population to his form of oral communication. On the outside, in relationships with the wider community, Rick finds his efforts to communicate orally, frequently ignored. Therapists in particular are inclined to say that in this environment Rick has no right to expect that people will stop and take time to listen. Therapists have said that if Rick really wants to communicate he ought to avail himself of assistive communication devices, such as printed signs, pictures, communication books, and electronic message devices.

The issue can be understood, as either one of pragmatics, or of ethics. From the pragmatic point of view, given the lack of power that Rick has to get his perspective across, Rick is seen to have very little option but to comply with this request, if he realistically wants to get anywhere in the wider social environment. It is thus considered socially expedient for Rick to utilize the communication technologies on offer. Historically, Rick has refused to accept this advice. In effect, what Rick has done is refuse to accept the boundary interaction offered from the side of professional communities of practice. He insists on presenting his own oral communication as the requisite boundary for professionals to adopt as part of their own practice. On this account Rick has been labeled 'difficult' and his behavior has been described as 'challenging'. We wish to explore this disqualification from an ethical point of view, for there is more to the situation involving Rick than simply a lack of willingness to fit in with professionals' expectations.

13.5 An Ethics of Enabling Occupational Community and Communities of Practice

One of the resources that David brings is his development of a model of Enabling Communities of Human Occupation (ECHO model, Turnbull 2012). This is a strategic model derived from combining the conceptual frameworks of Inayatullah (2002) and Isaacs and Massey (1994). The basic strategy is a process of writing that explores issues that arise from the narratives being offered. In this case writing is part of the process of enabling an occupational community that both upholds Rick's insistence on using oral communication, and takes seriously the claims presented by professional practitioners. Writing takes us through six levels of analysis. In brief these are: the silencing, the polemics, the social causes, the discourse, the myth/metaphor, and finally, the justification. Justification is effectively a new starting point since it is that at this point what Isaacs and Massey term the applied ethics agenda (see for a complete exegesis Clapton 2009) invites us into taking seriously the complexity of the ethical situation.

The silencing refers to the underlying experience that Rick has of a person being silenced, of not being heard, of being misunderstood and on occasion being willed to disappear from public view. Rick tells the story of attending the emergency department of the local hospital in considerable distress. The attending doctor asked rhetorically and dismissively: 'Why aren't you in a nursing home?' In effect this remark was a disqualification of Rick's appearing in a public space. To be placed in a nursing home is to be silenced, having no further part to play in public interactions.

The polemics refers the negative mode of communication sometimes being used towards Rick. The emergency doctor provides one example. Taxi drivers have been another source where Rick has been verbally abused because his message has not been understood. Rick has asked people in a shopping center for help and sometimes they speak rudely and dismissively.

The social causes refer to structural forces that limit the time people have to pay attention to another, or to the separation of roles such that people assume that Rick should either be accompanied by a carer at all times, or be kept out of sight and out of mind.

The discourse refers to the dominant modes of communication such that there are expectations placed on people to speak clearly, or otherwise to have someone speak for them, or to have some sort of mechanical message provided to give others a cue for knowing how to respond.

The myth/metaphor refers to the underlying sentiment or representation concerning Rick, for instance that he is diseased organism or a burden.

Separating the analysis into these aspects enables us to begin to consider at what level it is appropriate to respond. We find we are unable to respond effectively whilst being passive recipients of services and locked into organizational discourses that offer little hope for social change. What we wish to do is develop a way forward, through the use of various media of communication that enable us to construct a new discourse and a different understanding. If we were to passively go along with the pragmatic view, that Rick ought to use some form of assistive technology to enable his message to be understood, we would be in agreement with the myth that Rick is effectively a burden. It is up to Rick, on this account, for him to accept these technologies to reduce the burden he places on others.

This would be the easy way out. In justification of Rick's stance (and this is the sixth level of analysis) we argue that it is professional and organizational practices that need to change. Rick chooses to occupy the position of being someone who challenges dominant expectations. He has become accustomed to vilification, and as upsetting as it always is, he is prepared to accept this as the price he has to pay for sticking up for his right to communicate in a public space using oral speech. For David the inspiration to initiate a new beginning with Rick when the way seems hopelessly lost stems from his reading the works of Hannah Arendt (starting with Arendt 1958) and also readings about the social construction of humanness (for example Bogdan and Taylor 1992) and a persistent desire to address the systemic violence and abuse facing people with disability (well recognized by Sobsey 1994). These problems require unmasking, as they are difficult to detect amidst the daily hustle in which people with speech impairments are reduced to a status of liminality, a position of being neither in nor out of customary interactions (Ingstad and Whyte 1995) and this emphasizes our mutually recognized need for finding allies in emancipation: those who will openly discuss what others may wish to see buried (O'Brien and Murray 2005).

At a superficial level, Rick is merely constrained by a scarcity of opportunities to get his message out. In April 2013 an opportunity came by way of an invitation for Rick and David to speak at a forum on accessibility for wheelchair users in the transport system. The forum was organized by a group of rehabilitation engineers. Immediately prior to our session was a presentation by the local taxi company about the difficulties facing that industry. Prior to the forum Rick and David had discussed the exact location of the communication problem he encounters with wheelchair taxi drivers. The issue has to do with where Rick keeps his taxi fare. It is in a box on the side of the wheelchair. In the box is a wallet with a zipper pocket and inside that is the money. Rick has to communicate this information to people who are unable or unwilling to hear his words. The problem is compounded by an increasing number of immigrant taxi drivers for whom English is a second language.

We suggested in our session a reasonable solution to the difficulty. The problem would be partly solved, we said, if taxis had computerized information that showed exactly where (in Rick's case) the taxi fare is located. More generally, for individuals with speech impairments who regularly use taxis in specific locations, such information could be stored on a data base and brought to the screen of taxis as needed. To supplement this technical solution, we also suggested that taxi drivers needed to be trained in a specific oral communication technique. We offered to make a training video, tailored to the transport situation, so that all taxi drivers in the company could at least have the basics of the technique explained to them.

At the forum we invited the taxi company to engage with us afterwards. Phone calls were made and emails sent. At the time of this writing, the taxi company has still to get back to us with a time to meet.

We wish to make it clear that Rick is not resistant to the use of technology, if it can be used ethically. Rick uses a motorized wheelchair to get about in, and a computer at home. In sticking up for oral communication, we also recognize the time constraints and other difficulties of service providers. Rick is willing to make adjustments, so long as his basic point about the dignity of his own person using oral communication is acknowledged.

Rick says that it is only when people engage with him in oral communication that he feels that they are treating him as a person. If he uses a communication device he feels like he is allowing them to treat him only as an object. He senses that he is allowing them to treat him as if he has no inner life of thought and feeling. Rick's deepest motivation in his desire to communicate with others is to speak orally and be understood that way. It is through speech that his sense of being a person is realized.

This is Rick's stated justification. It is on the basis of this justification that we argue that the way forward for Rick is to be part of an expanding occupational community of people who enjoy facilitating oral communication and practical problem solving involving people with speech impairments. It does not require professionals or human services to be a member of this community. Retirees could be members of it, particularly people who now have considerably more time on their hands than when they were working full time. From our experience it only takes a couple of hours to become familiarized to Rick's speech and learn the communication technique he teaches. After that the role could be one of promoting Rick's public presentations and of facilitating various training or teaching events. It is not an onerous or extremely time-consuming commitment. Of greatest benefit would be people who understand the limitations of the human service system and have a political motivation to act to counteract its hegemony. However it does take professionals and managers of organizations to recognize the capacity and the justification that Rick has for teaching his form of oral communication. It requires people with authority, in hospitals, in universities, in shopping malls, in community venues where people gather and where people with communication impairments can be treated as the silent other, to open gateways for Rick to teach. These gateways are the type of boundary interactions that we support and promote between the kind of occupational community from which Rick comes, and the professional communities of practice that he seeks to influence.

The coaching future we envisage is through the use of digital media. Rick initially wanted to travel the country in a van teaching in various venues along the way. He has come to see this as unrealistic. Nowadays Rick is keen to use the expanding technologies of digital media and the internet to get his message across. We are both very excited about this prospect.

Editors' Postscript If you liked this chapter by David Turnbull and Rick Stoddart, and are interested in reading more about disability perspectives of occupation, we recommend Chap. 22 "Blindness and Occupation: Personal Observations and Reflections" by Rikki Chaplin and Chap. 24 "If disability is a dance, who is the choreographer" by Neil Marcus, Devva Kasnitz and Pamela Block.

References

Arendt H (1958) The human condition. University of Chicago Press, Chicago
Blackmore C (ed) (2010) Social learning systems and communities of practice. Springer, London
Blauner R (1960) Work satisfaction and industrial trends in modern society. In: Galenson W, Lipset SM (eds) Labour and trade unionism. Routledge and Kegan Paul, London, pp 339–360
Bogdan R, Taylor S (1992) The social construction of humanness: relationships with severely disabled people. In: Fergusen PM, Fergusen IM, Taylor S (eds) Interpreting disability: a qualitative reader. Teachers' College Press, New York, pp 275–294
Bulmer M (ed) (1975) Working class images of society. Routledge and Kegan Paul, London
Christiansen CH, Townsend EA (2010) The occupational nature of social groups. In: Christiansen CH, Townsend EA (eds) Introduction to occupation: the art and science of living, 2nd edn. Pearson Education Inc, Upper Saddle River, pp 175–210
Clapton J (2009) A transformatory ethic of inclusion: rupturing concepts of disability and inclusion. Sense Publishers, Rotterdam
Curtin M, Molineux M, Supyk-Mellson J (eds) (2010) Occupational therapy and physical dysfunction: enabling occupation, 6th edn. Churchill Livingstone Elsevier, Edinburgh
Davis DL (1986) Occupational community and fishermen's wives in a Newfoundland fishing village. Anthropol Q 59(3):129–142

Inayatullah S (2002) Questioning the future: futures studies, action learning and organizational transformation. Tamkang University, Taipei

Ingstad B, Whyte SR (eds) (1995) Disability and culture. University of California Press, Berkeley

Isaacs P, Massey M (1994) Mapping the applied ethics agenda. A presentation at the third annual meeting of the Association for Practical and professional Ethics. Cleveland, 24–26 February

Lee-Ross D (2008) Occupational communities and cruise tourism: testing a theory. J Manag Dev 27(5):467–479

Lipset SM (1956) Union democracy. Free Press, Chicago

Lockwood D (1966) Sources of variation in working-class images of society. Sociol Rev 14(3):249–267

O'Brien P, Murray R (eds) (2005) Allies in emancipation: shifting from providing services to being of support. Thomson Dunmore Press, South Melbourne

Oliver M (1996a) Defining impairment and disability: issues at stake. In: Barnes C, Mercer G (eds) Exploring the divide: illness and disability. The Disability Press, Leeds, pp 29–54

Oliver M (1996b) Understanding disability: from theory to practice. MacMillan Press, London

Pollard N, Sakellariou D, Lawson-Porter A (2010) Will occupational science facilitate or divide the practice of occupational therapy? Int J Ther Rehabil 17(1):40–47

Shakespeare T (2006) Disability rights and wrongs. Routledge, London

Snyder WM, Wenger E (2010) Our world as a learning system: a communities-of-practice approach. In: Blackmore C (ed) Social learning systems and communities of practice. Springer, London, pp 107–124

Sobsey D (1994) Violence and abuse in the lives of people with disabilities: the end of silent acceptance. Paul Brookes Publishing Co., Baltimore

Townsend E, Polatjko HJ (2007) Enabling occupation II: advancing an occupational therapy vision for health, well-being & justice through occupation. CAOT Publications, Ottawa

Townsend E, Whiteford G (2005) A participatory occupational justice framework: population-based processes of practice. In: Kronenberg F, Algado S, Pollard N (eds) Occupational therapy without borders: learning from the spirit of survivors. Elsevier Churchill Livingstone, Toronto, pp 110–126

Turnbull D (2012) The ECHO model: enabling communities of human occupation http://nodangerousthoughts.com/2012/02/08/the-echo-model-enabling-communities-of-human-occupation/. Accessed 23 May 2015

Wenger E (1998) Communities of practice: learning, meaning and identity. Cambridge University Press, New York

Wenger E (2010) Conceptual tools for CoPs as social learning systems: boundaries, identity, trajectories and participation. In: Blackmore C (ed) Social learning systems and communities of practice. Springer, London, pp 125–143

Wolfensberger W (1991) A brief introduction to social role valorization as a high-order concept for structuring human services. Training Institute for Human Service Planning, Leadership and Change Agentry, Syracuse University, Syracuse

Occupying Seats, Occupying Space, Occupying Time: Deaf Young Adults in Vocational Training Centers in Bangalore, India

14

Michele Friedner

Abstract
This chapter explores how sign language-using deaf young adults in Bangalore, India "occupy" vocational training centers set up for disabled people. Bangalore has many such centers and as disability has become a concept of great interest to both the state and civil society, additional centers are emerging. "Occupy" here has three meanings: the first relates to administrators' need for bodies to occupy seats in order to satisfy their funders' desires for high numbers of trainees. As the number of physically disabled potential trainees has decreased, deaf trainees have become a significant source of numbers at these centers. As such, deaf trainees "occupy" seats. The second meaning relates to the ways that deaf trainees "occupy" these centers and recreate them in ways unintended, and often below the radar of, administrators and teachers. As most administrators and teachers do not know sign language and are unaware of deaf values and moral orientations, deaf trainees create their own pedagogical spaces in which they teach each other, share news, and discuss ways of developing as deaf people. The third meaning has to do with "occupying" time: these vocational training centers are often spaces of urgency and anxiety as deaf trainees frantically try to learn something in the aftermath of primary and secondary school educational experiences that have failed them miserably. This time of trying to learn something is often a time of intense waiting as trainees wait to learn skills and then wait to find employment. Utilizing ethnographic data, this chapter argues for the importance of understanding the multiple registers of how vocational training spaces are utilized.

M. Friedner (✉)
School of Health Technology and Management, State University of New York,
Stony Brook, NY, USA
e-mail: michele.friedner@stonybrook.edu

© Springer Science+Business Media Dordrecht 2016
P. Block et al. (eds.), *Occupying Disability: Critical Approaches to Community,
Justice, and Decolonizing Disability*, DOI 10.1007/978-94-017-9984-3_14

Keywords
Deaf • Development • Futures • Vocational training • Neoliberalism

14.1   Circulating for an Occupation

Narayan is an earnest and shy deaf man in his mid-twenties from a village in Chikmaglur, Karnataka.[1] Chikmaglur is a region known for its coffee plantations located about an 8-h bus ride from Bangalore. Bangalore is Karnataka's capital and is known within the public imagination as India's "silicon valley." As a city, it is pioneering in its (neoliberal) creation of public-private partnerships, land reforms, and the preferential treatment given to private corporations; indeed scholars and activists have argued that Bangalore is being remade through the infusion of corporate capital and new forms of governance are emerging (which are not necessarily positive) (Goldman 2010; Nair 2005). Bangalore is therefore a very productive site for thinking about changes in deaf peoples' lives and employment trajectories. I first met Narayan in the summer of 2007 when he was a trainee at the Disabled Peoples Association's (DPA) vocational training institute in Bangalore. Narayan had moved to Bangalore after finishing his secondary school leaving certificate (SSLC) at a residential deaf school where he said that he did not learn anything. At the time that he had finished his SSLC, an older brother was living in Bangalore and had learned about DPA'a vocational courses and the possibility of reduced tuition because of the family's below-poverty-line status. After learning about this opportunity, Narayan traveled to Bangalore and enrolled in a welding course at DPA where he learned welding techniques with other deaf, physically disabled, and a few non-disabled trainees. Administrators at DPA told him that after he finished his 2-year course he would take a government exam and then he would get an apprenticeship in one of Bangalore's public sector companies. He was told that with his welding skills, his future would be good.

However, neither Narayan nor any of his fellow deaf trainees were able to get an apprenticeship or a government job. After working in private companies for a few months for extremely low wages, Narayan went to another non-governmental organization (NGO) offering vocational training and employment placement services for disabled people.[2] At this NGO, named Vision, he enrolled in a 3-month basic computer course. After completing this course, Vision found him a job placement as a data entry operator on the night shift with a subcontractor for a major Indian telecommunications company. After 3 months, this company shifted its offices to Delhi and Narayan was laid off. He then returned to Vision and to another disability

---

[1]The names of all individuals and NGOs have been changed.

[2]Going forward, I call each of the institutions that I am writing about an "NGO." They are also called training centers and job placement centers. Similarly, I call deaf young adults who frequent these NGOs "trainees" although they are also called students.

NGO called the Employment Center, which had recently opened, and asked them both for help finding a job. The Employment Center recommended that he take a basic computer course again at its center but Narayan was reluctant to do so because he had completed an identical course at Vision. And so, in search of employment, Narayan constantly circulated between both NGOs in the hope that one would find him another job placement that paid well. He also occasionally visited DPA, but less frequently.

Narayan's circulations between these three NGOs were not unique. During the 15 months that I conducted ethnographic fieldwork with sign language-using deaf young adults in Bangalore and other Indian cities, I observed that my interlocutors constantly circulated from NGO to NGO, sometimes individually, and sometimes as a group. They enrolled in identical courses at different NGOs, learning the same things multiple times, and they sought job placements from multiple NGOs. Indeed, this circulation between NGOs was made especially clear to me when a group of students from DPA's basic computer course showed up to register for the Employment Center's identical computer course just 2 days after the DPA course completed. Even though the course at the Employment Center was designed to teach them the same basic computer skills that they learned at DPA, they were still eager to enroll.

In this essay I want to think about the stakes of such circulations. In doing so, I will broadly discuss the current landscape of deaf education and employment in Bangalore and I will discuss why deaf people often see such circulations as the only option for finding livelihood. As this is a collection of essays about "occupation," I will frame my analysis by examining the multiple registers of "occupation" that take place during such circulations. That is, I will analyze how my interlocutors occupy seats, occupy space, and occupy time in NGOs offering both vocational training and employment placement. To be absolutely clear, I view the emergence of these NGOs as a product of neoliberal political economic restructuring that has benefited some people and not others and that has embedded deaf people within specific kinds of training and employment circulations.

14.2   Vocational Training: An "Opportunity" to Learn *Something*

My interlocutors were not always young adults and so in order to understand the stakes of vocational training and employment placement, I must provide a brief history and description of the present. To begin, primary and secondary schools for deaf children in India are widely seen as being failures (Bhattacharya 2010; Broota 2005; Zeshan et al. 2005). Schools are almost exclusively oral in ideology (although students often sign in between and after classes). The oral method, which posits that deaf children can learn to read lips and speak, is highly contested and does not work for all deaf children (Werner 1994). In addition, children are not provided with appropriate amplification (in the form of hearing aids or other technology) to make use of oral education nor are they provided with teachers with adequate training (Antia 1979; Broota 2005; Rehabilitation Council of India 2007; World Bank 2007).

The Rehabilitation Council of India (RCI), the government body which oversees and accredits special education teaching curricula and programs, currently does not permit deaf teachers to teach in deaf schools and so deaf children are learning from hearing teachers who, according to most of my interlocutors, often just write on the board and students copy down what is written without learning or understanding.

Most recently, as a result of India's ratifying the United Nations Convention on the Rights of Persons with Disability (UNCRPD) in 2007, which explicitly mentions the importance of sign language, the RCI started exploring the possibility of introducing sign language into deaf education. Previously, the government had not recognized or invested resources in research or teaching related to Indian Sign Language. In 2009, the RCI secretary convened a meeting to discuss multiple approaches to deaf education and for the first time, the council seemed interested in including sign language training into special education curricula and exploring possibilities for sign language-based deaf education. However, from what I have been told by both RCI's secretary and the former national disability commissioner, teachers will only have 15 days of sign language instruction, not at all enough time for them to establish fluency.

In many cases, deaf students graduate from secondary school and receive their SSLC without having learned much. Indeed, many of my interlocutors talked about either copying on this exam—they said that teachers came into the exam room and gave them answer sheets—or paying bribes in order to pass. Many of my interlocutors finished secondary school without being able to read and write properly in either their native languages or English and without proficient knowledge of sign language. Broota (2005) writes in her report on the current issues facing deaf people in India:

> ... it seems that oralism has left the majority of deaf people in the country without adequate modes of communication and education. If, for years, the auditory-verbal approach to communication has been followed and is claimed to be successful, then why do we not see graduates, doctors, engineers, civil servants, architects, lawyers who have hearing impairment? ... why don't we see deaf children in colleges? (Broota 2005, p. 6).

With this quote, Broota brings us to the heart of the matter: deaf children are not learning from their teachers in schools nor are they acquiring essential language skills. In interviews with advocates working to improve the education system for deaf children, I was told time and time again that deaf children often finish school without access to language development and that even teachers themselves do not realize the relationship between deafness, education, and language development. And so what happens when deaf children "pass" their SSLC without learning? What happens when they transition from childhood to young adulthood?[3]

As a result of state and private interventions, there is an increasing variety of options available to deaf young adults, especially those living in South India, where

---

[3]There are deaf children who emerge from school as fluent signers if they have access to sign language-using deaf peers, mentors, and/or family members.

higher education institutions for the deaf have emerged in Chennai and Madurai in Tamil Nadu, and Mysore in Karnataka. With the exception of JSS Polytechnic for the Physically Handicapped in Mysore where students receive diplomas after completing 3 years of education, the other institutions offer bachelor degrees. However, as with primary and secondary education, in the majority of cases teachers do not use sign language and students complain that they do not understand and so they copy and learn from each other or more advanced classmates. The numbers of deaf students pursuing higher education is miniscule at about 0.9 % of the known 307,600 deaf children in India (Rehabilitation Council of India 2007). [4]

As such in the aftermath of poor quality primary and secondary school education, vocational training is a key site for educating (and "rehabilitating") deaf young adults. The national government has required that government Industrial Training Institutes offer a 1 % quota to deaf students. It is important to note that both national and state governments have supported vocational training and that the number of government and private vocational training centers, and students enrolled in them, has increased significantly.[5] However, few deaf young adults choose to attend mainstream vocational training programs and instead they flock to where other deaf young adults are - at programs offered by disability-focused NGOs.

As vocational training focuses on manual and applied training, it is presumably possible to ignore deaf young adults' educational deficits and focus on imparting "technical" skills: more specifically welding and electronics skills, and increasingly over the past 8 years, basic computer skills. According to Deepa Patel, a community based rehabilitation and deaf education expert living in Bangalore, the problems that deaf young adults face are more difficult to ignore than the problems of deaf children. She writes:

> The child deprived of even a basic education having severely limited language and communication skills grows up without being able to get any kind of employment (unless its manual labour). This problem then becomes a very glaring problem and much more obvious than the problems of the deaf child. (Personal communication)

Patel pointed out that a focus on vocational training for deaf young adults was like "fighting fires or damage control" and that it was easier to find vocational

---

[4] According to RCI, these numbers are estimated from the 2001 census and are most likely inaccurate.

[5] Vocational training has been seen as a crucial program for creating a skilled Indian labor pool in general (International Labor Organization 2003; World Bank 2008). According to a 2008 World Bank report, there were 10,000 students enrolled in vocational training in the 1950s and this number has increased to more than 700,000 students now enrolled in 5,253 public and private institutions. This report noted that 60 % of students were still unemployed 3 years after finishing their vocational training course, there was not enough government oversight of private programs, and there were also ambiguous and competing government certification schemes. In addition, education provided was deemed to be too narrow in focus and there was not enough connection between actual industries and the vocational training centers. These factors combined with a general decrease in industrial sectors have resulted in increasing unemployment.

training teachers than deaf education specialists. It was perhaps easier to build and develop successful vocational programs than successful deaf education programs. All of this leads me to stress that vocational training is a critical space for deaf young adults—an "opportunity" to learn *something*. I place "opportunity" in quotes here because it is questionable whether or not deaf trainees actually feel that such NGOs provide them with true opportunities. It is also questionable whether courses that last between 3 months and a year can truly offer opportunities, especially in light of the significant structural barriers that exist.

14.3 Occupying Seats

While deaf young adults in Bangalore flocked to the three main vocational training and job placement NGOs that I discussed in the introduction—DPA, Vision, and the Employment Center—it is important to note that none of these NGOs were started with deaf students as their target population. These centers were not designed with sign language- using deaf young adults in mind and most NGO administrators were unaware of the specific needs and desires of deaf people. For example, DPA's director refused to permit a celebration or program for International Deaf Week because he said that deaf people should not be singled out or treated differently from other disabled people. Similarly, the Employment Center's director encouraged deaf trainees to write on individual white boards that she provided them with instead of using sign language as "[I]n the future they will be in the normal world where no one will know sign language and they will have to communicate." Both of these decisions, while presumably well meaning, were a rejection of deaf peoples' experiences and the importance of sign language within these experiences. In addition, while the NGOs physical spaces were designed to be accessible to physically disabled people, they were often not accessible to deaf students. Benches and seats in classrooms were arranged in set rows and teachers and trainers often stood in front of windows and were therefore drowned out by light. Communication policies were largely nonexistent. However, as I will discuss, NGO administrators were quite keen to enroll deaf students.

In order to discuss why enrolling deaf students was a priority, I would like to briefly outline the origin stories of each of the NGOs as well as their current relationships to funders. In addition, I provide background in order to make a distinction between DPA and Vision and the Employment Center as the latter two NGOs had very different approaches to what training and employment futures should look like. DPA, which occupies a campus in a formerly peripheral but now central neighborhood in Bangalore (due to constant building and construction in the city), sometimes feels like a relic of the past. An affluent family with a polio-affected daughter started DPA and due to this young woman's diligence and influential connections, it grew rapidly. Over the years it started a full-scale industrial training center, a self-contained manufacturing unit supplying parts to government industries, a primary school for disabled children, community based rehabilitation programs, horticulture training, and community health workshops. More recently, DPA started a computer-training program in an attempt to follow the current trend in vocational training. Both domestic and international funders fund these programs and DPA has become very well established in South India where it is known for providing a wide variety of services and training.

As polio incidence rates declined over the years and as access to physical therapy and mobility aids improved, DPA found itself with a declining student population for its industrial training center—until DPA was approached by deaf students finishing class ten at a local deaf school in 2002. At that time, Radhika, an electronics teacher, agreed to learn sign language. Through deaf networks, deaf students began flocking to DPA and Radhika became increasingly committed to learning sign language and teaching deaf students. She taught the other welding and electronics teachers sign language and as the numbers of deaf students grew, DPA instituted an informal policy under which *all* new students were required to learn sign language, in order to introduce an "inclusive" atmosphere (although in practice most non-deaf students were not so motivated to learn sign language). This policy has resulted in some tension, as the matriarchal founder believes strongly that DPA should prioritize people with physical disabilities and she told me that she felt that deaf people were taking over the space. However, most teachers and administrators do not sign fluently, if at all, and there is also high teacher turnover. And a few years ago, Radhika herself moved to the Employment Center where she is now the director.

In contrast to DPA which offers a variety of training programs, Vision and the Employment Center only offer computer and "soft skills," or personality development, courses to deaf trainees. These courses are free of charge to trainees unlike at DPA where trainees pay a nominal fee. Vision and the Employment Center also do not attempt to place trainees in government jobs: they are concerned solely with the private sector and often place candidates in multinational corporations and/or in India's emerging hospitality sector. Indeed, their list of placements is filled with prominent Indian and multinational corporations (many of which have received criticism by labor rights groups and anti-globalization activists). Both NGOs receive funding from these same corporations and from international disability organizations (some of which have been the target of criticism by Disability Studies scholars and disability rights activists who decry the internationalization of disability rights rhetoric). A husband and wife team started Vision in 1999; both formerly worked in the corporate world in the United States and India. As a result of personal experience with a disabled family member, they started offering computer training and job placement to blind people who they ultimately placed in corporate offices as transcriptionists, data entry operators, and business process outsourcing (BPO) workers. Similar to DPA, Vision was approached by a deaf person who they successfully trained and placed in a corporate environment. Subsequently, deaf people spread the word about its programs and flocked to Vision for training and employment placement. Vision is unique in offering a 3-month extensive BPO training to deaf trainees.

The Employment Center, which is attached to an international disability organization, is the newest NGO of the three. It opened its doors in 2008 and provides basic computer training as well as job placement services. It provides almost identical trainings and services to Vision although it does not offer BPO training. The Employment Center, unlike the other NGOs, actually has a deaf computer teacher and he is quite popular with his students because of his non-hierarchical teaching style and use of sign language. In addition, the basic computer-training program was open to anyone who wanted to take it, from bored housewives to manual workers hoping for new employment possibilities to students who just finished their SSLC and were not quite ready for employment. As such, there was a steady stream of deaf trainees who enrolled in this course.

During the 15 months that I conducted fieldwork in Bangalore, I observed that students often circulated between the three NGOs, often registering with all three, and sometimes enrolling in the same computer-training course more than once. When I spoke to NGO administrators about this circulation, they seemed concerned about the repetition in training on one hand but on the other hand they were happy to have students enrolled. Indeed, there was constant concern about having numbers: both sufficient numbers of trainees enrolled in courses and sufficient numbers of trainees placed in jobs. Such numbers were important because funders required them as "proof" that the NGO was doing its job. NGO administrators privately lamented to me that they found this numbers focus to be unrealistic due to the very real constraints around training and placing disabled people. However, they had no choice but to make numbers a priority. Deaf people, because of their ability to move through the city with relative ease compared to other disabled populations and the communicability of their social networks, became a key source of such numbers.[6]

This desire to recruit deaf students sometimes led to tension between the three NGOs. For example, I conducted fieldwork with one of Vision's BPO training cohorts. Many of the trainees had previously attended the Employment Center's basic computer course. One day, these trainees received a message, via text message, from the Employment Center telling them to come to the Employment Center for a job interview. Excited about the prospect of a job, these trainees were absent from their BPO training the next day. However, as we were later to learn, funders were visiting the Employment Center and so administrators wanted to stage mock interviews in order to impress them. And in the end, with nothing to show for their absence, Vision's BPO teachers were angry with these trainees for missing a day of training.

This focus on numbers also led to creative strategies: DPA often referred its computer students to a data entry/business process outsourcing corporation that was very keen to hire disabled workers because its chief executive officer believed that such workers did not attrite and were more productive. Students referred to this corporation often refused to work there because the pay was extremely low.

---

[6]In many cases, disabled trainees learned sign language and attempted to communicate with their deaf peers. Deaf trainees often told me that they appreciated this effort and they often relied on disabled peers for help when they did not understand their teachers. However, most of my deaf interlocutors considered deafness and disability to be two separate categories and they identified as deaf and not as disabled (although they of course benefited from government disability certifications and other government disability schemes).

However, DPA could say that it had placed trainees successfully after referring them to this corporation. Similarly, the Employment Center often counted giving a trainee an address for a potential job as a job placement even if the student was never actually hired. In conclusion, deaf trainees and candidates were therefore sought out to occupy seats, regardless of whether they were actually given job placements (or occupations).

14.4   Occupying Space

In the previous section I discussed how NGOs strategically sought to recruit deaf trainees in order to boost their enrollment figures, often ignoring deaf circulations and overlaps in training. In this section I turn to the question of *why* deaf trainees circulated and *how* they benefited from such circulations. What benefit did deaf young adults derive from attending courses at multiple training centers? How were vocational training centers key sites of both deaf sociality and aspiring towards deaf development? By deaf sociality I mean deaf peoples' orientations towards each other which leads to the creation of a distinct local moral world (Kleinman 1999). By deaf development I am referring to a concept used by my interlocutors and which refers to the creation of deaf-centered, and therefore sign language-centered, structures and institutions which will help deaf people develop social, economic, and moral skills for becoming successful deaf people.[7]

In answering these questions about what is at stake in circulations between NGOs, I introduce the concept of "unintended deaf spaces." I draw from Doreen Massey's (1994) work on place and space to think through how my interlocutors produced space in vocational training centers. According to Massey, spaces are constructed out of social relations; "the spatial is social relations 'stretched out.'" (p. 2). Massey also entreats us to see space as a simultaneity of stories-so-far and places as collections of these stories within a temporal moment. Places are not static and passive receptacles but they are actively produced and open processes that can be seen as temporary spatial-temporal events (pp. 130–131). In particular, Massey argues for an "alternative interpretation of place" in which "what gives a place some specificity is not some long internalized history but the fact that it is constructed out of a particular constellation of social relations, meeting and weaving together at a particular locus." (p. 154). In utilizing Massey's framework for approaching space and place, I argue that my interlocutors created deaf spaces that were unintended by those who created and administered these spaces. Thinking through Massey's take on space, these "unintended deaf spaces" were constructed out of, and through, deaf communicative, social, and moral practices. Deaf young adults often produced,

---

[7]In utilizing and highlighting the concepts of deaf sociality and deaf development, I am moving away from the concepts of Deaf culture, Deaf identity, and Deafhood as used by the Northern-based discipline of Deaf Studies (see Friedner and Kusters 2014 on the limitations of these concepts). Similarly, I do not use a capital D when writing "deaf" because my interlocutors did not do so.

learned within, and derived meaning from these spaces in ways unintended and unplanned by their founders and administrators.

As I noted, most NGO administrators and many of the teachers did not sign nor did they understand the needs of deaf students. Those who administered and taught at these training centers and NGOs desired, as one NGO director told me, to create responsible and productive deaf workers who "would be integrated into the mainstream and be productive and contributing members of society." While deaf young adults did occasionally learn how to be responsible and productive workers, they also learned *other* things, unbeknownst to these administrators and teachers. They learned how to be oriented towards other deaf people and to participate in deaf sociality. They learned deaf norms such as sharing information and helping each other and they created moral spaces for discussing both present day problems and ideas for the future with each other and with the deaf teachers and role models who occasionally came to visit or teach.

For example, I often sat and chatted with deaf trainees as they practiced new signs that they had learned from each other or asked each other for help with understanding a new English word or phrase. Deaf trainees also explained important computing, welding, or electrical concepts to each other as often there was much confusion about what teachers were actually teaching since there was poor communication access. In addition, trainees often shared information about the various NGOs, training centers, churches, and schools that they knew about and had experience with. They pooled knowledge about employment opportunities and shared what they had learned from other deaf friends elsewhere. Trainees also shared personal information and asked for advice about how to negotiate relationships with members of the opposite sex, health and hygiene, and manners. Indeed, in these spaces, deaf "communities of practice" (Lave and Wenger 1991) were created in which deaf people learned from each other.

However, unlike in Lave and Wenger's (1991) theory, which posits that there are peripheral learners who learn from experts or central learners, these were often "communities of practice" in which all members had the same level of knowledge. There were occasionally deaf role models who came to volunteer: at DPA, Chetan, a deaf government worker volunteered on Saturdays and taught trainees English, Sign Language, and personal development skills. Similarly, the Employment Center employed one deaf teacher who taught English and sign language. For the most part, however, trainees were left on their own during breaks in classes, when the power went out and prevented students from practicing typing, and when teachers were busy with other tasks. And during these times and after classes were finished for the day, deaf trainees collectively pooled knowledge, asked each other questions, and compared and contrasted their different educational, employment, and life experiences.

While these training spaces, at least for deaf attendees, came to take on deaf forms and structures of their own, I do not mean to imply that they were spaces of resistance. To the contrary, deaf young adults made no claims against these spaces nor did they actively attempt to reorder or change them to make them more representative of the needs and desires of deaf people. Program administrators and teachers were therefore unaware of how deaf young adults used these spaces and often complained to me that they saw their deaf students as "lazy," "pampered," "immature," "emotional and prone to gossiping," and "not capable of making good decisions." There was often tension between administrators and teachers on one hand and deaf trainees on the other. (And of course in most cases, NGO administrators and teachers had no idea what their students were chatting about since sign language was not legible to them.)

And so why did deaf trainees continue to circulate among these NGOs and why did these NGOs continue to be "unintended deaf spaces?" In the absence of other kinds of institutions where deaf people could learn from each other and in the absence of employment that was seen to be meaningful and sustainable, deaf young adults gravitated towards vocational training centers as they were seen as places where deaf people could hopefully learn something. Indeed vocational training centers have replaced other social spaces such as deaf clubs in Bangalore. They have become intense social spaces in their own right; indeed, deaf people repeatedly returned to centers to practice typing, hang out, and just to pass time. In addition, the existence of such NGOs has changed the structure of searching for jobs in Bangalore. Many deaf people told me that in the past they found employment through kinship, neighborhood, and friendship networks.[8] I was also told that in the past, deaf people, alone or with the help of their families, visited companies and applied for jobs on their own. In contrast, deaf people told me that they now go to NGOs to register and then wait for the NGOs to find them a job. In the following section, I discuss such practices of passing time and waiting.[9]

14.5   Occupying Time

As I noted, most of the welding students at DPA did not get their desired government apprenticeship or job. There was a sense too that these kinds of jobs were no longer attainable, especially with the shrinking of public sector industries and the (neoliberal) expansion of the private sector in Bangalore and in India more broadly (Nair 2005). These trainees quickly learned that they needed to do something else— study computers and/or work in the hospitality industry (as a kitchen worker in Kentucky Fried Chicken or as a "silent brewmaster" at a Café Coffee Day outlet for example). And so they flocked to Vision and the Employment Center in pursuit

---

[8]These training centers do not exist in all Indian cities and the existence of three large centers is rather unique to Bangalore. When I spent time in Coimbatore, a second-tier city in Tamil Nadu, I observed that such NGOs did not exist and that deaf people therefore depended on their families, neighbors, or extended social networks to find employment. As such there was a different structure of opportunity that existed: deaf people actively looked for employment instead of waiting for an NGO to find them a job.

[9]Many of my interlocutors had stories of never receiving employment placements and of waiting indefinitely. However, those participating in Vision's BPO training were usually given jobs within a few months.

of computer training and hospitality jobs. In addition to these trainees, there were many other students with slow typing speeds and poor English skills who enrolled in computer courses but they were unable to find computer jobs. Yet they kept on coming to these organizations to practice their typing, meet their friends, and to wait together for jobs. There were also those who were too young for employment—16 and 17 years of age—who came to these NGOs because their families were too poor to pay for higher education or they did not want to study anymore and so they continued a routine of typing practice even after they had finished their basic computer courses.

And then there were trainees who moved to Bangalore in order to wait for Vision's BPO training to start or who, upon finishing this training, waited for employment placements. Indeed, some of my key interlocutors were trainees who I followed through Vision's BPO training and I also spent time with them when they waited for Vision to place them in a BPO job.[10] During this period of waiting, their teachers told them to continue to practice typing and to be diligent in continuing to improve their typing skills; they were told to be patient. They waited for 3 months, sitting in rented rooms that they shared with each other and/or traveling through the city to hang out and pass time. Many these interlocutors echoed what they were told by Vision's trainers and spoke of the importance of being "patient;" they also spoke of having faith in Vision's ability to find them good jobs. Yet others were concerned, especially after having less than good experiences with other NGOs that promised to find them jobs yet failed to deliver on this promise. There were constant stories about the need to "adjust" and manage expectations and there were concerns about what the future would bring.

My interlocutors were aware that the field of deaf employment was shifting and that the future was unknown: again, the previously taken for granted government job was now a thing of the past and fortunes were to be found in the private sector, a source of much uncertainty. Indeed, there were few, if any, older deaf role models working in BPO offices or in the hospitality sector, and my interlocutors did not know if these positions would be sustainable in the long run "for life." These concerns were especially prominent for those working in the hospitality sector because some of the coffee chains did not hire workers who were older than 30 and as such it was not clear what would happen to these workers in the future. I encountered a few deaf people who had been laid off from such chains due to their closing and they were unable to get other jobs in the hospitality sector because of their ages (see Friedner (2013) for more on deaf workers' ambivalence towards working in the hospitality sector).

While these NGOs were meant to be spaces that deaf young adults moved through—a stopping point between finishing school (either an SSLC, a diploma,

---

[10]Many of these interlocutors did not actually want BPO jobs. They wanted to be artists, designers, teachers, and autocad engineers. However, when they went to Vision to register, they were told that because they were deaf, they should work with computers and that a BPO job would be good for them.

a certificate course, or a bachelor degree) and employment—in practice these organizations became produced spaces of waiting, typing, and socializing; they were dwelling spaces for the meantime (of waiting). Time, through circulations between training centers and everyday practices of waiting for employment placements (for 1 month, 2 months, 3 months), became stretched out. I suggest that this slowing of time represents a different experience of modernity than David Harvey's (1990) theorization of modernity as characterized by space-time compression in which there are fewer boundaries and time moves very quickly. Time here is stretched out, ironically, mocking the deaf typer's race against the clock to improve her typing score.

However, I want to stress that such practices of waiting were productive for deaf sociality and deaf orientations. As deaf trainees spent time together on a daily basis at multiple training centers, they learned from each other and shared knowledge and news. They learned new ideas of "deaf development" and they collectively imagined futures in which such development would take place. Training centers became "unintended deaf spaces" and there was a way that each training center blended into another: this was made clear to me one afternoon while sitting at the Employment Center with a small group of trainees. One young woman had her notebook out and I asked if I could see it. As I flipped through it, I saw notes and vocabulary words from a Vision training that she had also attended and on another occasion, I noticed her teaching some of the vocabulary to some of the young women with whom she was sitting. As Erica Bornstein (2005) suggests, NGOs are often overlapping in terms of those who work for them, the work that they do, and who they serve. Bornstein's observation rings true for NGOs working with deaf young adults in Bangalore. Such overlaps help to create local moral worlds (Kleinman 1999) in these spaces.

14.6   Conclusion: NGOs as Deaf Occupations

NGOs such as DPA, Vision, and Employment Center are very much a part of the social fabric of deaf young adults' lives in Bangalore: they are spaces of occupying seats, occupying space, and occupying time. Such NGOs are so ingrained in deaf presents and futures that wealthier and/or deaf young adults who were successful at finding well-paying jobs often told me that they hoped to help other deaf people by starting their own training programs. These training programs would have deaf teachers and feature sign language as the medium of instruction. Many of my interlocutors who were not so wealthy, successful, or lucky also told me that they wished that they could become teachers in NGOs because they wanted to help other deaf people. However, I was also told that NGO employment would not pay well and that in many cases deaf people would not be paid a salary equal to what non-deaf people were paid in these spaces. While I do not know if this is true, I am interested in what this says about deaf trainees' mistrust of hearing administrators at these centers. Indeed, returning to Narayan, the young man with whom I opened this essay, DPA had offered him a job as a welding teacher but he refused because he said that it would not pay well enough.

And in the meantime, the experience of modernity for deaf NGO trainees is about circulating through spaces of waiting, cultivating patience, sharing skills and news, and helping other deafs. While some deaf young adults do learn technical and marketable skills in these vocational training centers such as computer skills, welding, and electronics skills, I argue that the values and orientations that deafs learn in these spaces are more important for everyday life; deafs use these values and orientations to create an everyday marked by desiring deaf development. These values include an orientation towards other deafs, a collective sense of responsibility towards sharing and pooling information in pursuit of improving deaf lives, valuing sign language, and desiring better deaf futures. And whither an occupation based upon these values and practices?

Editors' Postscript If you enjoyed reading this chapter, we recommend both Melanie Yergeau's Chap. 6 "Occupying Autism: Rhetoric, Involuntarity, and the Meaning of Autistic Lives," which looks at misinterpretations of autistics' communication, Chap. 24 "If Disability is a Dance, who is the Choreographer? A Conversation about Life Occupations, Art, Movement," by Neil Marcus, Devva Kasnitz, and Pamela Block, as they all explore non-normative communication. Akemi Nishida in "Neoliberal Academia and a Critique from Disability Studies," Chap. 10 takes a similar approach. Chapter 22 by Rikki Chaplin "Blindness and Occupation: Personal Observations and Reflections" makes an interesting comparison with Friedner's on deafness.

Acknowledgements I would like to thank all my interlocutors as well as the NGOs mentioned in this chapter for their generosity in allowing me to occupy their centers. I also thank Stefan Helmreich, Mara Green, and Annelies Kusters for thoughts and comments on different versions of this paper. And much appreciation to editors Pamela Block, Nick Pollard, Devva Kasnitz, and Akemi Nishida.

References

Antia SD (1979) Education of the hearing impaired in *India*: a survey. Am Ann Deaf 124(6):785–789

Bhattacharya T (2010) Re-examining issue of inclusion in education. Econ Polit Wkly 45(16):18–24

Bornstein E (2005) The spirit of development: protestant NGOs, morality, and economics in Zimbabwe. Stanford University Press, Stanford

Broota S (2005) Concerns of people with hearing impairment in India. Draft Report prepared for the National Centre for Promotion of Employment for Disabled People, New Delhi

Friedner M (2013) Producing "Silent Brewmasters": deaf workers and added value in India's Coffee Shops. Anthropol Work Rev 34(1):39–50

Friedner M, Kusters A (2014) On the possibilities and limits of "DEAF DEAF SAME": Disability Stud Q 34(3). Accessed at http://dsq-sds.org/article/view/4246

Goldman M (2010) Speculative urbanism and the making of the next world city. Int J Urban Reg Res. Retrieved from http://onlinelibrary.wiley.com/doi/10.1111/j.1468-2427.2010.01001.x/full. On 27 Mar 2011

Harvey D (1990) The condition of postmodernity: an inquiry into the origins of cultural change. Blackwell, Cambridge

International Labor Organization (2003) Industrial training institutes of India: the efficiency study report. Prepared by Sub Regional Office for South Asia, ILO New Delhi. Retrieved from: http://www.ilo.org/public/english/region/ampro/cinterfor/news/gasskov.pdf. On 15 Mar 2011

Kleinman A (1999) Moral experience and ethical reflection: can ethnography reconcile them? A quandary for "the new bioethics". Daedelus 128(4):69–97

Lave J, Wenger E (1991) Situated learning: legitimate peripheral participation. Cambridge University Press, New York

Massey D (1994) Space, place, and gender. University of Minnesota Press, Minneapolis

Nair J (2005) The promise of the metropolis: Bangalore's twentieth century. Oxford India Paperbacks, New Delhi

Rehabilitation Council of India (2007) Status of disability in India-2007: hearing impairment and deafblindness, vol 1. New Delhi: Rehabilitation Council of India. United Nations Convention on the Rights of Persons with Disabilities. (2006). Retrieved from http://www.un.org/disabilities/documents/convention/convoptprot-e.pdf. On 15 Mar 2011

Werner D (1994) Disabled village children. Voluntary Health Association of India, New Delhi

World Bank Human Development Unit South Asia Region (2007) People with Disabilities in India: From Commitments to Outcomes. The World Bank, Washington, DC

World Bank Human Development Unit South Asia Region (2008) Skill development in India: the vocational education and training system. The World Bank, Washington, DC

Zeshan U, Vasishta M, Sethna M (2005) Implementation of Indian sign language in educational settings. Asia Pac Disabil Rehabil J 16(1):16–40

Nick Dupree

Abstract

This chapter is an autobiographical essay written by activist, writer and artist Nick Dupree. Dependent on mechanical ventilation for survival, Dupree worked to change Alabama Medicaid policy to allow him to live at home after he turned 21. Up until that time, ventilator-users in Alabama were routinely forced to move to out-of-state institutions once they reached adulthood. Dupree describes his experiences in higher education at Spring Hill College, and his decision to move to New York City in hopes of a more open, connected, loving existence. He moved into an institution in order to establish New York State residency and to qualify for community-based housing. Dupree concludes by recounting his experiences with the Occupy Wall Street Movement and how we can go further.

Keywords
Occupy Wall Street • Mechanical ventilation • Medicaid reform • Activism

I started out and made my name as a Medicaid reform activist in the foggy port city of Mobile, on the Alabama Gulf Coast, where I spent the entirety of my childhood, teen and college years inside or near Jesuit higher education at Spring Hill College. Martin Luther King praised Spring Hill in his *Letter from Birmingham Jail*[1] for

---

[1] The 1963 *Letter from Birmingham Jail*, a defense of direct action and confrontational nonviolence or the cause of civil rights, catalogued the ideas behind the Birmingham march and subsequent demonstrations, many of which were met with police brutality, including the use of fire hoses and attack dogs, infamously deployed by Birmingham Commissioner of Public Safety Eugene "Bull"

N. Dupree (✉)
VENTure Think Tank, Stony Brook University
e-mail: nick@nickscrusade.org

© Springer Science+Business Media Dordrecht 2016
P. Block et al. (eds.), *Occupying Disability: Critical Approaches to Community,
Justice, and Decolonizing Disability*, DOI 10.1007/978-94-017-9984-3_15

225

being the first university in the Deep South to integrate, to enroll black students. Growing up around Spring Hill College, where my mother taught studio art, I was exposed to the new ideas being discussed and developed in Jesuit thinking at that time (the mid-to-late 1980s) which included the struggle against dictators, death squads and associated authoritarian policies in Central America. During my time as a student in the opening years of the new millennium, formative moments included writing for *The Springhillian* college newspaper as the 9–11 terrorist attacks and subsequent two "land wars in Asia,"[2] first in Afghanistan, then Iraq, changed everything. The early months of "Nick's Crusade," my campaign to end Alabama Medicaid's policy of cutting off home care when people turn 21, made it into my *Springhillian* column as well. During the Crusade, I also used occasions when state and local leaders spoke on campus to introduce myself, ventilator and all, and tell them about the age 21 cut-off and its effects, that it would remove me from my home, my community, my college, and shove a flyer I'd written with bullet points on the *Olmstead* decision[3] into their hands. Later, in February 2003, Federal judge Mark Fuller in Montgomery oversaw a settlement in our favor without a trial, days before I was to lose coverage on my 21st birthday. The settlement included a new waiver program that allowed continued funding for vent-dependent Alabamians turning 21, allowing those like me who were "aging out" of coverage to maintain home care.

Unfortunately, because of flaws in the Medicaid system as a whole in Alabama and many other states, that it requires licensed nurses care for "ventilator patients" but doesn't pay enough to attract new nurses—Alabama pays just over half what New York Medicaid does—I found myself without nurses that could take me back and forth to campus. The contradiction of "victory" on the one hand, speaking and getting awards for activism at conferences dotting the East Coast and Midwest, while on the other hand, supports were disappearing beneath my feet and I was unable to sustain classes at the college I love, triggered a sort of "slow implosion" in my will to continue. At the time, I even felt that continuing might send a dishonest message—that the system is fixed when it is anything but. The physical and emotional exhaustion after fighting for the better part of 3 years, frantically writing and speaking against the 21 cut-off, was difficult enough. The fact that I faced the natural "comedown" after "victory" on top of my supports crumbling, that

---

Connor. Written by Rev. Martin Luther King Jr. on April 16, it preceded the "I Have A Dream" speech delivered on the National Mall on August 28 later that year.

[2]"Never get involved in a land war in Asia"—the most famous of the "classic blunders" mentioned by Vizzini in the film *The Princess Bride*.

[3]Olmstead v. L.C., 527 U.S. 581 is a landmark Supreme Court decision, issued June 22, 1999. In a majority opinion written by Ruth Bader Ginsburg, the court held that under the Americans with Disabilities Act, individuals with disabilities have the right to live in the community rather than in institutions if, "the State's treatment professionals have determined that community placement is appropriate, the transfer from institutional care to a less restrictive setting is not opposed by the affected individual, and the placement can be reasonably accommodated, taking into account the resources available to the State and the needs of others with mental disabilities."

I ended up with something worse than the status quo I'd been fighting for, and my college career evaporating in front of me, broke my heart.

I certainly pushed those around me for help, and there were a couple of near-misses with the advocacy community in Alabama trying to help me solve the problem of *after the crusading, what next?* Some proposals didn't miss; I worked with the ILC of Mobile[4] for a time and took part in some very fruitful collaborations. I still spoke publicly about my experiences with the 21 cut-off, the concerns of vent users, and the *Olmstead* decision, and I even had the chance to speak at Martin Luther King's church in Montgomery. My last major presentation was given in summer 2005 in Minneapolis.

In the 18 months or so following my "victory" I tended to ditch my nurses, or take a gap between nurses, and pile into the family van with Spring Hill friends and go to a movie or concert or just hang out on campus. In retrospect this was super dangerous, given ventilator technology's reliance on flimsy plastic tubes that tend to blow themselves off, though I did try to educate friends on the tubes and emergency bagging protocol. I got lucky and didn't die, though the first time I went out without a nurse the tube came off of the humidifier and Sarah Jane the 18 year-old freshman and Frankie the unlucky neighborhood guy with a mullet put it back on. Growing up on a ventilator means isolation. You must try to become a man (or woman) while many milestones of psycho-social development are delayed or blocked by the unusual levels of medical supervision required to maintain survival on a ventilator. Knowing that many of the milestones and rites of passage of young-adulthood are largely off-limits to you, would you give up on extraordinary efforts to interact with peers? If not, how far would you go for opportunities for human contact? Sometimes breaking the isolation is more important than avoiding risk. Despite the rule-bending involved and an acute awareness that the bulk of college life would be out of reach, I judged opportunities to connect with others as worth a lot of risk. Human connection is what makes life worth living, and without it it's difficult to justify continuing the daily battle that is living with mechanical ventilation.

I ended up learning that while Catholic students easily understood that I'm a living soul, and that being pro-life easily led them to the idea that helping disabled people *live* is a good thing, a few personal connections and understandings don't necessarily translate to the will, time, resources or ability necessary to form a "circle of support" that can drive you around and help you access the community and achieve goals. I learned about the concept of the "circle of support" at the two TASH[5] conferences I attended, the idea being that even in states without much funding for supports, family and friends can share the load. But after over a year trying to build a mini-version of this, I had succeeded only sporadically. Living off campus was a constant barrier. Though some of them did a great deal with me, every last one of my Spring Hill friends left the city after graduation. With the last threads of my lifetime connection with the Jesuit learning environment suddenly gone I slid

---

[4] Independent Living Center of Mobile (Mobile, Alabama).

[5] An international disability advocacy organization, see http://tash.org/about/

deeper and deeper into despair. Inner resources aren't inexhaustible. Lacking a plan
B or plan C, I really shut down. Finding no path out and little "fight" left inside me,
I avoided struggle and confrontation as much as I could and became very secluded.
Especially after 2005, after two category 5 hurricanes in as many years (Ivan and
Katrina) wreaked havoc on my city, I went into a bitter hibernation of sorts, and
illness followed the despair like a running back follows openings in the defensive
line. I needed the system to understand the needs beyond the body, my drive to see
and do and learn. It seemed the thing I'd fought so hard for, the nursing and the
waiver with all its assumptions that the best thing for me and the others breathing
on ventilators was to be stuck at home with a nurse for the rest of our days, was
running counter to what I really wanted, to create a better life. Leaving my family
and all my connections on the Gulf coast behind, despite being really aware that I
was more privileged than nearly any vent-dependent person in the South and would
be seen as spurning my own victory, was the most difficult decision I've ever made.

We need a Medicaid system that understands that there's a human spirit. Failing
that, we need communities, religious and otherwise, that understand that there's
a human spirit. Failing that, or preferably, in addition to that, we need small
groups of dedicated people who understand that there's a human spirit, groups
that can form the foundation of a new movement. I propose a new, deeply human
movement, that is built around the human dignity inherent in the disabled person
and all mankind, and, in the spirit of *Occupy Sandy*, will "be the change,"[6] leading
empathic actions on the ground and in person, communicating and connecting with
the most marginalized and disconnected, taking their stories "viral." We must strike
the empathic chords within the human spirit, remind people of their humanity. In
speeches, Chris Hedges often references the violinist that appeared in the subway
during the worst ethnic cleansing of the Bosnian conflict in the 1990s, playing
beautiful classical pieces, reminding everyone that there are other things to listen
to besides Slobodan Milošević's warmongering state TV and hate radio, and that
we can still be human. These small acts of resistance should be the main aim of
our new movement beyond Occupy because they're so powerful. In a situation
where both national political parties have embraced an economic system that
rewards institutionalized lack of empathy, wherein the CEOs that prey on subprime
mortgages, lay off the most workers or pull off the worst leveraged buy-outs always
end up on top, it's a time when alternate cultural narratives are badly needed. When
the culture itself is increasingly lack empathy, we desperately need a movement
that is more social and cultural in its direction. And providing another *way to be*
can be as simple as an internet meme or youtube video that demonstrates empathy,
kindness or our human love for the arts.

---

[6]This Gandhi quote, "Be the change you wish to see in the world," turns out to have been massaged
for bumper stickers. What Gandhi really said "If we could change ourselves, the tendencies in the
world would also change. As a man changes his own nature, so does the attitude of the world
change towards him. ... We need not wait to see what others do." http://www.nytimes.com/2011/
08/30/opinion/falser-words-were-never-spoken.html

I moved to New York City in August 2008 in hopes of a more open, connected, loving existence, which despite many difficulties and unexpected complications, has succeeded. Despite all the speeches I'd given against institutions, I put myself in a state rehab hospital, directly from LaGuardia Airport to unit A-13, because Medicaid rules required this so I could establish residency, eligibility and eventually obtain the needed home care. I've learned a lot since moving to the big city. Less than 30 days after I landed in New York City, the economy began to go belly up, and I saw every aspect of the world change. The financial crisis of late 2008 changed everything, a rare off-road swerve from our historical trajectory, a move that was especially devastating in New York City. City hospitals began to crumble in a serious way. Several important hospitals closed. The crisis is obvious at a glance at the population of Bellevue, where overcrowding is increasingly visible in every department as alternate public hospitals disappear.

I was in a state hospital on the island in the East River named after President Franklin Delano Roosevelt (the 1940s US President who had polio) realizing that everything had changed.

A few months later, when I applied for affordable housing, I got a rejection letter. It said that the Section 8 (subsidized) housing benefit list had been closed since 2006, and "your application has been destroyed." In the United States government's "Fiscal Cliff" Bill that came together at the end of 2012, the investment giant and demonic "great vampire squid"[7] Goldman Sachs got subsidized housing for their building in Manhattan (triple tax exempt, no local, state or federal taxes, plus they got Liberty Bonds, that were only supposed to be used for the reconstruction of the World Trade Center complex). Even in a time of supposed austerity.

If it weren't for a series of serendipitous and bizarre events that made it possible to move in with Alejandra (my partner), who has affordable housing through a different, local, program, I'd still be in the facility. I've lived here since September 10th 2009, in Lower Manhattan. I am bizarrely lucky, and know it. And I'm very grateful. Living in the facility, the fact that most of my fellow patients had no hope of ever getting out, that the system is never going to respond, that I got out due to LUCK, was very clear to me.

We live very close to Zuccotti Park, so we observed the Occupy Wall Street 2012 movement closely. Alejandra and I are part of the Occupy "disability caucus," trying to bring disability issues to the attention of the wider movement. Just holding meetings where people with disabilities can talk openly about their predicament following the collapse of the economy has been very valuable; our concerns never see the light of day in media and political circles, but we have the beginning of a movement that expresses the realities of the problems we face.

---

[7]*Rolling Stone*'s Matt Taibbi once famously described Goldman Sachs as "a great vampire squid wrapped around the face of humanity, relentlessly jamming its blood funnel into anything that smells like money." Taibbi's description inspired Occupy to pioneer a new form of creative protest—"Squidding," the act of protesting Goldman Sachs HQ with giant squid props or squid costumes.

Occupy Wall Street is a reaction to the economic system dying, its apparent murder via mismanagement, malfeasance and predation shoving it off the cliff. There's no complex list of demands. It's a protest of the crimes of the bad actors of Wall Street, the resulting collapse of the economy and the attendant suffering, and our political system's inability to respond effectively aside from aiding the bad actors. The worst elements in our economy received generous corporate welfare programs like TARP—"Troubled Asset Relief Program"—plus "reforms" with obscure passages that enshrined certain banks by name as "Too Big to Fail," and the Affordable Care Act, which requires every American to buy health insurance from select companies. These things cry out for a protest movement to oppose them. I see Occupy as a breath of fresh air, a healthy immune response to injustice, a sign society is still alive. And the grievances highlighted by the movement resonate deeply with me and many other young people who have fought to circumvent systems that confine them, who yearn for more.

The security establishment (NYPD [New York Police Department], FBI, etc.) seemed to respond to Occupy's protests against the obviously harmful practices of corporations like Goldman Sachs as a direct attack on the state itself. Though it was called Occupy Wall Street, the NYPD never let the protesters get near Wall Street around the New York Stock Exchange (NYSE). They cordoned off the area around the NYSE building and sent a very clear and violent message whenever Occupiers tried—in non-violent marches—to get past the barricade. Several times, I saw Occupiers, by the thousands—amazingly strong numbers—cross in front of our apartment building to get closer to Wall Street. The most violent responses from the NYPD came in these moments, that's when the tear gas and rubber bullets came out, officers breaking heads and mounted police blocking streets with highly coordinated Roman-style formations. I learned a lot from this. It seemed very important to the police that they protect the people in and around the NYSE from even seeing the protests. They also—in the final weeks of the occupations in Lower Manhattan— had a new satellite-dish-looking technology that disabled cell phones, cameras, and other digital devices, so the more violent incidents couldn't be photographed or documented in any way. I shudder to guess what these devices would do to a digital ventilator like mine. I was texting a friend when one of the jamming devices blocked her phone at a protest near Trinity Church.

But we clearly have much more to do. Something is very wrong when the Affordable Care Act, which, at its core is *$400 billion* in subsidies to the dying private health insurance industry, is embraced as "liberal." When people buying private insurance online—and, in many instances, spending more on insurance than they ever had previously—is heralded as a *once in a lifetime* progressive victory on the left and derided as a socialist plot on the right, you know we've fallen through the looking glass into a new and bizarre political unreality. For me, the most frustrating part of the Affordable Care Act and the ugly legislative sausage-making that birthed it is its failure to prioritize the most disabled and most vulnerable, leaving those who are in poverty because of serious disability and/or chronic illness to make due with increasingly underfunded Medicaid and Medicare systems. The "middle class" is targeted for subsidies, though even the subsidized folk must fork over big money to buy insurance on the exchanges, the most needy get the cold shoulder. We watch helplessly as Medicare and Medicaid are hit with sequester cuts and new restrictive regulations. Meanwhile, ill-informed pundits oppose ObamaCare because it has supposedly given people free health insurance or helped the poor too much. The Affordable Care Act doesn't address any of the long-term care problems and Medicaid issues I have fought to bring to light over the years. Instead, it is almost solely about federal cash propping up zombie health insurance, as jobs increasingly no longer provide health insurance.

Occupy gives voice to the true concerns of those hit hardest by the financial crisis, who are disproportionately Americans with disabilities, a desperately needed counterpoint to an administration that has been largely silent on issues of poverty. But we need to go further, and challenge the corporate culture and the commoditization of everything that underlies our skewed economic and social system. A system that grants subsidized housing to Goldman Sachs while denying it to people with disabilities suggests a deeper problem than corrupt politicians. It suggests a cultural sickness. The messages coming in via mass corporate culture are usually the exact opposite of the inherent value of human life, humans having inherent value and sanctity and dignity. Instead, the only value on display is what you produce, your income, or how ruthless you are. It bombards us constantly like the TVs in Orwell's Nineteen-Eighty-Four you can never turn off. The messages we've become acculturated with, have resulted in our loosening our grip on the moral imperatives we must hold fast to . . . .

I would argue that disability activists, and on a deeper level, the disabled person, provide a powerful counter narrative to the prevailing messaging. That we participate in society, that even the most disabled and those of us on ventilators are active in the public sphere in-and-of-itself implies that there is more to life than the external, that the soul and human dignity exist outside of the material, outside of the typical notions of success or the newest consumer goods. Our success shifting the culture to a healthier state will depend upon how broadly we can extend the tent of human dignity, how well we provide an obvious, powerful alternative that grants refuge from the corrosive waters of the mainstream. Protestant existentialist theologian Paul Tillich, in his essay *The Person in a Technical Society*, provides an example of the moral thinking our new movements need:

> The person as a person can preserve himself only by a partial non-participation in the objectifying structures of technical society. But he can withdraw even partially only if he has a place to which to withdraw.
> . . . It is the task of the Church, especially of its theology, to describe the place of withdrawal.[8]

Without discounting the important role "the Church" and religious life can play in providing space outside of the dehumanizing forces of mass, technological society

---

[8]Tillich. "Christian Faith and Social Action: A Symposium." *The Person in a Technical Society*, Edited by John A. Hutchinson, 137. Scribner, 1953.

and the positive push for change preachers, priests, rabbis and Buddhist monks can lead, I'd propose that the disability community already offers a certain special social space, a place of refuge from the "objectifying structures of technical society," and thus we would make an ideal core to build new regional and national movements around.

Occupy Wall Street successors need to come into the streets, there have to be outlets for the real grievances of real people, but much more is needed. Beyond Occupy, we need the kind of movements that articulate the true concerns of the poor and disabled in language that flows from the conscience and moral imperatives that can't be denied. Movements with human dignity behind them, like Solidarity in 1980s Poland or the Arab Spring, that "go viral" across broad swaths of society or entire regions became they tap into some intolerable affront to human dignity or some universal value, are what's needed.

In the case of the Arab Spring, a poor Tunisian fruit vendor self-immolated after harassment and disrespect from a corrupt policewoman pushed him too far, sparking protests that, further fueled by leaked diplomatic cables published through WikiLeaks exposing U.S. knowledge of and complicity with the corrupt Tunisian regime, forced the government to resign. What went "viral" following the dramatic events of December 2010, the self-immolation, the protests, the ouster of Tunisian President Zine El Abidine Ben Ali, was what I see as almost an "Islamic liberation theology." The Arab Spring erupted when the friction between Islamic values and the realities of life under the corrupt regimes in the region became too great, the depredations of dictators and their cronies increasingly irreconcilable with Islam, shared beliefs too threatened. The contradiction finally became unsustainable when the affront to Islamic values struck chords within every segment of society, unearthing grievances everywhere, from poverty and hunger to calls from more conservative Islamist-oriented factions about traditional gender roles—the Tunisian policewoman triggered a cultural backlash that resonated with Islamist groups across the Arab world—concerns that seem incompatible with Western values but nonetheless proved pivotal within the Islamic societies involved. Society wide uprisings like the ones seen at some early moments of the Arab Spring are incredibly rare. We should be sensitive to the fact that the Arab Spring sprung from many of the same issues that caused revolutions in the Arab world centuries ago—regimes and cultural excesses perceived as gone too far—and thus its effect on women, religious minorities and other vulnerable groups is questionable in many instances. But without erasing our concerns over the deeply problematic side effects of Islamic revolutions, we can learn important lessons from the Arab Spring.

One of its most important lessons is the pivotal role cultural narratives play. Multiple regimes were forced out because, at root, they contradicted the narrative people heard at their local mosque. The West needs a viral narrative that contradicts our corrupt regimes, something that resonates across all segments of society with values we share. Those values may have to be rebuilt as a counter-culture of sorts, an alternative to the materialistic, anti-empathy mainstream. And people with disabilities should be part of the new narrative, as we offer proof that existence outside of mainstream notions and materialistic norms is possible just by continuing to actively participate in our communities.

Editors' Postscript If you liked this chapter by Nick Dupree, and are interested in reading more about disability, protest and activism we recommend Chap. 2 "Krips, Cops and Occupy: Reflections from Oscar Grant Plaza" by Sunaura Taylor with Marg Hall, Jessica Lehman, Rachel Liebert, Akemi Nishida, and Jean Stewart; Chap. 4 "Movements at War? Disability and Anti-Occupation Activism in Israel" by Liat Ben-Moshe, and Chap. 21 "Black & Blue: Policing Disability & Poverty Beyond Occupy" by Leroy Franklin Moore Jr., Lisa 'Tiny' Garcia, and Emmitt Thrower.

Beyond Policy—A Real Life Journey of Engagement and Involvement

16

Stephanie de la Haye

Abstract

Despite the presence and growth of the service user (ie those who have experienced mental health and physical disabilities) movement health and social care, people with lived experience of disabilities still have limited involvement in delivery policy, research or development. So how do people who have multiple disadvantages influence health policy when professionals and policy makers have not grasped the importance of inclusion? This chapter describes some of the author's experiences gained from campaigning for user engagement and involvement in the UK health system and university cultures.

Keywords

Service user movement • Policy • Research • Inclusion

16.1 In Context

There is nothing more unequal than the equal treatment of unequal people. (Thomas Jefferson, US President)

How do we as people who have multiple disadvantages have a real say and influence health policy at all levels? The service user movement has been gaining strength for some years and is now starting to develop a real momentum, but with one important caveat—health and social care professionals and policy makers in the main continue to create a "tick box" type of involvement culture. Many, although without malice, do not really understand or place the importance of a person with

S. de la Haye (✉)
Independent User Consultant, Educator and Researcher in Mental Health, Sheffield Hallam University, Sheffield, UK
e-mail: stephanie@bbn.uk.com

lived experience of disability, both mentally or physically, being included in all aspects of delivery, policy and development. This has improved over time, but tends to be found in silos rather than within general practice, which would give so much more fundamental empowerment to individuals.

One recent example is of a research lead not having a basic grasp of why they should create equality within a research team when users are a "core" part of the group. They are not, and indeed are somewhat treated as if they should be grateful to be there. Where does this come from? In the main, and in this instance, institutional inequality and a lack of understanding of the principles and practice in which individuals can make a full and marked difference within academia predominates.

Many sections of our society have had to campaign and fight for their rights over the centuries from slavery, to gay, lesbian, bisexual & transgender people to mental health issues and physical disability, and why? Well, because of the range of attitudes describing them as 'being different' within society or just 'not fitting in,' everything from a lack of understanding or education to outright prejudice and vilification. Of course some people do not necessarily have an outward appearance of say physical disability, so the hidden types of illnesses which cause the individual a great deal of pain and suffering can go unnoticed by the general population but still cause a multitude of potential hurdles the person has to 'jump' over to receive treatment and understanding.

16.2   Journey

My personal journey began when I was 17 and developed post viral chronic fatigue syndrome, which also led to other mental health issues. I was thrown into a world of unknown treatment, discrimination, and fighting to gain support which continued for 25 years. As an athlete in my early days most of my time was taken up with training and my life was a daily regime of exercise and strict diet. Until one day after two rather nasty viral infections, my body stopped working while riding my bike and I collapsed. This event transformed my life. (As I write this the Paralympic Games are currently under way and I think about those people who are now competing after gaining a disability after being abled bodied). So, I had no diagnosis as Chronic Fatigue Syndrome, or Myalgic Encephalopathy as it's now known, was not really in the headlines during the early 1980s within the UK. Then it was called "yuppie flu" and the like, with no real understanding of the condition. There has been a great deal of acceptance by medical professionals and the National Health Service that the condition is real but currently it has no real cure. People with the condition continue with ongoing treatment by specialist practitioners.

So I had a real fight on my hands to cope with something people did not understand or even see as an illness. Mental health issues then developed and so created more stigma and discrimination around my condition. My life seemed to be a battle, in and out of hospital, lack of support from even the medical professionals in whom I had trust. I did come across professionals who seemed to go beyond their roles as clinicians. This gave me some hope that I had a future and would not just be cared for.

When you have condition/s for which the "cure" does not exist, as there is not one, what is highlighted is the sometimes futile efforts you make in trying to manage and move forward. Acceptance of the condition, by yourself and others who are supporting you is key at this point, and this took some time after being so physically active. Many people have this experience, but some don't accept they have to adapt and change their lives to create something they can believe in and make inroads into their condition. There is no doubt that doing this is no easy task. Having to then rely on the local health services, and seemingly hitting those walls of ignorance and misunderstanding does take some effort. An example of this was when consulting with my general practitioner at the time, whose idea of recovery was to say to me "you should get a job that will sort you out." While I agree that work in all its forms improves your well-being, to say this to a person who needs support does not create a recovery. Another example of practitioners' fears around mental health was to be asked about my physical issues, but then when mentioning the dreaded words, "mental health issues," she looked at me and shrugged her shoulders and said "well, what do you want me to do?"

Not even a tissue when I burst into tears!

When you're unwell trying to negotiate the "care system" can seem an impossible task, with the bureaucracy, red tape, form filing, poor policy and just people seemingly against you every way you turn. My personal policy was to fight my way through this maze, and I was determined to get the support I needed, even *expected,* and not be left on the shelf. This battle lasted for some 15 years and I gained much in the way of positive outcomes as well as negative ones! I now understand that for me this was going to be my life's work in supporting others and developing, influencing and changing policy and professional practice. This was certainly not a route I expected after still managing to study at university.

16.3   What Is Policy?

According to the World Health Organization's (2014) web site health policy

"refers to decisions, plans, and actions that are undertaken to achieve specific health care goals within a society. An explicit health policy can achieve several things: it defines a vision for the future which in turn helps to establish targets and points of reference for the short and medium term. It outlines priorities and the expected roles of different groups; and it builds consensus and informs people." (www.who.int/topics/health_policy/en)

And according to the Department of Health's (2010) web site in the United Kingdom –

"Making and implementing policy is a key strand of the Department of Health's work. Their policies are designed to improve on existing arrangements in health and social care, and turn political vision into actions that should benefit staff, patients and the public. They aim to ensure services funded or supported by the Department are delivered in the most responsive, flexible and patient-centered way."

Underpinning this are the articles taken from the universal declaration of human rights (UN 1948), *Article 25*:

"Everyone has the right to a standard of living adequate for the health and well-being of himself and of his family, including food, clothing, housing and medical care and necessary social services, and the right to security in the event of unemployment, illness, disability, widowhood, old age or other lack of livelihood in circumstances beyond his control."

Health policy generally starts from the national government of the country and the concepts are drafted by politicians and civil servants, with "robust" consultation with professionals, carers and users of the services as well as the general public. The use of robust consultation can be deemed by some as a point of tension in that many policy decisions seem to be a "done deal" and further discussions will not in fact change the decision already made at a higher political level. In theory and on paper this may be the ideal way of developing or changing current policy drivers to create a better health service.

Some inroads have been made in the past decade to involve and include people in real and meaningful consultations, sometimes these individuals or groups can be the same ones that always get involved and the people who don't get a voice miss out. This tends to be minority groups, those who are the ones using the systems and those who the new policy will affect the most. One useful example of this within the mental health field is the fight to have advocacy within the English Mental Health Act. After many years of campaigning by individuals and an alliance of charity groups the role of Independent Mental Health Advocates is now a legal right for a person who is detained under the Mental Health Act 1983 (amended 2007) (UK Government 2007).

Another national example is of the National Survivors User Network (2014) who have members on the ministerial mental health advisory committee, who help to advise the government on all matters related to mental health policy and development. Carr (2004) asks whether service user participation has made a difference to social care services? Efforts to involve people in the planning and development of the services they use are taking place across the UK. However, the impact of that participation on the change and improvement of social care services is yet to be properly monitored and evaluated. Much progress has been made in establishing the principle of service user participation and developing ways of doing this. There is now a second stage that will entail looking at how organizations, systems and practice need to change in order to respond to participation.

16.4 Influencing Policy

My theory on how to influence policy and create real meaningful participation must include the 3 levels of development: national, regional and local drivers. Currently in the UK the government is driving towards local community empowerment and has reduced regional influence but with accountability to national policy. Being involved with all the levels of development is very much a spinning plates type of concept as it's not the easiest thing to do, and you could just focus on say local policy within your health trust or elected council. I wanted to gather the whole picture and how the national policy developments then effect the local actions in health and social care.

I placed myself within boards nationally and regionally and then became involved with the local mental health National Health Service (NHS) trust. I did this by applying to sit on, for instance, the national mental health board in order to have a voice, and from that I was elected onto the local mental health trusts Service User & Carer Council which gave me a seat on the main board. This gave me not only influence but the ability to disseminate views from other users of the service and to make sure people who did not have a voice were able to give views and opinions. I was elected and as a representative of many individuals' views and frustrations, I was able to present these to the managing board. There is a continuing problem that the loudest voice gets through and those who are isolated or do not have the confidence will be silent. The picture is not of perfection but one of trying to create equal opportunities and gaining views from all of the diverse members of the community.

In rather an extreme example, I know of one person who was asked to sit on a panel made up of consultant health professionals discussing very complex issues such a medication and therapeutic models. She was thrust into this panel without training or real support and as a result found it completely impossible to be an equal, rather than a token user of the service parachuted in.

My experience of national boards and committees has been less than positive due to a tick box culture and the feeling that I was not actually being taken seriously. Do we just include people with disability in talks only to create a less than favorable environment to gather vital information they can bring to the table? One particular example of this was an individual who was asked to attend a high level group within the mental health field to give their views as a user of services. Without a real induction or training the person was thrust to a table with clinicians and academics and the outcome was for the person to walk out in tears as they were not able to deal with the nature of the discussions and the environment. Society does not want to set people up to fail at the first hurdle and then put them off being involved again. So why did this happen? Ticking the box comes to mind, and lack of insight and understanding around the needs of someone who could have given so much to the debate.

With the correct support, training, possible mentor or buddy this could have been prevented and the outcome very different indeed. Personally I have had positive experiences as well, but these tended to be down to one individual who went beyond their normal duties to create and develop a package of support and understanding that ultimately gave me more choice and control over what I did. At all levels, but in particular nationally, the system itself tends to put pressure on how involvement is conducted. National guidelines have a mixed picture in their accuracy and are not focused on what happens on the ground. Many are just put off being engaged or involved as people bring very complex issues. In addition being involved can affect welfare benefits.

Claiming payments can be a real issue that affects the individual, it puts people off. People come from different backgrounds and some will be happy to volunteer through to individuals who are self-employed. They should be getting paid as anyone else who is involved to share their views and real understanding of what it's like to live with a particular disability or health issue. Something you cannot learn from academic literature and lectures is the "expert by experience" skills and knowledge. Having lived through a particular experience creates an understanding that while you may read about it cannot be replicated by another. Each personal journey is unique and while they may have common threads, personal characteristics that someone can express within the development of policy or participation are important, this person is an expert in their own right and should be treated as such.

While I have said the three tiers of policy/participation are all critical, I will focus on local development. This is a major issue now in the UK with the new Health & Social Care Act (UK Government 2012) and the government's devolution of power to local communities. NHS trusts have become foundation trusts[1] which are meant to have more autonomy and can use the money they receive within the local drivers rather than the more top down drivers of the past, i.e. Central government.

New clinical commissioning groups led by general practitioners (GP's) who will have 80 % of the NHS budget should have started by April 2013. These and others will affect the involvement of users of services locally both within the NHS trusts and the local authority. Sadly the changes in health structure have created an even more complex set of health bodies than before. The only way that robust, real engagement will happen is to make sure the people know and understand what is happening and how it will work (or not, as the case may be!) At the time of writing the new health commissioning bodies are only just starting to publicly show their new regimes and policies. It is not yet clear how people will be involved across the health sector and there are concerns that some best practice may be lost due to lack of funding and other priorities taking precedence. Another development in the UK health environment is the rise in private companies winning tenders for work previously carried out by the NHS or the voluntary sector. This can be deemed a "privatisation" of the health service, which many people do not agree with, due to the undercutting of services, so potentially reducing the level of care. Of course we cannot say all private organizations are just out to make a fast buck!

As an example of local policy change, while being involved with the local NHS trust some years ago I received a letter from the trust explaining that I had an appointment to see a health professional but this was for 5 months ahead. My thoughts were, "well what if I was not involved in other aspects of mental health support, how would I feel about this? If the person needed support now not in 5 months, what can they do in the meantime?" The letter offered no other options, or signposting to a support group in the community sector or similar in the meantime. I was very surprised and indeed angry. So I recorded my frustration by calling a

---

[1]Foundation trusts were first established in 2002 and were intended to bring about patient led structures within the NHS in the UK, some of them adopting co-operative structures.

lead health professional and gained a meeting with the appropriate head of service who agreed that the trust needed to send some details and contact numbers with a standard letter of this type. This has now been part of the policy since and although very simple to do was highlighted by a user of the service.

I have talked about policy and involvement within service providers or national policy generating groups, but another area which should involve users of service is research. This of course has influence on policy and a good example is the Increasing Access to Psychological Therapies (IAPT) (Department of Health 2008). This mainly uses a cognitive behavior therapy base which is supported by research data.

My experience of being part of a university health research team is mixed, but one positive example is with a national review of independent mental health advocacy. The process in the first instance was of inclusion and equality and this came across from the academic team and principle investigator.

An induction for the whole research team included in-depth paperwork and training in which I was asked to deliver in part as I had previous experience training the mental health advocates with the department of health. Procedures were very clear and although the university's protocol in general can be complicated and not very flexible, many issues were discussed and sorted with the academic team at an early stage. Universities tend to have very complex systems and this does not always help the expert by experience navigate the system. Support must include being an equal within teams and with proactive work on sorting systems out beforehand to make for a smoother working relationship. A good example of this was the associate staff card. One of the academic leads had already created an agreed system for experts to be granted a card with no red tape getting in the way.

As the project progressed the communication was good and this made sure everyone knew their roles and how they were progressing. With regular team meetings and reflection people were well engaged and felt supported. Many of the service users of the team led parts of the research, such as interviewing and focus groups, which created a stage for inclusion. During dissemination stages of the research individual service user members were asked what they would like to do and be lead on in terms of writing in journals, workshops etc. The principal research lead took a step back, which for some lead academics is a challenge indeed.

In comparison, with another university, when I was engaged part way through the research I did not have a robust induction with no real paperwork to refer back to. I found it very difficult to access some of the aspects which I had automatically been able to do in other research. Some of this was due to global university policy (which varies greatly across establishments) and some due to managers not creating a full and equal framework for individuals to access and feel more supported. This can happen for many reasons such as pressure of the deadlines and budgets to managers just not understanding issues faced by their fellow service user researchers. I was indeed on the verge of stepping back from the research.

A positive resolution to this came about with a meeting to discuss the issues, such as access to a university ID card and then to create an action plan to resolve as much as possible within the department. The ID card was a university-wide issue as I did not fit into its neat sections of employment. This needed higher influence to reconfigure. The key points about this process were that at least managers were listening and developing action points. This solved many of the problems I faced around communication, inclusion, and equality within the team, an example being access to resources such as the journals on line and library.

It can't be underestimated that relatively minor points can cause the service user researcher to feel less than equal in this situation and this is why all teams must be prepared to labor and resolve the key points.

16.5   Beyond Policy

The polices which we follow and are guided by are ever changing and must be seen as a fluid and adaptable item, which may or may not have had robust consultation with users of service. They should not be deemed to be written in stone and have a fixed non movable nature. Fixed policies do not respect the needs of individuals, and most people have individual needs. It's quite likely that they will fall outside the scope of narrow or inflexible provision in which organizations and individuals have to follow, potentially creating less of an equal playing field or clarity around the engagement of people who are experts by experience. I remember one of my professors at university who said "books, journals and publications are only someone's view of the world and are not necessarily right" the same of course goes for policy.

The question then arises how do we create a culture of equality for people who have some disadvantage in life? We start at the beginning and to make sure people are included in the initial concepts of policy development not just at the final process. Organizations must have the common thread of involvement & engagement embedded within all aspects of the institution or government body, where from the Chief Executive Officer and chairperson to the front line staff all have a passion and drive for inclusion. Making sure it's real, not just a shiny publication that looks great, but sits on the shelf gathering dust. This is a job for everyone and the culture may need to shift which can be very challenging for individuals and organizations as a whole, but can be made real if the drive for change is apparent. To give an example, a mental health trust had a historical lack of involvement and procedures in engaging with its users and carers. A new CEO and Chairman on the board both had a real commitment to turn this around. They considered the need for a user and carer council in which the trust would invest. This was not only set up, but from it a sense of culture change was apparent which was fed down to all areas of the trust. It was not without its issues but gave a real voice to people who were not only isolated but their illness meant their health fluctuated and found it challenging to engage. So both culture and investment were initiated by key people within the organization.

People are the experts not only in their own disability or health issues, and also know what is needed to create an environment in which they would feel happy to contribute to debate, policy, and service reform. Many of these aspects are not actually difficult to do and just need some thought and reflection of making sure they are applied. A very good example if this are the payment systems for service users that are used by some organizations. These may well have options such as being involved as a volunteer, making a small one off payment or indeed paying by invoice as someone may be freelance or self-employed, down to making sure people have the taxi fare in cash to get to a venue. This may seem very simple but in many organizations people have had to wait a month or more and go through the accounts system to receive the £5 it cost for travel. While many organizations policies do not allow them to do this, some voluntary organizations can give cash on the day. This comes down to organizations being more flexible. While accounting systems may be complex and have to follow national legislation and guidance, if the will is there it can be managed and changed.

16.6   What Works?

Of course engaging experts by experience to deliver training within organizations around inclusion and equality is the gold standard and many examples of this have been found. One very interesting case involves a NHS trust who had some involvement but a was long way from best practice. By creating new policies for people to be involved with the induction process for new staff, training teams, being part of the training of health professionals it created, if but slowly, a culture where staff expected input by the ex/users of the service. When given a lecture by a mixture of presenters they said it was in fact the users' talk which provided the most powerful and thought provoking stories and gave them better understanding of the issues people really face.

Top ten tips for inclusion and collaboration I believe are:

1. Involvement from the start of any research (ideally).
2. Creating an equal platform with users and academics/managers.
3. Clear and robust induction.
4. Getting the communication right.
5. Getting the payment systems correct before you start.
6. Creating a team that works- regular team meetings and development-collaboration is key.
7. Addressing issues as you go and not leaving to fester.
8. Academics & Managers letting go a bit more.
9. Service users/researchers being able to adapt and not expect everything will go right.
10. Being open and transparent.

So its takes drive and a willingness to create the procedures and policy to develop the inclusive and supporting environment people must have to be able to contribute effectively and to sustain this engagement. Individuals need to feel that they are not just a tick in a box and that their involvement will make a real difference. This applies to everyone in the health and social care setting whether social workers or occupational therapists to clinical psychiatrists to managers and chief executives.

Everyone has a part to play in the creation of a system that automatically refers and includes the users of services. The more we do this the more it becomes ingrained in the culture of organizations and individuals. With one caveat though, to make sure that continued development and drive for best practice is carried out and not to become complacent.

On reflection, in my own personal experience these initiatives can work and people can influence policy. Why should we have to resort to marching down the streets and demonstrations to get heard or our views across? While this may be of use when pushed into a corner and indeed long term radical action may be needed to actually change for the better, we should not have to do this. Making sure people are seated at the table and are included in discussions, and people listen and create action that individuals can see actually happening is vital. We also must remember the fine line we tread when dealing with government policy- while we need to be a critical friend we do not cross the line to become just another part of the establishment. Having the independence is a critical feature in all this potential change. I have seen people and organizations that start off with the best intentions but then get absorbed in the system and then their credibility is lost.

For my own personal journey I have come across many negative attitudes and stone walls which needed knocking down. Saying this, those organizations and individuals who actually engaged and went beyond their roles to create the positive change made such a difference. Recovery can also be a part of this process if implemented in the right way and helps with healing and management of health conditions.

There is a huge resource of people out there who have gained experiential knowledge of their own health and disability. Make sure that the core part of any policy and practice is to involve and engage these people in order to develop the core needs of health professionals' research projects and training. Not everyone will want to be involved but give them the choice and they will take you from textbook theory to real life and beyond.

Editors' Postscript If you liked Chap. 16 by Stephanie de la Haye, and are interested in reading more about psychiatric rights, we recommend Chap. 8 "Artistic Therapeutic Treatment, Colonialism & Spectacle: A Brazilian Tale" by Marta Simões Peres; Francine Albiero de Camargo; José Otávio P. e Silva; Pamela Block. If you are interested in reading more about grassroots action to influence policy, read Chap. 12: "Refusing to Go Away: The Ida Benderson Seniors Action Group" by Denise M. Nepveux. If you would like to read more about forms of psychiatric survivor empowerment, we suggest you read Chap. 23: Surviving Stevenage, by Stevenage Survivors. If you would like to read more about mental disabilities and changing institutional cultures, read Chap. 6: "Occupying Autism: Rhetoric, Involuntarity, and the Meaning of Autistic Lives, by Melanie Yergeau."

References

Carr S (2004) Has service user participation made a difference to social care services? Social Care Institute for Excellence, London

Department of Health (2008) Improving access to psychological therapies commissioning toolkit. Department of health, London

Department of Health (2010) Policy development. http://webarchive.nationalarchive.gov.uk/+/www.dh.gov.uk/en/aboutus/howdhworks/dh_074362

National Survivors User Network (2014). www.nsun.org.uk. Accessed 31 July 2014

UK Government (2007) Mental health act 2007. http://www.legislation.gov.uk/ukpga/2007/12/contents. Accessed 31 July 2014

UK Government (2012) The health and social care act 2012. http://www.legislation.gov.uk/ukpga/2012/7/contents/enacted. Accessed 31 July 2014

United Nations (1948) Universal declaration of human rights. http://www.un.org/en/documents/udhr/index.shtml#a25. Accessed 31 July 2014

World Health Organization on Policy. http://www.who.int/en/. Accessed 31 July 2014

Self Advocacy and Self Determination for Youth with Disability and Their Parents During School Transition Planning

17

Eva L. Rodriguez

Abstract

This chapter provides a critical account of legal, policy and practical ways that US school systems prepare children for transition to adulthood. School transition processes are meant to support students as they move from secondary education (high school) to university-level education, vocational training, employment or community placement. Rodriguez writes from the perspective of a parent of a child with a learning disability and a pediatric occupational therapist with decades of experience in the United States school system at primary, middle and high school levels. She discusses current systemic practices which are lacking, and offers suggestions of ways to encourage self-advocacy and self-determination for students and parents.

Keywords

Special education • Office of Special Education Programs • Individualized educational program • Committee on special education • Parent advocacy • Self-advocacy • Self-determination

In this chapter, I will be discussing legal, policy, and practical aspects of how children with disability are prepared by school systems to transition from secondary education (high school) to university-level education, vocational training, employment or community placement. I am writing both the parent of an adolescent child with a learning disability and a pediatric occupational therapist with decades of experience in the United States school system at primary, middle and high

E.L. Rodriguez (✉)
Occupational Therapy Program, Stony Brook University, Stony Brook, NY, USA
e-mail: eva.rodriguez@stonybrook.edu

© Springer Science+Business Media Dordrecht 2016   247
P. Block et al. (eds.), *Occupying Disability: Critical Approaches to Community, Justice, and Decolonizing Disability*, DOI 10.1007/978-94-017-9984-3_17

school levels. I assert that the systems currently in place to support students and parents do not encourage self-advocacy and self-determination and I will be making suggestions as to how this can change.

In 2004, the Office of Special Education Programs (OSEP) at the U.S. Department of Education required the New York State Education Department (NYSED) to develop and submit a 6 year State Performance Plan as per the requirements of Public Law 108-446, the Individuals with Disabilities Education Act (IDEA) 2004., (http://www2.ed.gov/policy/speced/guid/idea/idea2004.html) OSEP had identified three major areas of priority:

• Free Appropriate Public Education in the Least restrictive Environment;
• Disproportionality (evaluates the proportion of racial and ethnic groups in special education to prevent inappropriate identification in specific disability categories and special education services); and finally,
• Effective General Supervision Part B (these are the Child Find and Effective Transitions) (Public Law 108-446).

Each of these three priority areas contains additional indicators that must be tracked and reported. There are a total of 20 indicators that must be monitored, and if there is failure to demonstrate improvement within the school districts, a report of explanation is required. Examples of indicators include: Graduation rates, Dropout rates, Identification and Correction of Non-Compliance, Mediation Agreements, Secondary Transition, and Parental Involvement.

Before going into further details, it is important to explain some terminology that may not be universally recognized or understood. An Individualized Education Plan (IEP) is the legal binding contract established between the school district and its representatives and the family of the student requiring any special education or accommodations to support the child's success in the learning environment. The IEP identifies the accommodations or services that will be provided by the school educating the child, so that the child can be successful in that learning environment. In the United States, the school district is responsible for providing educational accommodations and/or services that will support the child's learning needs, starting the year the child turns 3 years of age and lasting until the child reaches 18 years of age. IEP Transition Planning refers to particular stages in the child's life when the child will "move" into a different learning environment, for example when the child is transitioning from preschool age into school age environment pre-kindergarten to kindergarten and beyond) as well as when the child moves from middle school to high school and then again when the child transitions from high school to post high school. With the new regulations in place, school districts must develop a plan for the child for after high school graduation and for successful integration into the community. This transition is the central theme of this chapter.

The indicator for Parent Involvement was and still continues to be measured by having parents complete a 25-item survey (New York State Education Department [NYSED] State Performance Report). The instructions on the survey indicate that this information will be used to help parents be involved in their children's special education programs by having the parents rate different ranges of agree to disagree on such items such as whether the school:

- Allows participation in the decision making process;
- Respects cultural heritage;
- Personnel help parents feel more confident in their parenting skills, and;
- Encourages them to suggest changes in school programs or services that the parents believe would benefit their child or other children with disabilities.

The parent survey does not inquire about parent and student involvement during transition service planning. Nor was there a survey for the child to complete if he/she attended Individualized Education Plan (IEP) meeting to evaluate whether this IEP is helping the child understand the transition process and whether the child is learning to identify whether their own needs were supported or met by the IEP team members. This last point is important especially when the child is at or near, the point of transition during his/her secondary education level. As a parent with a young adolescent child with learning disabilities who requires special education services, and as an occupational therapist working with youth who have disabilities, it is also important to me.

The mandates of the Individuals with Disabilities Education Act (IDEA) 2004 requires all states to establish measurable post-secondary goals and recommendations for transition services and activities to be in effect when the student reaches age 15. The federal law also mandates that the students must be invited to these IEP meetings (commonly referred to as CSE meetings- Committee on Special Education). This is so that the student will participate and engage in the planning process that will facilitate his/her movement from secondary school to post-secondary school activities within the larger community in the role of a young adult. This recommended practice is derived from research-based best practice models (Landmark et al. 2010; Lubbers et al. 2008; Martin et al. 2006). Through this engagement, the student is expected to self-advocate for their needs, and for the future goals they wish to pursue. Other members on this planning team (Special Education Teacher, General Education teacher, School Psychologist, School Administrator, and Parents) are supposed to provide guidance and support on achieving those goals.

As a parent of a child with learning disabilities, I have always been sensitive to the concept of "too much help" passively given to my son because he needs "help" to learn. I am also sensitive to the message being sent to him. Would he consider himself not good enough, or would he learn to be helpless, because someone else decided what kind of help he needs, as opposed to having him figure out what he needs for himself? After all, isn't that what we do as adults? We know what needs to be in place in order for us to do a job well. If you need something built, and carpentry isn't your personal strength, what do you do? You figure out what you need, and you hire a carpenter. If the student is attending their own IEP meeting, they should be able to learn how to express what they need and why they need it. It should help them be comfortable recognizing and stating what they need to do a job successfully and to demonstrate competence in a school environment. Yet, current research on self-determination, self-advocacy and the participation of youth with disability in the transition planning process indicates that schools are inconsistent and often ineffective in helping the youth learn these skills and integrate them into their sense of selves (Lubbers et al. 2008).

Starting in the 1980s, and continuing into the 1990s, the Office of Special Education and Rehabilitative Services (OSERS) sponsored research on how to promote changes in the special education system and to transform how Committee of Special Education (CSE) meetings are held. OSERS sought to identify the barriers that limited the collaboration between school personnel, parents and the student. The list of barriers included items such as:

- A lack of opportunity for people with disabilities to lead;
- Insufficient opportunities for individuals and their families to assume generic leadership roles; and,
- Limited opportunities for leadership development of underserved people and communities.

These and the other barriers limited a disabled person's ability to exercise their own control and choices. Research shows that limiting control and choice selections undermines the development of self-determination, leadership, and advocacy. To combat this, OSERS supported programs to develop self-advocacy for these students. Beginning in the 1990s and continuing into the early 2000s, the researchers were able to identify the barriers that provided negative transition services outcomes and they were able to implement practices that would create positive outcomes in the coordination of transition services planning (Lubbers et al. 2008; Greene and Kochlar-Bryant 2003; DeStefano et al. 1997; Guy and Schriner 1997; Johnson and Halloran 1997; Rusch et al. 1992). Research outcomes changed policy procedures to ensure that students and their families have more active roles in the transition planning process; established model programs; improve collaborative partnerships with various community and state organizations that would support the student's transition goals; and most importantly, increase stakeholder knowledge about the transition process and services available (Lubbers et al. 2008).

These research outcomes prompted many states, including my home state of New York, to develop Regional Special Education Technical Assistance Support Centers (RES-TASC), each with one or more Transition Specialists, whose role is to provide districts with professional development and technical assistance for effective transition practices and strategies. These measures of assistance, in theory, should provide adequate training for all CSE members in helping the student develop the necessary self-advocacy and self-determination skills needed to enable him or her to be actively engaged in developing goals and outcomes for transition planning at his/her IEP meeting. Unfortunately, current research findings report the same barriers that existed 30 years ago are still present today (Banks 2013;

Wehman 2013; Landmark and Zhang 2013; Landmark et al. 2010; Woods et al. 2010; Lubbers et al. 2008; Martin et al. 2006). If the same barriers still exist, why then are parent surveys still being distributed as part of the IEP meeting process and why are students not completing any surveys at all? Why are Parent surveys still not reflective of any transition planning areas? What other areas can be evaluated to help address continued presence of these barriers and provide consistent best practice of student-focused transition planning services?

The resistance to student-focused and driven transition meetings may originate in an antiquated behavioral learning paradigm that has dominated the field of education for many decades (Martin et al. 2006). Overwhelmingly the educational preparation for these professionals is underpinned by a behavioral view of learning (Cochran-Smith and Dudley-Marling 2012). The foundational influence of behavior psychology defines learning and the process of learning as a behavior that can be divided into a sequence of step or a finite set of component skills and sub-skills and this can also be applied to the special education process as well, since special education under this model addresses the deficits within the component skills or in the sub-skills (Cochran-Smith and Dudley-Marling 2012). This model creates the role of the education professional as the authority on learning, and places the student in the role of the passive recipient of the skills and sub-skills being taught. Although many education programs are now incorporating more interactive, critical review models such as social injustice models, these changes are not consistent and have not been in place for a long period of time (Cochran-Smith and Dudley-Marling 2012). Although is it beyond the purview of this chapter to delve too far into history of education, it is interesting to consider if the behavior learning model as the paradigm in teaching has created a barrier in student-focused transition planning, because it creates an authority role for the school professionals, placing them as the experts in the learning process and all non-professionals, such as family members and students, into the role of service recipients. If this is the case, then I would advocate for a different model to be adopted within university academic programs for school professionals, or there may always be inconsistency in transition service provisions (Lubbers et al. 2008).

A paradigm explains the collective perspectives, ideas and values that shape a common vision for a profession (Kielhofner 2009). According to Kielhofner (2009), it defines the practice of a profession and identifies beliefs about how to practice. The paradigm (models of practice) is the culture of that profession; it defines common beliefs and values that are used to guide a professional action, allowing the professional to understand what they are doing when they practice (Kielhofner 2009). Implied in this perspective, it also identifies not only a mindset of how to observe and identify necessary information to work with, it also includes utilizing a "language" or the use of a particular expression of communication that identifies the application of a model of practice (Turpin and Iwama 2011). Applying Kielhofner's definition of what a model of practice is and how it drives the actions and beliefs of a professional could also be applied to the "culture" of a school. If the model of practice of the school is that the school professional is the expert in all learning, then it would be difficult for the student to be the "leader" in a student focused transition planning meeting.

The history of the occupational therapy profession highlights practices in which the development and application of models of practice has been and continues to be important. Core to the various models of occupational therapy practice is the relationship of occupation (human action) to the development of self -actualization, health, and quality of life in an individual (Turpin and Iwama 2011, p. 8). A few of the models of practice that occupational therapists use are based in explaining the relationship between a person, their choice of occupations and the environments where those occupations exist. Although emphasis in the areas of the relationship between these three factors may vary in these paradigms, the commonalities across these models of practice are that performance of the human action (occupation) is the result of the complex process of a person's perceptions, goals, responsibilities, and desires. These will change over time and influence how they think about themselves and how they can influence their environments (Turpin and Iwama 2011, p. 107). This dynamic type of model is more helpful in facilitating self-advocacy and self-determination in students and families.

In addition, I wish to note the role of occupational therapy and the value it brings in facilitating self-determination as part of the therapeutic process between the occupational therapist and the client. In the literature of occupational therapy, facilitating self-determination is often done when the therapist uses person-centered therapeutic approaches. These types of therapeutic models utilize empowerment theory elements in occupational therapy practice. Fleming-Castaldy (2009) explains that these person-centered approaches applied to the therapeutic use of occupation, enables choice, develops personal control and increases self-determination in a person. Fleming-Castaldy (2009) continues to explain that empowerment theory compliments the core values of occupational therapy, as both the values of the profession and of the theory recognize that the empowerment of the self occurs when a person has self-control, collaborates with others to attain goals, and is cognizant of their own strengths and weaknesses as they make decisions. Occupational therapists engaging in school-based practices can help model such approaches during transition planning meetings with youth, their families and school professionals.

For example, during an eighth grade IEP transition meeting, a young male adolescent had prepared, according to his state's best practices for youth involvement in these type of meetings, a powerpoint presentation of his desires, interests, goals and a list of what he would like assistance with from the teaching staff that would attend the meeting. When the time for the meeting came, the lead school representative started to present his own perceptions and thoughts of what the youth should be doing, and his statement was followed by the reports of the rest of the school professionals. The youth quietly put away the flash drive that held his powerpoint presentation and just sat there passively. When the presentations of the school professionals had concluded, the youth was asked to present his information, but he denied that he had anything to offer. After the meeting, I asked the student privately what his thoughts were about the outcomes of the meeting, although I was not the therapist treating him, I did consult with both the youth and his mother (a personal friend of mine) on how to prepare the powerpoint presentation. He replied, "Well, they think they have a better idea what I need for school, and maybe so, especially if I decide to go to college, but honestly, I'm not sure I want to go to college. I like hanging out with my uncle who owns an automobile repair shop and sometimes I think I like the idea of becoming a mechanic. I always have fun there, learning how to fix things and understanding how cars work." When I asked why he didn't say anything, the student replied, "Well, they're experts in what I need for college, so I decided to go with that. With the mechanic thing, I can hang out with my uncle during the summers and my other days off from school, and between him and my parents, I'll know what I need if I decide to go that route."

My heart sank, here was this young man who wanted to communicate his needs and learn how to self-advocate, and was ready to accept the support of adults he viewed as his mentors, and he left the meeting feeling as though he had no voice at the meeting. Later in the day, I ran into the mother and asked her for more details. She explained that she had asked the lead school representative to have the youth present first, the lead school representative replied that this was not the way these meetings were to be conducted and that if he allowed every student to speak, the meetings would run more than the allotted hour. The school representative then felt that he would compromise and stated that the student may present at the end of the meeting, with time permitting. I asked the mother why didn't she speak up and explain to the representative that this procedure undermined the intent of the transition meeting, her reply was: "His reaction (the representative) was so strong that I felt as though what we were asking was so unacceptable and so violating the educational process, that I myself shrank back. I clearly got the message of 'We are here to tell you what is the best plan for your son regarding his educational needs because we are teachers, you are just his mother.' She then expressed regret about having me convince her and her son that he could run his own meeting, stating how embarrassed she felt and when she looked at her son she felt he was embarrassed as well.

An occupational therapist hearing this conversation could apply a person— occupation—environment model, and ask: what did the input from all the instructors mean to the student? What similarities existed between the students' abilities, experiences, perceptions and those of the instructors and parents? What combination of interventions could be applied to increase the similarities between the student's own perceptions of his occupations, and those of the school professionals? An example of these supporting viewpoints occurred with my son, also, attending that particular school and grade; and, also in the special education process of transition planning for high school and beyond. I worked with my son in preparing a similar powerpoint presentation for his transition meeting, which was held later in the same day as my friend's son. Once again, the head of the committee started to open the discussions for the meeting, but, this time, I intervened and insisted that my son open the meeting with his own presentation. Although, the head of the committee was not pleased with this change in routine, he did allow my son to present first. Why? Because I advocated for him, I cited the law and the intent of the law and stated that as his parent and an active member of this committee, I was recognizing another committee member, (my son), to open the meeting. The lead school representative was quite angry and the other teachers there looked as uncomfortable as my son, but my son opened the meeting by presenting his needs and wants. At the end of the meeting, I asked my son how he thought the meeting went, and he replied, "At first, I got really annoyed with the Team Leader, you know after all, it's MY LIFE, MY PLANS! But then, you just encouraged me to go ahead and present so I did, and then I felt, like, WOW! I am really changing everyone's perception of me. I am really able to share with my teachers my ideas and plans and they're listening! I really felt that when I told them that I have so many ideas about different careers, but wasn't sure if any of them would fit my skills, that they actually came up with a plan to help me be more exposed to different careers in those industries. When I talked about being either a lawyer or police officer, they identified the industry as law enforcement, and suggested I be shown all the many careers involved in that area, they even mentioned ones I didn't know about. It was helpful and I felt empowered!"

My presence as his mother, who happens to be an occupational therapist and on the team, meant that the role I played was as the "bridge" between the instructional staff and my son simply by using a person-centered model, changed the environment and culture of that IEP meeting. The roles of the instructional staff went from a behaviorist model of "experts" presenting the stimulus to attain the "correct response" from everyone, including the student, to a collaborative team model, where the professionals applied their knowledge to ideas presented by the student. Subsequently, I asked the special education teacher what she thought of my son's meeting and she replied: "It was such a delight to see him engaged in his future. He really advocated for himself and we were there to guide him and support him. I think that is what an IEP meeting should be all about." When I explained to the special education teacher the difference between the two meetings, and how I applied a person-centered model onto the team dynamics, the special education teacher became aware of how that model changed the entire dynamics of the meeting and provided more relevant outcomes for the student.

Weeks later, in his English class, the teacher wanted my son to read a passage from a novel and describe the meaning of the dialogue between two characters. My son is dyslexic, and on his IEP there is a mandate that the school must provide him audio books, it happens that this English teacher neglected to order an audio book for my son. During that particular lesson, the teacher insisted that my son read from a book, stating to my son that it would be a disadvantage to the other students for him having an audio book since it would be easier for him to interpret the dialogues due to variations in the speech patterns of the readers, and besides, my son must learn how to read, he couldn't possibly spend the rest of his life "getting out of reading activities." My son, after years of participating in his own IEP process, and being taught what an IEP is and why it is important, explained to a high school teacher why he needed audio books in a very matter of fact tone. He explained to the teacher, "Yes, I can read simple things, but reading more complex novels, where you ask me questions about meanings and plots, well, in order for me to give you a thoughtful response, I will need to hear it. This way, I put all my talents and skills to recognizing patterns or concepts within that story. If not, I can use all my talents and skills in trying to make sense out of words that visually have no meaning to me. The choice is up to you." The teacher's response was to allow him to use an audio book he was able to download with the classroom computer, and he was so taken with my son's deep, and complex interpretations of the stories, that he often had my son lead a discussion group with the other students in the class after that experience.

Occupational therapists are trained to recognize, honor and collaborate within cultural values and beliefs of person, and also to reach out to other organizations/agencies that can help a person achieve their goals. The use of person-centered models and language, helps us understand and recognize that how a person thinks of themselves and how the things they do also influences their environment, and culture of that environment. This type of thinking and use of models, helps recognize that people with disabilities are competent and are fully capable of self-determination. Occupational therapists must take a more active role in the process of Individualized Transition Planning for youth with disabilities to ensure that best special education practices are implemented and supported. By doing so, the occupational therapist can help school professionals move away from behaviorist model that are no longer useful for working with youth with disabilities. We all should be asking, "what does this person need or want to do in the context of his or her life?" As a school professional, what should I suggest or provide that would support the interrelationship between person, environment and occupation so that this student can grow into a mature, self-sufficient and self-advocating adult? As a school professional, what do I need do to help the parents teach their child to become an insightful reflective adult? Letting go of the behaviorist model and working in a model that uses language, and a mindset that puts the person with disabilities at the center and in control of coordinating their future planning will create a culture where they can be viewed as a person who is expert in their own life and not someone who needs help because they "can't do it." As an occupational therapist working in a school setting, that is what I work towards, and as a mother, that is what I wish for my son to have.

Editors' Postscript   If you liked Chap. 17 by Eva Rodriguez, and are interested in reading more about the empowerment of youth who are transitioning to adulthood, we recommend Chap. 14 by Michele Friedner: "Occupying Seats, Occupying Space, Occupying Time: Deaf Young Adults in Vocational Training Centers in Bangalore, India," and Chap. 16 by Nick Dupree: "My World, My Experiences with Occupy Wall Street and How We can go Further." If you are interested in how occupational therapists have engaged with disability studies across the lifespan, we recommend Chap. 11: "Soul searching occupations: Critical reflections on Occupational Therapy's Commitment to Social Justice, Disability Rights, and Participation" by Mansha Mirza, Susan Magasi and Joy Hammel and Chap. 12: "Refusing to Go Away: The Ida Benderson Seniors Action Group" by Denise M. Nepveux.

References

Banks J (2013) Barriers and supports to postsecondary transition: case studies of African american students with disabilities. Hammill Institute on Disabilities, Austin
Cochran-Smith M, Dudley-Marling C (2012) Diversity in teacher education and special education: the issues that divide. J Teach Educ 63:237–244
DeStefano L, Hasazi S, Trach J (1997) Conceptualizing an evaluation of system change. Career Dev Except Individ 20(2):123–140

Fleming-Castaldy RP (2009) Activities, human occupation, participation, and empowerment. In: Hinojosa J, Blount ML (eds) The textures of life: purposeful activities in the context of occupation. AOTA Press, Bethesda

Greene G, Kochlar-Bryant CA (2003) Pathways to successful transition for youth with disabilities. Pearson Merrill Prentice Hall, Upper Saddle River

Guy B, Schriner K (1997) Systems in transition: are we there yet? Career Dev Except Individ 20:141–164

Johnson D, Halloran W (1997) The federal legislative context and goals of the state systems change initiative on transition for youth with disabilities. Career Dev Except Individ 20:109–121

Kielhofner G (2009) Conceptual foundations of occupational therapy practice. F. A. Davis Company, Philadelphia

Landmark LJ, Zhang D (2013) Compliance and best practices in transition planning: effects of disability and ethnicity. Remedial Spec Educ 34:113–125. doi:10.1177/0741932511431831

Landmark LJ, Ju S, Zhang D (2010) Substantiated best practices in transition: fifteen plus years later. Career Dev Except Individ 33:165–176. doi:10.1177/0885728810376410

Lubbers JH, Repetto JB, McGorray SP (2008) Perception of transition barriers, practices, and solutions in Florida. Remedial Spec Educ 29(5):280–292

Martin JE, Van Dycke JL, Christensen WR, Greene BA, Gardner JE, Lovett DL (2006) Increasing student participation in their transition IEP meetings: establishing the self-directed IEP as an evidenced-based practice. Except Child 72:299–316

New York State Education Department (NYSED) State Performance Report. http://www.p12. nysed.gov/specialed/lawsregs/

Public Law 108-446, The Individuals with Disabilities Education Act (IDEA) (2004) http://www2. ed.gov/policy/speced/guid/idea/idea2004.html.

Rusch FR, Kohler PD, Hughes L (1992) An analysis of OSERS-sponsored secondary special education and transitional services research. Career Dev Except Individ 15:121–143

Turpin M, Iwama MK (2011) Using occupational therapy models in practice: a field guide. Churchill Livingstone Elsevier, New York

Wehman P (2013) Life beyond the classroom: transition strategies for young people with disabilities, 5th edn. Paul Brookes Publishing Co., Baltimore

Woods L, Sylvester L, Martin J (2010) Student-directed transition planning: increasing student knowledge and self-efficacy in the transition planning process. Career Dev Except Individ 33(2):106–114

Part III
Struggle, Creativity and Change

Editors' Note: For an introduction to Part III see Sect. 25.3

Should Robots Be Personal Assistants?   18

Katherine D. Seelman

Abstract

Modern technology is generating ethical problems relevant to all of us. It sounds almost laughable, but should robots become personal assistants? Do electrodes implanted in the brain with internet communication capability have implications for personal identity and control? Should care mean monitoring people? If a prosthetic limb gives a runner an advantage should he/she be permitted to compete against those without the advantage? This chapter will present a look at ethics in using technology in a few case studies of technology-generated problems of particular interest to the disability community and examine them using ethical tools drawing on a Common Morality approach to ethics.

Keywords

Disability • Advanced technology • Bioethics • Robots • Sensors • Human enhancements • Identity

18.1   Introduction

Ethics may once have been associated with Aristotle but today advanced technology is generating ethical problems unique to our own age. Should robots become personal assistants? Should they have human rights? Under what conditions should we monitor Grandma? If human enhancements using prosthetic limbs, steroids or genes give an athlete an advantage, should he/she be permitted to compete in the same event against those without these enhancements? What if enhancements

K.D. Seelman (✉)
School of Health and Rehabilitation Sciences, University of Pittsburgh, Pittsburgh, PA, USA
e-mail: kds31@pitt.edu

© Springer Science+Business Media Dordrecht 2016   259
P. Block et al. (eds.), *Occupying Disability: Critical Approaches to Community, Justice, and Decolonizing Disability*, DOI 10.1007/978-94-017-9984-3_18

relieve the necessity for institutionalization but the trade-off is compromising identity?

We live in an age of technology. In our age, ethical questions often arrive wrapped in complex technologies. This chapter focuses on three categories of advanced technologies, robotics, sensors used to monitor and track people, and human enhancements. While Disability Studies has critically analyzed Bioethical problems such as those relating to abortion, suicide, pre-natal screening and genetic testing (Ash et al. 2008; Wasserman and Asch 2009), it has been less attentive to discourse leading to a disability perspective on the development and use of these and other advanced technologies (Seelman 2001). While both assistive and advanced technologies can be enabling, only the latter can change the nature of what it is to be human. The impact of their use can obscure the boundaries between human beings and machines and render obsolete current distinctions between cure and independent living and therapy and cosmetic interventions. Participation by citizens in decisions about the design, development and use of the artifacts of science and technology is a major concern for democracy (Jasanoff 2011). Consciousness of the nature of advanced technology and the scope of its impacts, both existing and potential, can make us very uncomfortable. Nonetheless, people with disabilities have both rights and responsibilities as citizens and in the case of advanced technologies as targeted markets of end users. This chapter is a preliminary exploration of the need for more broad based participation by the disability community in critical analysis of science and technology development and use.

A number of intellectual movements and approaches are relevant to these problems. The Transhumanist movement (Bostrom 2005), for example, affirms the possibility and desirability of fundamentally transforming the human condition and therefore eliminating aging and by association, disability. The Ableism approach (Cambell 2008; Siebers 2008) operates in the here-and-now, taking aim at discrimination on the basis of physical or mental differences, and attitudinal and physical barriers to equal opportunity. Finally, more phenomenological and subjective approaches akin to Feminism, direct us to focus on our own experiences as people with disabilities (Shakespeare 2006). A scientist with a seemingly renaissance mind, Gregor Wolbring, the son of a parent who used thalidomide, counsels us to focus more on citizenship (Wolbring 2012). People with disabilities should join the discourse.

While a comprehensive critique of advanced technology would require exploration of vast unmapped and unexplored intellectual and experiential terrain, this chapter has more modest dimensions and more concrete aims. Advanced technologies are examined within the context of ethics, especially values important to people with disabilities such as self-determination and human rights and related principles in Bioethics. The advanced technologies which are introduced later have been chosen more on the basis of their relevance to the here-and-now than on science fiction. They are on the market or soon to be introduced into the marketplace (Chen 2012). They include robots for kids with autism and brain- computer interfaces for those with Amyotrophic Lateral Sclerosis (ALS). Advanced technologies such as robotics, sensors used to monitor and track people, and human enhancements are not routinely covered through Medicare and Medicaid. However, they may be available in the course of research projects using as research subjects people with disabilities and older adults, in out-of-pocket sales direct sales transactions and as educational tools.

Popular culture and the scientific literature provide interesting representations and evidence about the social "nature" of these technologies and the experience of people with disabilities who use them. Technical factors include new materials such as those used in prosthetic feet, design processes which may or may not enable consumer choice options, and introducing genetic materials into the body that may alter human intelligence. Social factors involve acceptance by the individual and adoption by society. Cultural representations in film and evidence from scientific studies are culled to describe the technical and social characteristics of robots, sensors and human enhancements. Applying values such as self-determination and human rights from disability rights and related traditional ethical principles in western bioethics (Beauchamp and Childress 2009) to actual case studies, we then move on to identify and examine some of the ethical problems experienced by users in order to discern the contours, if not the core concepts of a disability perspective.

18.2 Significance

Advanced technologies have more profound, long-lasting effects on human beings and society than their predecessor assistive technologies. As later sections of this chapter will illustrate, they can substitute for human judgment and affect the way people think and feel. Ethical dilemmas (Hamric et al. 2000) arise from the options generated by the enabling features of advanced technology. An individual may choose to supplement a malfunctioning memory by borrowing memory and accepting support from a robot even if the robot is controlled by undetermined sources outside the end user's network but within the robot's communication network. The other option available to the individual is often institutionalization. Ironically, this non-medical intervention for supplementing and supporting a person with a disability may lead to cure if enough memory is borrowed so that the functioning that is enabled approximates that of someone without memory loss. What is the line between maintaining one's identity while using the memory of another and inadvertently taking on the identity of another or at least succumbing to the control of an unknown other? These problems blend well with colonization and identity which are themes of our book. Colonization involves absorbing and assimilating people into the culture controlled by a more dominant group and thus destroying any remnant of the less powerful culture. Depending on scale and other factors, experiences such as borrowing memory may or may not severely harm the disability community and compromise the identities of for example previously free persons with disabilities. The disability studies community may find problems such as these worthy of further critical analysis.

18.2.1 Advanced Technology and Health Care

Advanced technologies have been introduced into health care to enhance quality of life. (Helal et al. 2008; Seelman et al. 2014; Stephanidis 2009). These assistive technologies may be used for therapy and support or they may be cosmetic and aimed at a level of performance which, without them, would be impossible to achieve. People with disabilities are considered an important market in health care and advanced technologies (Chen 2012; "Wheelchair Toyota's Robot" 2012; Wolbring n.d; O'Reilly 2012). Industries actively advertise enabling features of products, describing their positive impact on the quality of life of older adults, people with disabilities and their caregivers. Government makes decisions about the safety and effectiveness of many of these products. However, the implications of these technologies for the quality of life of people with disabilities await the advent of widespread discourse in the disability community.

18.2.2 Human Rights, Bioethics and the Challenges of Containing New Technology in Old Wineskins

Self-determination, human rights and justice are fundamental values for the Disability Rights Movement. The right to universally designed and available technology is widely accepted by the disability community. These values are incorporated in the UN Convention on the Rights of Persons with Disabilities and serve as the moral foundation of the Independent Living Movement. Human rights laws and conventions are the first line of defense against discrimination. Bioethics, related laws, regulations and codes of practice in the health professions form a second line of protection.

The Hippocratic Oath may be the most familiar application of ethics in science and technology. The Hippocratic Oath is an enduring example of the value placed on beneficence as a foundation of modern health care. Beneficence counsels that the basic responsibility of the clinician is to do good for his patient. Bioethics is rooted in human biology and provides guidelines for the ethical behavior of human beings. The Oath assumes that only humans are moral agents, therefore, robots are excluded but as an example provided later from the movie *Robot and Frank* suggests, robots may struggle with human dilemmas such as choice. Over the centuries the health professions have developed a comprehensive biomedical ethics framework of patient protection, well-being, and confidentiality of information. Informed consent, for example, is the process by which a fully informed patient can participate in choices about her health care. It originates from the legal and ethical right the patient has to direct what happens to her body and from the ethical duty of the physician to involve the patient in her health care. Institutional Review Boards approve, monitor, and review research involving humans. Researchers and clinicians have adopted basic principles to guide them in protecting research subjects and as a basis for professional codes for ethical practice. They include: respect for persons and autonomy, beneficence, non-maleficence or do not harm and justice (National Commission for the Protection of Human Subjects of Biomedica and Behavioral Research 1979). These principles augmented by self-determination and human rights will be used to examine the case studies presented later.

Adoption and use of advanced technologies has breached the framework of Bioethics and governmental regulation so that the flow of risks and benefits associated with them are largely undirected. Today, with the introduction of advanced technology and globally competitive industries into health care and the influx of engineers and other non-health professions, the field of Bioethics no longer provides a comprehensive framework to guide behavior and decision making. Ethics relevant to health care has diverged into many subfields including bioethics (Beauchamp and Childress 2009), computer ethics (Johnson and Miller 2009) and human machine ethics (Veruggio and Operto 2008). There is no integrated ethics with which to approach a disability perspective on the use of robotics, sensors and enhancements. Nor have ethicists and governments taken head-on the problem of cultural differences within the context of advanced technology. Other parts of the world and corporate culture may be more pragmatic and less identified with Western ethical standards. On the one hand, criteria for technology design, adoption and use decisions may be reduced from ethics to technical standards for safety and effectiveness of a device (Veruggio and Operto 2008). On the other, the Disability Community has enshrined the human right to universal design of technology in the UN Convention.

18.3 Method

Two approaches are used to identify and examine the ethical dimensions of advanced technology—outside-in and inside-out. Using popular culture and scientific literature, the outside-in approach introduces some of the technical and social characteristics of robots, sensors used for monitoring and tracking and of enhancements. Ethical concerns about personhood, identity and subsequent colonization and discrimination are identified.

Applying the inside-out approach, we turn to a process of identifying and examining ethical problems within consumer case studies, using a principle-based Common Morality approach from Bioethics (Beauchamp and Childress 2009). A common morality community is formed based on acceptance of principles such as respect for persons (autonomy), beneficence (non-maleficence) and justice. Common Morality assumes that only human beings can be moral agents, denying agency to those with artificial intelligence such as robots. While principles such as autonomy are content-thin, the case studies are content-rich; the combination of both provides a basis for fixing the contours of the ethical dimensions of problems generated by these technologies. The common morality approach encourages adaptability. If the results from examination of the case studies suggest that existing norms for ethically obligatory behavior are insufficient, then additional guidelines may be proposed. This adaptability is particularly important when involved with new technologies such as robotics, tracking and monitoring and enhancements, because standards governing their use and limiting their impacts may not have been developed or are evolving.

As the previous discussion suggested, Bioethics is a pail full of holes and a can full of worms. While no longer sufficient to contain and guide human decisions about advanced technology, it is a necessary tool. Rooted in Western culture, Bioethics may yet be enhanced to construct an adequate ethical framework for the design and use of advanced technology used in health care and independent living.

18.4 What Are Advanced Technologies: Implications for the Disability Community?

Advanced technologies almost always involve information and communications technology and computers, standing alone or embedded in other products and networked into global transmission systems. They are also characterized by sophisticated electronics, software, robotics and artificial intelligence (Seelman et al. 2014). Guided by algorithms, rather than human beings, software routinely instructs these technologies on what to do (Peterson 2011.). Algorithms are step-by-step problem-solving procedures for decision making. For example, algorithms may bar, limit, or enable end user options to control technology such as those that can be incorporated into a robotic mobility device. These mobility devices—the next generation electric wheelchair—are introduced in the first case study.

18.4.1 Robots

Robots can be viewed as only being machines, as having a moral dimension, or even evolving into a new species (Veruggio and Operto 2008). They are stand-alone or embedded in other technology. Exoskeletons, for example, use robotic systems, advanced battery technology and materials. People, who otherwise could not walk, slip into them for mobility support (Chen 2012).

Movies such as *Blade Runner* have acquainted us with bad robots that illustrate the conflict between robotkind and humankind. Perhaps less ethically challenging are good robots such as a little robot named Bandit whose purpose is to help children with autism better understand social cues and emotional behavior (Conley 2011). Movies such as *Robot & Frank* introduce us to the complexities of distinguishing a good robot from a bad robot. The robot's cognitive and communication capabilities are more in the realm of Science Fiction; nonetheless, it provides a robotic rendition of a future personal assistant.

In *Robot & Frank,* Frank is an aging former petty thief with progressive memory loss who lives alone but has a family who cares about him. Against Frank's wishes— but better than the other option of living in a facility—Frank's family responds to their concern about his welfare by providing him with a robot health aide. The robot is referred to as Robot. Neither a human being who by birth receives a name and social security number nor an anonymous machine which often remains nameless, Robot reflects moral ambiguity in valuing an advanced technology characterized by both human and non-human features. At first, Frank regards the health aide as a stupid appliance. However, Robot is a very personable robot who assumes a role akin to a buddy, but not always an empowering buddy. He does not provide Frank with a "turn-off" switch. No information is provided about who controls the Robot or has access to its memory. Frank accepts the robot even though he has not been protected by informed consent which is routinely required for research subjects and patients in medical settings. Informed Consent is closely aligned with medical services. However, the services provided by Robot are categorized as non-medical.

Robot supplements Frank's memory and "lends a hand" around the house. He helps Frank with personal and housekeeping activities such as eating, cleaning and routinizing schedules and healthy behaviors such as rising in the morning, exercising and eating vegetables. While Robot is diligently and sociably performing his tasks, Frank discovers that the robot does not have software, which would provide ethical guidance such as that *thou shalt not steal*. Frank regains a sense of his youthful self when he realizes that with the aid of Robot he once again can engage in petty theft and robberies. However, after executing these robberies and because of his past criminal record, Frank comes under suspicion by a tech savvy victim who realizes that the evidence to prove Frank's guilt lies in the memory of Robot. Will Robot provide Frank with the secret to wiping out his memory; will Frank push the erase button? Well, see the movie! However, even without viewing the end of the film, we are made aware of the ethical problems involved with establishing boundaries between human beings and machines, sustaining individual identity in face of the threat of colonizing the human mind as well as invasion of privacy. Thus, independent living for Frank is, at best, a matter of shared decision making with those who may supersede his choices or fabricate his choice options. At what stage should the Robot's own narrative be given more than technical and economic value? Some of these problems involve self-determination and ethical principles such as autonomy and non-malfeasance which instruct us to respect personhood and do no harm. Others await the development of a new dimension in ethics.

18.4.2 Sensors Used to Monitor and Track People with Disabilities Across the Age Span

The second case study catapults us into applications of sensor technology in the life of an older adult. Sensors are devices capable of detecting and responding to physical stimuli such as movement, light, or heat. Sensors can be located within the body, on the body and in the environment. The U.S. Food and Drug Administration, for example, recently cleared a tiny ingestible sensor used with a companion wearable patch and mobile app to improve medication adherence (Pogorelc 2012). Sensors collect and transmit information, such as blood pressure and about falls or going to the bathroom, often wirelessly to external devices such as smartphones which, in turn, may transmit this information to clinicians, family members and caregivers.

Perhaps the most familiar use of sensors is for monitoring and tracking older adults. Modern home automation and communications systems often provide a visual interface that makes it easy to stay connected with aging or disabled loved ones from anywhere in the world. Sensors can be installed on entryways, chairs, medicine cabinets, cupboards so that a family member or caregiver can be notified automatically of any unusual activity or patterns which should cause concern. They can make life safer by alerting occupants to phones ringing and someone at the door. If they are coupled with the use of locational technology, such as a geographic information system (GIS), then information about location also becomes available. Sensors may also be coupled with video technology. Again there are ethical dilemmas. Just how much autonomy and privacy are you willing to trade-off for independent living?

18.4.3 Human Enhancements

The scope of human enhancements is expansive incorporating many individual advanced technologies and combinations. Robots, for example, can be categorized as memory enhancements. Therefore, they are difficult to categorize and encapsulate in a brief description. The impact of enhancements on human beings can be profound, encompassing a broad range of changes in human nature and function. They are used to temporarily or permanently overcome the current limitations of the human body through natural or artificial means. Enhancements range from the familiar, such as prosthetics and steroids to the less familiar, brain and gene implants (Hamilton et al. 2011; Hanna 2006). Their impacts range from no long-term effects on the body and mind as in most limb prosthetics to effects that make someone not just well, but better than well, by optimizing attributes or capabilities – perhaps by raising an individual from standard to peak levels of performance using genetic enhancements.

Bioethics has been used as a platform for debates involving the ethics of advanced technology in therapy versus their use for performance and cosmetic enhancement (Resnik 2000). On the one hand, brain implants, for examples, have considerable potential for pinpointing and shutting down seizures caused by epilepsy (Stimson 2011). On the other, an international movement called Transhumanism affirms the possibility and desirability of fundamentally transforming the human condition by developing and making widely available technologies to eliminate aging and to greatly enhance human intellectual, physical, and psychological capacities (Bostrom 2005). People with disabilities would no longer exist.

The products of popular culture reflect various ethical concerns about human enhancements. The film *Gattaca* features the genetically superior *valids* and normal humans, known as *invalids*. The valids get all the high-paying jobs, and practically run the country, while the invalids are shown as janitors and other menial workers. In other words, the direction of discrimination runs against normal humans. A two-tiered system positions normal humans as outcasts and valids as dominant. We shall return to this concern for fairness and justice in the case study of the South African runner, Oscar Pistorius.

18.5   The Case Studies

The case studies that follow are composites of real experiences of people with disabilities. Acceptance or rejection of the technology is influenced by their own medical and functional status as well as the concerns of their caregivers and family. The case studies introduce technologies that are more assistive in nature, so that their impacts do not involve changes in what is generally regarded as human nature. Dilemmas arise when trade-offs provide no easy and highly desirable option.

18.5.1 A Young Man with Spinal Cord Injury; Let's Call Him Jake Adams

Jake Adams sustained a serious spinal cord injury in an automobile accident and uses a power wheelchair for mobility. He has limited use of upper extremities and some cognitive involvement. Jake has been involved in research to develop a robotic mobility product ("Quality of Life Technology Engineerng Research Center"). The robot will be equipped for mobility and manipulation so that Jake can use the robot's arms to open doors, including refrigerator and microwave doors enabling him to eat independent of human assistance. The research is being conducted at a university setting well known for its commitment to participation by people with disabilities and universal design.

The designers have set a goal aimed at producing a device in which there is a person-system symbiosis. The mobility device components will be designed to enable independence. Users can operate the device in multiple control modes:

- Autonomous control mode in which the user can specify an activity of daily living (ADL) task, such as where the mobile base should go and what object the robotic arms should manipulate;
- Local control mode in which the user can fully access the control of both mobility and manipulation;
- Remote control mode, a remote user, for example, the caregiver, is able to remotely complete ADL task for the local user;
- Cooperative control mode, in which the amount of work provided by the user in the wheelchair and the amount of work provided by the caregiver through remote operation.

The range of control modes provides Jake and his caregivers with incentives for independence and for cooperation. The remote control mode will require communication and other capabilities to provide a service not unlike the remote telephone relay services which provide deaf, hard of hearing and speech-impaired customers with telephone service. However, these control options and other features generate privacy issues. The robotic mobility device utilizes cameras, sensors, WiFi and other technology which collect data for physical location (GPS), and from visual and auditory recordings. Who has access to the data—caregivers, clinical providers, insurance, and for what purpose? Is the vast information transmission system secure so that the data is held confidential? Safety issues also emerge in the use of the remote control mode. For example, a remote user could open the front door to allow a robber to enter.

In this case study, the engineers have adhered to the principles of autonomy and beneficence and malfeasance by designing technology that enhances independence and seems to be good for the individual. The end user can decide who controls what. If Jake receives training in use of the device and if he is apprised of the privacy and safety risks involved in the use of the various video, locational and communications system and agrees to accept them, then the researchers have met their ethical responsibilities. Justice, involving both ethical distribution of risks and benefits, is not within the authority limits of research but nonetheless, the research team should regard themselves as advocates for fair reimbursement policies.

18.5.2 An Older Woman Who Is at Risk for Falling and Is Sometimes Forgetful; Let's Call her Eve Jones

Mrs. Jones is a fiercely independent 85-year-old who is determined to continue living in the home in which she and her husband, now deceased, raised their children. She has a heart condition and arthritis for which she takes medications when she remembers. The meds sometimes makes her feel dizzy, affecting her balance.

Her children are worried about her. They, and her physician, have tried to convince her to move into a more protected environment but she has refused to budge even though she has a number of conditions which put her at risk of injury. Mrs. Jones' older daughter has pleaded with her to accept some surveillance equipment. The daughter's investigation about costs shows that the family can afford the equipment. Human tracking equipment is now affordable and available without restriction for $200 plus a monthly service fee of $20. The equipment is often marketed as "kid-tracking" devices, though some ads also mention pets and senior citizens. ("Human tracking: Big Brother goes mainstream" 2005). This equipment, which does not involve a prescription and which is located in the home is not regulated so as to require privacy protections akin to informed consent in research and health care.

Mrs. Jones views video cameras as particularly repugnant because they are ubiquitous and highly invasive. She rejected video cameras outright, especially for the bedroom and bathroom. She does not want images of her intimate activities captured and shared. Mrs. Jones claimed that her occasional memory lapses do not justify the use of GPS and ingestible sensors. However, she did acknowledge that she might receive comfort by some sensor monitoring, especially for falls and also alerts to incoming telephone calls and people at the door. Her family, however, wanted her to accept more extensive surveillance.

The question of who has the right to choose is made more complex because Mrs. Jones is at risk for physical injury. However, she is mentally competent. These problems correspond to the principle of respect for persons and autonomy. However, under conditions of considerable risk of injury, negotiations among the parties are necessary and justified. Does justice require that society place restrictions on the adoption and use of the equipment and on the content of advertising?

18.5.3 Human Enhancements: The Case of the Long Distance Runner

Oscar Pistorius was born in 1986 in South Africa, with congenital absence of the fibula or calf bone in both legs ("Pistorius, Oscar" n.d.). When he was 11 months old, his legs were amputated halfway between his knees and ankles. Nonetheless, he became a world class runner, capturing his first gold medal at the Paralympics in London in 2006 when he helped South Africa win the 4x100m relay in a world-record time at the Olympic Stadium. Pistorius uses high energy-storing prosthetic feet products known as Cheetahs. Viewing Cheetahs as providing an advantage over another athlete not using such a device, in 2008, the International Association of Athletics Federation banned him from competing in the Olympics. The ruling was overturned after Pistorius challenged the Federation because of lack of evidence.

Evidence, and some would argue, fairness, may support the admission of Oscar Pistorius to Olympic competition. However, the impact of high tech prosthetic feet presents a vivid contrast to the seemingly dangerous impacts of genetic enhancements and their impact on human nature. What conditions and criteria justify the individual acceptance and societal adoption and use of these enhancements? Can these criteria harmonize with principles of respect for persons, beneficence, maleficence and justice?

18.6   Conclusions

Should Robots be Personal Assistants? Clearly criteria must be predicated on response to one or the other of two categories of advanced technologies. Technologies in category 1 provide support but do not make fundamental changes in human nature. These technologies, for the most part, correspond to and are embedded in an ethical framework of disability rights and Common Morality. Technologies in category 2 may change human nature and exist in a context without a widely accepted ethical framework. Decisions about technology in category 2 are market driven. People with disabilities should be involved in questions of who defines the good or sanctions the bad for these technologies. They have a large stake in who loses and who gains.

Technologies in category 1, such as the robotic mobility device, the surveillance equipment and the Cheetah prosthetic feet introduced in case studies generate many unresolved ethical problems. While not widely acknowledged in Ethics, technology has social dimensions as in adopting a process of designing technology to incorporate user choice into a robotic mobility device or impacts of a device on privacy. While individuals who are subjects of research and patients in the health care system have privacy protections such as informed consent, no equivalent protections exist for people who want to live independently but must choose between surveillance equipment in their homes or facility-based living. Rarely, does the scientific literature report findings of studies of personal assistance which includes human personal assistants as an option equal to that of technology.

Tier 2 involves technology for which the ethical contours are emerging. As with the robot in *Robot and Frank* and genetic enhancements, these advanced technologies do not fit comfortably with currently accepted values. Self-determination, human rights and principles of Bioethics were developed to apply to human beings—not to those entities which have human, super human and non-human attributes. Tier 2 technology involves trade-offs between identity and colonization of personhood and realization of medical cure and cognitive, physical and sensory functioning and super functioning. Some adults and parents of persons with disabilities may desire or require increments of support, as in the case of borrowed memory, which may cure symptoms but colonize minds. This is not self-determination and independent living as we understand it today. Perhaps through the lens of a person with dementia or the parent of a child with cognitive disabilities, the option should be made available. If so, the framework for dispensing this advanced technology must involve strict criteria for use within a context resembling the health professionals.

Disability theory has used the social model of disability to explain disability. Ableism theory has provided impetus for the important work of dismantling discrimination. Perhaps, theory should be developed based on disability narrative which could inform experience with some of these advanced technologies. Under what conditions do harsh terms such as colonization apply as descriptors of the impact of these technologies on the lives of people with disabilities? New theory must emerge to explain why and under what conditions we should or should not accept, adopt and use Tier 2 advanced technology. Therefore, the question, "Should Robots be personal assistants?" remains in the active file for follow-up!

Editors' Postscript If you enjoyed Chap. 18 by Katherine Seelman "Should Robots be Personal Assistants?" about the development of assisted technology, you may find the theme technology versus human help in chapters about communication such as Chap. 13 by Rick Stoddart and David Turnbull "Why Bother Talking? On Having Cerebral Palsy and Speech Impairment: Preserving And Promoting Oral Communication Through Occupational Community and Communities of Practice." Chap. 22 "Blindness and Occupation: Personal Observations and Reflections" by Rikki Chaplin also explores the gentle balance between help and independence or interdependence.

References

Ash A, Jeffries T, Taylor J (2008) Prenatal testing. Touchstone, New York

Beauchamp TL, Childress JF (2009) Principles of biomedical ethics, 6th edn. Oxford University Press, New York

Bostrom N (2005) A history of transhumanist thought. J Evolut Technol 14(1):1–25

Cambell FK (2008) Refusing Able (ness): a preliminary conversation about Ableism. M/C J 11(3). http://journal.media-culture.org.au/index.php/mcjournal/article/viewArticle/46 Last accessed 25 July 2014

Chen BX (2012, September 12) Robots in all walks of life: machines that help disabled people and make soldiers stronger, New York Times, pB1

Conley M (2011) Robots to help children with autism. ABC News. http://abcnews.go.com/Health/robots-children-autism/story?id=14780741. Accessed 25 July 2014

Hamilton R, Messing S, Chatterjee A (2011) Neurology: rethinking the thinking cap. Neurology 76:187

Hamric AB, Spross JA, Hanson C (2000) A framework for resolving ethical dilemmas in health care. From http://learn.gwumc.edu/hscidist/LearningObjects/EthicalDecisionMaking/index.htm

Hanna KE (2006) Genetic enhancement. National Human Genome Research Institute. http://www.genome.gov/10004767. Accessed 25 July 2014

Helal A, Moktari M, Abdulrazzak B (2008) The engineering handbook of smart technology for aging, disability and independence. Wiley, Hoboken

Jasanoff S (2011) Constitutional moments in governing science and technology. Sci Eng Ethics 17:621–638

Johnson DG, Miller K (2009) Computer ethics. Prentice Hall, Upper Saddle River

National Commission for the Protection of Human Subjects of Biomedical and Behavioral Research (1979) Belmont report: ethical principles and guidelines for the protection of human subjects of research. U.S. Department of Health & Human Services, Washington, DC. http://www.hhs.gov/ohrp/humansubjects/guidance/belmont.html. Accessed 25 July 2014

North Jersey Record (2005, February 21) Human tracking: big brother goes mainstream. North Jersey Record. http://www.infowars.com/articles/bb/tracking_human_tracking_bb_goes_mainstreeam.htm. Accessed 25 July 2014

O'Reilly D (2012) The Colbert report's take on proteus digital health. Colbert report. http://www.behance.net/gallery/The-Colbert-Reports-Take-on-Proteus-Digital-Health/4796295. Accessed 25 July 2014

Peterson M (2011) Colloquium: is there an ethics of algorithms? 3TU Centre for Ethics and Technology, Enschede. http://www.ethicsandtechnology.eu/news/comments/colloquium_is_there_an_ethics_of_algorithms/. Accessed 25 July 2014

Pistorius O. (n.d.) Official website. http://www.oscarpistorius.com/. Accessed 25 July 2014

Pogorelc D (2012b) FDA clears first smart pill that senses when it's been taken. Med City News. http://medcitynews.com/2012/07/fda-clears-first-smart-pill-that-senses-when-its-been-taken/. Accessed 25 July 2014

Quality of Life Technology Engineering Research Center. From http://www.cmu.edu/qolt/Research/index.html. Accessed 25 July 2014

Resnik DB (2000) The moral significance of the therapy-enhancement distinction in human genetics. Camb Q Healthc Ethics 7:365–377

Seelman KD (2001) Science and technology policy: is disability a missing factor? In: Albrecht GL, Seelman KD, Bury M (eds) Handbook of disability studies. Sage Publications, Thousand Oaks, pp 663–692

Seelman KD, Hartman LM, Yu DM (2014) When cutting edge technology meets clinical practice: ethical dimensions of e-health. In: Pimple R (ed) Emerging pervasive information and communication technologies (PICT). Springer, Dordrecht, pp 101–148

Shakespeare T (2006) Disability rights and wrongs. Routledge, Florence

Siebers T (2008) Disability theory. University of Michigan Press, Ann Arbor

Stephanidis C (2009) The universal access handbook. CRC Press Taylor & Francis Group, London

Stimson D (2011) Ultrathin flexible brain implant offers unique look at seizures in NIH-funded research. NIH News. http://www.nih.gov/news/health/nov2011/ninds-13.htm. Accessed 25 July 2014

Veruggio G, Operto F (2008) Roboethics: social and ethical implications of robotics. In: Rus D (ed) Human-centered and life-like robotics, Section G. In: Siciliano B, Khatib O (ed) Springer handbook of robotics. Springer, Berlin, pp 1499–1522

Wasserman D, Asch A (2009) Informed consent and prenatal testing; the Kennedy-Brownback Act. AMA Virtual Mentor 11(9):721–724

Wheelchair Toyota's Robot. (2012, February 5). Disabled & disability. http://www. disabilityinaction.com/wheelchair-toyotas-robot.html. Accessed 25 July 2014

Wolbring G (n.d.) Scoping Document on nanotechnology and disabled people for the Center for Nanotechnology in Society at Arizona State University. Retrieved from http://cns.asu.edu/cns-library/documents/wolbring-scopingCDfinaledit.pdf

Wolbring G (2012) Citizen education through an ability expectation and "Ableism" lens; the challenge of science and technology and disabled people. Educ Sci 2:150–164

Crab and Yoghurt

19

Tobias Hecht

Abstract

"Crab and Yoghurt" mixes ethnographic interviewing with street children in Northeast Brazil with fiction, taking the form ultimately of a short story. Leaving aside the borders between what was and wasn't observed and what is and isn't fiction here, disability forms part of the notions of power held even by homeless children, who themselves are subject to ineffable discrimination. Disability renders adults closer—literally in this case—to the stature of children, at least from the vantage point of the thumb-sucking, pistol-wielding protagonist of the story.

Keywords

Street children • Brazil • Exploitation • Disability

Conceição wondered how the man would ascend the steep, narrow staircase. He wasn't old, not nearly so old as João Defunto whom she met from time to time at the Chantecler nor half so frail as Seu Dário, the watchman at the post office. She could even discern the muscles that bristled tentatively around his shoulders and forearms. He did not falter from side to side because one leg was made forever childlike from polio. Nor did he lurch like the old ladies in the favelas who drag a bloated foot at the end of a leg, thin and tired but spared as yet from elephantiasis. The man simply stopped in the middle. He had no feet. He had no legs.

The street urchins called him Carangueijo, because he moved like his namesake the crab. Through the veil of inhaled glue, it seemed to the children that when the man slid along the sidewalks, one hand thrust before the other, he had not one pair

T. Hecht (✉)
Independent Scholar
e-mail: hecht.tobias@live.com

© Springer Science+Business Media Dordrecht 2016   273
P. Block et al. (eds.), *Occupying Disability: Critical Approaches to Community,
Justice, and Decolonizing Disability*, DOI 10.1007/978-94-017-9984-3_19

of hands but several. He would weave along the sidewalks among Recife's languid strollers, surprising those he passed that the top half of a man could not only move of its own accord but was possessed of an urge to move faster than they. Some of the children even thought the man suspended his body in the air an inch above the ground with the reluctant strength of his arms. But Conceição knew otherwise.

She discovered his secret when once he had passed quite close to her. Conceição was sitting along the wharves. She realized that Carangueijo did not bob in the way one would imagine fitting for a man who walked with his hands and carried his torso. His body remained at a steady elevation above the earth, never descending fully to slap the hot pavement. As he approached, Conceição heard the pained cry of metal.

Carangueijo's hands propelled him, but the wheels nailed to the board below his torso were the key to his movement. It was difficult to know where the man ended and the contraption began. He would tuck his shirttails under the board, uniting the ends of the fabric with a pin, leaving no part of the wood or the wheels beneath exposed.

Carangueijo surveyed the stairs, planning his ascent. His calculating gaze reminded her of the look she had seen many times in the eyes of Seu Zé, her sometimes step-father. Before he would thrash out against Conceição or her mother or a figment of his drunken imagination, he stopped to consider his tactics. His eyelids would widen, his brow furrowed. His body would tense like a frightened rodent. He required several moments to decide whether to clasp an empty bottle, to unfurl his belt, to lift a chair by its back. She remembered how once he had grabbed a light bulb dangling from the ceiling on a thin wire. He wrapped his hand around the bulb and socket and yanked. Before the cord snapped from the ceiling the bulb popped in his hand. He noticed the splinters of glass in his palm, the red drops falling. His weapon, the wire, listless on the floor. Angry that his plan had been foiled, he forgot that he had planned to hit Conceição and instead grabbed the plastic relic of Preto Velho from the pantheon. He threw Preto Velho on the floor, pounding his heel into the saint.

"You ugly nigger! You never looked my way. Marinefa's a whore, so why do you listen to her? And she gave birth to more whores and knaves than I can count." He lifted the saint, thrust its plastic head in his mouth and clamped his teeth. He pulled on the body, but it would not separate from the head. He bit harder and saliva bubbled from the corners of his mouth.

Carangueijo raised his left hand and grasped the rail. He held his right hand behind him, then thrust it violently counter-clockwise. At the same time he heaved his torso upward and hopped onto the first step. He repeated the movements many times, pausing at each step, never loosening his left hand lest he sail backwards. Conceição stood at the top of the stairs, arms akimbo, as the crab ascended. He looked only as far ahead as the next step, never at Conceição. The rusted wheels gave him an uncertain perch.

Conceição began imagining what she would do with the money she would get off the crab. She wanted to fill her mother's refrigerator with new things that came in plastic containers, like Danon yoghurt. She wanted to surprise her mother with all sorts of food. She wanted a few of those pills that only Come-Rato knew how to get. She wanted sweetbread and Coca Cola, a tank-top and sunglasses, shoes and a colorful knapsack. She wanted all of those things.

The crab took a long time to climb the stairs. When he was about half way up, Conceição remembered Bochecha—for no apparent reason. He lost his crank to a bottle of glue. There he was, his bare toes clasping the back bumper of a bus, one hand through an open window, the other wrapped around the hot tail pipe. Conceição imagined the wind blowing through the boy's hair as the driver accelerated. Bochecha stretched his neck around the corner of the bus to take in more of the view. The bus lurched from side to side. A group of children at one stop taunted him—"glue sniffer." He spit in the wind, even knowing his cob would never reach them. As the bus left the stop, Bochecha took another look back at the kids. He felt his right hand burning on the tail pipe and released it. He aimed to grab a piece of trim on the corner of the bus but before he had a chance to get a solid grip, the bus swung around a sharp curve, sank to the right onto its tired shocks. Bochecha lost his hold on the windowsill where his left hand clasped and spun into the air, then onto the pavement. His torso settled into the pavement to the crackle of glass and ribs. The bottle that once bore honey but that Bochecha had filled with carpenter's glue and placed inside his shorts had shattered. When he awoke in the corridors of the Restauração, he no longer had a wick. He pissed through a hole they made in his belly. Conceição had seen it.

Afterwards the kids would tell him, "Bochecha, you should give in to death, you can't go on living like that. How are you going to screw a girl?" He said, "no problem, with my finger or my tongue."

When the man reached the penultimate step, Conceição retreated. She let her arms fall along her flat hips. She noticed the beads of perspiration that had gathered across his forehead and she felt tall for the first time as she looked down at the bearded crab. Usually she had to tilt her neck upwards to look at Johns. Sometimes she would stand on a box or a bed so they could rub their lips across her face, breathe into her ears.

When she was alone, sometimes Conceição sucked her thumb, the left one. She had recently wrapped the same thumb around the handle of a Mauser. Matuto, with whom she roamed sometimes, had showed her the pistol. It was so much heavier than she had ever imagined. But even though it was difficult for her to lift it into the air, she liked the feeling of grasping it in her hand, the crisscross pattern of the grip against her palm. Now she raised her thumb and hooked it through an empty belt loop. Carangueijo skated into room seven. Conceição, who had gone up first and been standing on the landing in the boarding house, followed.

The grimy window in room seven faced east and caught no wind. It looked out on a police station, boites, and a church whose only visitors were toothless, men who pestered Father Rogério for a sip of wine, a taste of wafer. The Father usually obliged. He knew of no other way to attract parishioners, and he didn't want to be transferred to the backlands where he hated the dust and feared the parching sun and empty sky.

Now it was Carangueijo who bent his neck backwards to scale Conceição's body
with his eyes. She smirked and he didn't know why. It was not the smile of shame
and fear he would have welcomed. It was the look he saw a hundred times a day.
How could half a man move? How could half a man fuck? She wondered if the crab
was like Bochecha, if he peed through his belly and screwed with his tongue.

"I don't do this for nothing," Conceição said.
"I know. You told me already, two hundred thousand."
"Yeah, and next month it'll go up. It goes up every month. Everything goes up
    every month."

He said nothing. He reached inside his shirt pocket and pulled out four crumpled
bills of 50,000. He stretched out his arm to lay them on the bed. Conceição saw
that the spot from which he had removed the bills wasn't empty. Carangueijo rolled
closer to her. His hands propelled him gently. The wheels squeaked. Another sound
intermingled with the crying of the wheels. Carangueijo stopped and turned his
head. He saw Matuto stepping toward him, Mauser in hand. Matuto knew even
more about the crab than Conceição did. He'd been watching him, following him
from a distance.

"It's in his shirt," Conceição said.

The crab's eyes opened wide, his brow furrowed. Just like Seu Zé. Only she knew
he could not pick up a chair, unfurl a belt he'd never worn. The smirk remained on
Conceição's lips. The crab didn't move. He was still, like a mechanical doll whose
spring had suddenly run out. Matuto handed the Mauser to Conceição. She looked
at it. It really was big inside her hand. She pointed it at Carangueijo. Matuto ripped
off the crab's shirt. Carangueijo, no longer attached to his board, tumbled to the
side, writhing to steady himself against the bed. He was naked without his shirt.
The crab grasped at Matuto's legs. Matuto kicked him, once in the ribs. The second
time in the jaw. And again in the ribs. The crab fell flat, and Matuto stepped on his
neck. He meant to hold the man down like that for a moment, but he realized that if
he kept his foot there and raised his body so that all his weight rested on the crab's
neck, the half man would soon stop writhing. Conceição wondered if the crab's neck
was as strong as Preto Velho's. From his back sprouted stiff black, hairs. His arms
thrashed, his eyes opened even wider, and the sounds from his mouth were of both
of fury and defeat. He became almost quiet before his entire body arched, just like
with the other men who paid her. Then it all stopped. He was as limp as the cord
Seu Zé had yanked from the ceiling. Matuto picked up the rest of the money that
had fallen from the crab's shirt pocket.
    Conceição went to see what was in the refrigerator. It was a tiny refrigerator, no
taller than the crab himself. She pulled open the door. He had beer—in those little,
tiny bottles. Conceição removed two of them and let them roll onto the floor. In the
back she saw a plastic container of yoghurt. She picked it up. "Danone," she said,

unable to read the blue letters. It was famous. She held it in one hand and wondered what her mother would think when she received the gift.

Editors' Postscript   If you liked this chapter by Tobias Hecht, and are interested in reading more about disability in Brazil, we recommend Chap. 20 "Occupying Disability in Brazil" by Anahi Guedes de Mello, Pamela Block, Adriano Henrique Nuernberg, which contains a discussion of Hecht's story and its relationship to disability studies in Brazil and internationally. Another chapter about disability and occupation in Brazil is "Artistic Therapeutic Treatment, Colonialism & Spectacle: A Brazilian Tale" by Marta Simões Peres, Francine Albiero de Camargo, José Otávio P. e Silva, and Pamela Block. If you are interested in intersections of disability, race, ethnicity, class, and violence consider Chap. 4: "Movements at War? Disability and Anti-Occupation Activism in Israel" by Liat Ben-Moshe and Chap. 21 "Black & Blue: Policing Disability & Poverty Beyond Occupy" by Leroy Franklin Moore Jr, Lisa 'Tiny' Garcia, and Emmitt Thrower. Other chapters that feature disability in the global south and legacies of colonialism include Michele Friedner: "Occupying Seats, Occupying Space, Occupying Time: Deaf Young Adults in Vocational Training Centers in Bangalore, India," Chap. 5 "Landings: Decolonizing Disability, Indigeneity and Poetic Methods" by Petra Kuppers, and Chap. 9: "A Situational Analysis of Persons with Disabilities in Jamaica and Trinidad and Tobago: Education and Employment Policy Imperatives," by Annicia Gayle-Geddes.

Block and Lilian Magalhães (faculty in the Occupational Therapy Program at Western Ontario University) used this short story very effectively when teaching a class on disability in the global south to occupational therapy students. Magalhães found images of Crab's mobility device, also images of Recife and even the neighborhood where the events in the story took place. Students were reminded that although this is a work of fiction, the events in the story actually took place and were documented in ethnographic interviews that Hecht collected. Magalhães discussed temporality and risk as experienced by poor people in Brazil, and also the desire to do good for loved ones, as evidenced by Conceição's desire to bring home something nice for her mother. This was a very powerful mechanism to discuss the intersectionality of gender, race, class, sexuality, disability and violence and the relevance of all of these to occupation.

Occupying Disability Studies in Brazil

20

20

Anahi Guedes de Mello, Pamela Block, and Adriano Henrique Nuernberg

Abstract

The objective of this paper is to present a historical overview of the field of disability studies in Brazil. The approach takes into account the background of social models of disability and precursor scholarship in Brazil leading to the emergence of disability studies in the 2000s. It emphasizes the influence of key international scholars on their Brazilian counterparts and current research challenges for Brazilian disability studies.

Keywords

Disability studies • Intersectionality • Race • Poverty • Sexuality • Disability • Brazil • Social models of disability

Spoiler Alert We recommend you read Tobias Hecht's short story (chapter 19) before reading this chapter. This chapter reveals plot elements from Hecht's story.

A.G. de Mello (✉)
Graduate Program in Social Anthropology, Federal University of Santa Catarina, Florianópolis, SC, Brazil
e-mail: anahi.mello@posgrad.ufsc.br

P. Block
Disability Studies, Health and Rehabilitation Sciences, School of Health Technology and Management, Stony Brook University, Stony Brook, NY, USA
e-mail: pamela.block@stonybrook.edu

A.H. Nuernberg
Graduation and Postgraduation Program in Psychology, Federal University of Santa Catarina, Florianópolis, SC 88015-310, Brazil
e-mail: adriano.nuernberg@ufsc.br

© Springer Science+Business Media Dordrecht 2016
P. Block et al. (eds.), *Occupying Disability: Critical Approaches to Community, Justice, and Decolonizing Disability*, DOI 10.1007/978-94-017-9984-3_20

20.1   Introduction

Here we introduce critical reflections on occupation in Brazil as they intersect with anthropology and disability studies and explain why we chose the short story, "Crab and Yoghurt" written by Brazilianist anthropologist Tobias Hecht. Hecht was not a scholar of disability studies, and nor was he even Brazilian, he was based in the United States. Yet, since encountering this work of ethnographic fiction, we found our thoughts returning to it repeatedly. Although the piece was fictional, it was based on actual events as retold and documented while Hecht was engaged in anthropological field work in a Northeastern Brazilian Favela. It became a reference point, for us, an unconventional guide for understanding what Brazilian disability studies has been and might become and to illustrate the theoretical debate around the oppression of the disabled body as it relates to other oppressions. It provided a Brazilian scenario where gender, race, sexuality, social status and violence intersected with disability.

Expected power relationships and notions of freedom and constraint were inverted in this story. Crab was a man without feet and legs who hires a child prostitute. The story unfolded from the perspective of the girl as she sets up Crab to be robbed, bludgeoned, and ultimately, killed by her pimp. Crab was a man with missing lower limbs, but he moved with seeming effortlessness through the streets on his skateboard-improvised mobility device. From the perspective of a child prostitute he was rich and free. The greatest wish of the girl was to steal a yogurt, perceived by her as the height of luxury, from Crab's refrigerator to give as gift to her mother. With the use of assistive technology that provided function and the "better position" of gender and social status, Crab was able ascend to a level of social, material, and spiritual status that the prostitute and pimp could never have. It was only through the use of violence that the pimp put Crab "in his place"— the accustomed place where the disabled body repulsed with its strangeness and vulnerability—and could be abused and discarded.

This short story provided an opening for us to discuss the academic dimensions and politics of occupying disability studies in Brazil. We did this not just in terms of a disciplinary field of academic investigation and of the professional work of many researchers, but also in material terms of who "occupies," as social actors, a prominent place in theoretical debates in this area of knowledge. We considered that reflexivity (Clifford and Marcus 1986; Geertz 1973; Giddens 1990) was a trademark of contemporary anthropological theory and research, associated with what George Marcus defined as a movement of "self-critique, the personal quest, playing on the subjective, the experimental, and the idea of empathy" (Marcus 1998, p. 193). This work understood reflexivity to be the focus of analysis. Thus we focused upon our analytic trajectories and individual experience as activists and researchers in the field of Brazilian disability studies.

20.2   Personal Trajectories

Moving between various activisms in different moments of her career, Anahi became a "deaf-rights activist" in 1992 and a "disability-rights activist" in 1998 when she was a Chemistry student at the Federal University of Santa Catarina (UFSC). In 2008, when she was a Social Sciences student at the UFSC, Anahi identified herself as a lesbian activist. She participated in the founding, in 2004, of the Center for Independent Living of Florianópolis (CVI-Floripa), the first in the state of Santa Catarina, and was its first president for two consecutive terms (2004–2006, 2006–2008). In this way she became the first deaf person to officially join the Independent Living Movement in Brazil (MVI). Another influential experience was her participation in the preparation and approval of the Brazilian disability access law Decree 5.296/2004, which regulates Law No. 10.048/2000 and No. 10.098/2000, known as "the laws of accessibility."

In her academic career, Anahi was always strongly influenced by her "activist capital," in terms of Pierre Bourdieu (1986), a form of social capital. This was evidenced through her active participation, since her youth, in social movements for the rights of people with disabilities, and her participation in important national and international events in the construction of public policies for people with disabilities, especially those focused on accessibility issues, gender and sexualities (Torres et al. 2007; Mello and Nuernberg 2012; Mello and Fernandes 2013). Her theoretical approach and definitive adherence to guidelines and feminist disability studies research was shaped by anthropologist and bioethicist Debora Diniz's (2003) "Social Model of Disability: a feminist critique." This theoretical work was considered one of the first examples of the interface between disability studies and feminist theories in Brazil. As a disabled woman, Anahi was intellectually, emotionally and existentially involved in discussions on women's and gender studies and disability studies. She went on to develop her research in two academic spaces[1] which articulate in different, but complementary ways, gender, sexuality, violence and disability.

One of the many contributions which Brazil had to offer the international disability studies community was a grounded intersectional approach to social problems (a unique approach to race, gender, sexuality and social status) and participatory research methodologies. When Pamela went down to Brazil in the 1990s for her doctoral research, she had planned to study intersections of race, gender, class and sexuality but at the last moment decided to include—and privilege—the category of disability. She compared eugenics movements and their legacies in the US and Brazil.

None of Pamela's US mentors had any expertise in disability and she did not begin to connect to the United States disability studies community until after she

---

[1]The Nucleus of Gender Identity and Subjectivities (NIGs) coordinated by anthropologist Miriam Pillar Grossi, and the Nucleus of Disability Studies (NED) coordinated by psychologist Adriano Henrique Nuernberg.

defended her dissertation and received her doctorate in 1997. Thus her primary mentors when she conducted her research in Brazil were Brazilian disability researchers.[2] These people may not have called themselves "disability studies" scholars, but functionally their research meets the criteria for what constitutes disability studies with a focus on socio-cultural, narrative and historical perspectives. Pamela expresses her gratitude for having the opportunity to learn disability studies in the Brazilian context by doing everything possible to promote Brazilian disability studies both in Brazil and abroad.

As a researcher and professor in the area of disability studies, Adriano Henrique Nuernberg participated in a diverse range of academic and political events relevant to this theme. He was introduced to disability studies by the book *O que é deficiência?/What's disability?*, authored by Debora Diniz (2007). In his work Adriano used a social model perspective to explain the importance of removing barriers to social participation of people with disabilities. He developed several studies aimed at promoting equal access to knowledge for students with disabilities (Nuernberg 2008, 2009). As a teacher, Adriano guided research and extension work that resulted in the better inclusion of children and youth with disabilities. He was recognized with three national awards for his work related to disability and human rights perspectives. Currently he is interested in the field of disability studies in Education as a powerful field to support his research related to inclusive education.

20.3 The Precursors of Disability Studies in Brazil

Disability studies and social model approaches in Brazil was introduced quite recently and was still limited to a small number of scholars, as Adriano's experience underscores. Under the aegis of social integration, the Brazilian disability rights movement, mostly headed by disabled women, began in 1979 during the military dictatorship. At this time, major disability rights associations formed a social movement and began to contest control of disabled people by the State, family and experts in the fields of health and rehabilitation. This movement was formed to lobby representatives in the Constitutional Assembly in 1987, and in 1988 this group wrote the early draft of sections of the current Brazilian Constitution that refer to specific

---

[2]They included: Dr. Olivia Pereira, who advised Pamela in research methodology, guided her to consider the Pestalozzis to the APAEs in a historical perspective, and directed her to study the legacy of Helen Antipoff (Block 2007). Dr. Rosana Glat, whose 1989 book "Somos Iguais a Vocês" ('We are equal to you') was ahead of its time, incorporating analyses of gender and power in the personal narratives of women with intellectual disability. Dr. Glat also spent hours with Pamela explaining the differences between US and Brazilian service systems for people with intellectual disability. Lastly Dr. Annibal Coelho de Amorim, whose research compared the self-advocacy movements for people with intellectual disability in Brazil, the United States and Japan. His example of creating communities through participatory research was very significant. Additional influences include: Rosangela Berman Bieler and Lilia Pinto Martins for introducing me to Brazilian disability rights history and the Brazilian approach to independent living movement. Sueli Satow brought her theoretical personal narrative approach.

and general rights for disabled people. This movement also staged a campaign called "Rehabilitation Decade (1970–1979)" as part of an effort promoted internationally by the United Nations (UN), for the establishment of more rehabilitation centers and educational opportunities (Brasil 2010).

Parallel to these political events, in late twentieth century Brazilian academia, the theme of disability drew the interest of a few sociologists, anthropologists, social workers, and historians. The Brazilian social science academics had long neglected this area of study, leaving research related to disability in the realms of medicine, education and psychology. In the context of the redemocratization process of the country and the emergence of various social movements from the 1970s, the first Brazilian researchers to include social model formulations of disability came, with a few exceptions, from the fields of education and psychology. Most of these researchers were not disabled, did not affiliate with the disability rights social movements, and were greatly influenced by foreign disability studies scholarship.

We noted in particular the contributions of Sadao Omote and Rosana Glat to the areas of Psychology and Education. These authors provided the first arguments and conceptualizations of social models of disability in Brazilian Portuguese, pointing to the sociocultural context as a constitutive element of disability. Although the concept of disability was not as radical in these as it is in subsequent models, we propose that these early works had an important role in mobilizing the Brazilian academic community towards disability perspective more focused on human rights.

Sadao Omote, Professor of the College of Philosophy and Science at the State University of São Paulo, campus of Marilia (Unesp/Marilia), was noteworthy for his historic contributions, in the 1980s and 1990s, to scholarship on the social dimension of disability (Omote 1994, 2010). He wrote about stigma and stereotypes in relation to disabled people, especially in the context of education (Piccolo et al. 2010). His scholarship represented a disability studies perspective, highlighting the importance of the uniqueness of disability experience as a social category, citing authors influential to the field of disability studies in the United States, such as Erving Goffman (1963). Rosana Glat, Professor and Dean, College of Education at the State University of Rio de Janeiro, was the author of "Somos Iguais a Vocês"/"We are Equal to You" (Glat 1989), a book with conceptual and methodological elements that make it a foundational work of disability studies in Brazil. We would argue that only language barriers prevented this book from receiving the international attention it deserves. By giving voice to 35 women with intellectual disability, valuing their perceptions and perspectives about sexuality, affectivity and their family and social interactions, Glat conceptualized disability in ways previously articulated with other social categories, such as sex differences and/or gender. In the 1980s Brazilian context of scientific development during which disabled people were usually reduced and objectified as the focus of assessment and intervention procedures, Glat's focus on the narratives and experiences of these women through interviews and life stories was methodologically innovative. Her writing about women with intellectual disability using a disability studies perspective was also unique, for in the 1980s very few disability studies scholars internationally were doing this. Moreover, her arguments pointed to the social nature of the phenomenon of disability, as the author says:

> [...]I think it important to point out that my choice, for the purpose of analysis, of the social model of disability is not due solely to a theoretical preference, but primarily due to nearly 15 years of clinical experience in this area. I believe that, at least in people with mild or moderate disabilities (who represent the population of this research), socio-educational factors are the main determinants of their overall functioning.[3] (Glat 1989, p. 22)

Rosana Glat's research emphasized the singular dimension of the experience of disability, and criticized conceptualization and classification models that homogenize people with intellectual disabilities. To do so, she relied on primarily anthropological and sociological scholarship to analyze of the social production of disability. Rosana Glat received her master's degree training in Psychology in the United States.

We could cite several other authors, such as Suely Harumi Satow (2000) and Lígia Assumpção Amaral (2004), and a thorough genealogy of perspectives leading up to the establishment of disability studies in Brazil should be conducted someday. Although there are examples, they were not well known in the context of the early Brazilian disability studies, and we do not have the space here to explore these in depth. Our goal was to document that the early presence of critical approaches to the phenomenon of disability in Brazil arose primarily within psychology and education. These precursors made a conceptual leap by providing alternatives to biomedical models and prepared the way for the subsequent emergence of disability studies from a social model perspective in multiple fields within the Brazilian context.

20.4   The Emergence of Brazilian Disability Studies or Who Occupies Disability Studies in Brazil?

The 2003 publication of "Social Model of Disability: a feminist critique" by anthropologist Debora Diniz (University of Brasilia, UnB), was a turning point for the emergence of definitive disability studies in Brazil. This landmark publication introduced a disability studies social model approach which intersected with feminist theories. Diniz asserted that disability is governed under the same theoretical-epistemological frameworks used in studies of gender and feminism, since:

> [...] It considered inequality as immoral and fought against oppression. The analogy between the oppression of the disabled body and sexism was one of the pillars that supported the thesis of "the disabled" as a social minority. Just as women were oppressed because of sex, the disabled were oppressed because of the body with injuries—this was a rhetorical approach that facilitated the task of de-essentializing inequality.[4] (Diniz 2007, pp. 58–59)

---

[3]Free translation.
[4]Free translation.

The twenty-first century inception of disability studies in Brazil took place when Debora Diniz returned to Brazil from New York in 2002 after participating in a 3-week National Endowment for the Humanities Institute organized by two prominent theorists of gender and disability studies: Eva Feder Kittay and Anita Silvers. In Brazil, the field of feminist disability studies grew out of research produced by Anis—Institute of Bioethics, Human Rights and Gender, including Debora Diniz and other scholars whose work engaged the intersection of disability studies, feminist theory, and theory of justice. Anis was the first non-profit organization in Latin America dedicated to research, advisement, and training in Bioethics. Based in Brasilia and staffed by an interdisciplinary team of professionals from different fields, Anis also developed training activities and materials around the issues of bioethics and disability, in partnership with the research group led by two social workers, Cristiano Guedes and Lívia Barbosa Pereira: "Ethics, Health and Inequality" at UnB. Researchers at the institute have produced scholarship of national significance, as represented in the edited collections of articles published as books: "Deficiência e Discriminação"/"Disability and Discrimination" (Diniz and Santos 2010) and "Deficiência e Igualdade"/"Disability and Equality" (Diniz et al. 2010). Each volume included a reprinted article by renowned foreign authors in the field of Theory of Justice, such as Amartya Sen (2010), who won the Nobel Prize in Economics in 1998, and Martha Nussbaum (2010), translated into Portuguese.

Other recent works that emphasized the experience of disability from the theoretical disability studies perspective included: Santos (2008), Ortega (2008, 2009), Mello (2010), Bernardes et al. (2009), Nicolau et al. (2013), and Gesser et al. (2012). Wederson Santos (2008), from the same group as Debora Diniz, provided an overview of the condition of persons with disabilities in Brazil, identifying from a critical perspective two major currents inside these models, (ie, medical and social models) of disability. His text was one of the first published in a Brazilian journal to discuss the hegemony of biomedical models in the analysis of Brazilian disability issues.

Francisco Ortega (2008, 2009) examined the innovations and contradictions of the neurodiversity movement, mostly led by autistic people, usually those with the "high functioning" characteristics of Asperger syndrome. This movement did not consider autism as a disease, but rather an aspect of the diversity of humanity, and therefore rejects the attempts to cure, and opposes aversive behavioral therapies that seek to eliminate or hide inherent behavioral characteristics of autism. Neurodiversity movement activists sometimes opposed parent groups over treatments and parenting techniques and provided a strong recommendations in the areas of education, treatment, and public policy for autistic people. Interestingly, these arguments against a cure for autism found a parallel in the anti-cure rhetoric of the Deaf Pride movement.

Liliane Bernardes et al. (2009) used a social model of disability to assess bioethical aspects of public health access by persons with disabilities, and to analyze the relationship between the disability experience and the condition of vulnerability. In a related work, Stella Nicolau et al. (2013) assessed the dual vulnerability of women with disabilities in access to basic health care in São Paulo, based on a feminist analysis linking gender and disability.

Marivete Gesser et al. (2012) provided a theoretical study that emphasized the relevance of social psychology in considering disability as a category of analysis in psychosocial research and praxis. For the authors, the focus of social models of disability was linked to the critical social psychology, especially in its commitment to human rights.

Using qualitative ethnographic methods, based on participant observation, interviews, and informal conversations with disabled people with a history of activism, Mello (2010) discussed the constitution of the social experience of disability. Her approach focused on the issues of construction of the person, body and subjectivity in order to understand how these categories were articulated in the production of disability as a social identity. For Anahi, disability acted as a *mode of subjectification*[5] in the contemporary world. The specificity of this process of subjectification was linked to the concept of resilience, i.e., the ability of a human to overcome their limitations, adapt and build positive attitudes from the adversities of life. Thus, as corroborated by Charles Gardou (2006), the experience of the disabled body revealed new dimensions to the anthropological approach of body and corporeality. In other words, the embodiment of the experience of disability, to subvert the stigma of the disabled body, highlights the condition of the person, or disability was "also a way to be like a certain type of subject—in this case it is the body, or more specifically, a particular corporeality, that builds a particular person"[6] (Maluf 2001 p. 96).

20.5   Contradictions in the Field

Due to the difficulty of separating socio-cultural from disease/pathology approaches to disability, it was not uncommon to find both conceptualizations mingled in most Brazilian disability studies research, with biomedical perspectives predominating. This was because its proponents have neither separated nor even indicated their understanding of the difference between disability research (based in medical, educational, and psychological principles) and disability studies research (based on a socio-cultural framing). While the first emphasized the perspective of medical treatment and the notion of disability as a "personal tragedy" or anomalous condition that needs be corrected, the second provided a perspective of disability as a facet of human diversity. This was a tension present in discussions at International Symposia of disability studies at the Institute of Social Medicine, State University of Rio de Janeiro (IMS/UERJ) on May 23–24, 2011, and at the Convention Center Hotel Novotel São Paulo, June 19–21, 2013. In general, this

---

[5]According to Foucault *regimes* or *modes of subjectification* are "the different modes by which, in our culture, human beings are made subjects." (Foucault 1983, p. 208).

[6]Free translation.

was always a challenge in interdisciplinary academic studies on disability. There was both a bit of everything, and everything in excess: the voice of suffering, life histories marked under the label of "narratives of personal tragedy," many awkward silences, not enough critical social analysis, and a significant amount of biomedical conceptualization. The 2011 symposium lacked basic physical and communication access and included only a limited number of researchers.[7]

In the 2013 symposium there was a much larger number of people attending the event, with a commensurate increase in diversity of approaches to what constituted "disability studies." This symposium included activists, academics, artists, performers, managers and teachers of special education, and rehabilitation. This resulted in various tensions based the diversity of approaches: partial inclusion vs. full inclusion; Deaf culture versus oral deaf and hard of hearing people; use of technology versus acceptance of an unmodified condition; "research on disability" versus "research in disability studies," etc. Many audience-members had disability experience, but no academic training, which meant that discussion at times devolved into political arguments and rejections of presentation content which conflicted with understandings based on personal experience. This relativization or subjectification of academic focus inspired Anahi (first author of this chapter) to intervene at times, using her dual position of researcher/activist to bridge the gap between activist social experience and academic social theory. Examples of this tension include questions raised by two blind male activists about the relationship between gender and disability. For them the role of gender had nothing to do with people with disabilities. Anahi intervened in the debate, first clarifying that although she was an activist-academic, her focus in that moment would be scholarly. She then explained how disability studies was derived from the same epistemological premises as feminist and gender studies, and related to classic dichotomies such as nature and culture, universal and particular, society and the individual: the dichotomies of sex(nature)/gender(culture) is to women's and gender studies what the dichotomy impairment(nature)/disability(culture) is for disability studies. She also explained that care is a point of intersection between the two fields, hence the political catchphrase: we are all "some mother's child" (Kittay 1999, p. 24).

The audience was mostly female, mostly nondisabled women, educators or managers of special education, which also pointed to the misconception of the field of disability studies as a sub-category of special education. A significant number

---

[7]Several scholars from Brazilian universities were invited to present their research and discuss the "state of art" of disability studies in Brazil by event co-organizers Francisco Ortega, philosopher and teacher of IMS/UERJ, and chapter co-author (and former president of the Society for disability studies) Pamela Block. Invited keynotes included bioethicist and prominent Brazilian disability studies scholar Debora Diniz, Devva Kasnitz (who was President of the Society for disability studies at the time), and psychiatrist and historian Fernando Ramos. Several Brazilian universities including the State University of Rio de Janeiro, the Federal University of Rio de Janeiro, the Federal University of Santa Catarina, University of Brasilia, the Federal University of São Carlos, and the University of Campinas, among others, all of these having groups, centers, or research lines connected with disability or accessibility.

of abstracts on the topic of special education were approved for presentation at this event, which was consistent with this trend. Very few disabled Brazilian researchers working in the field of Brazilian disability studies attended and presented. Most attendees were not disabled and some prominent disabled scholars attended but did not present. All but one of the international guest researchers[8] were men, and only one was disabled. In addition to the excellent physical accessibility of the conference center and the accessibility features for deaf and blind (captioning, sign language interpretation, and audio-description) the main lectures and presentations were simultaneously translated in English and Portuguese. This was available due to the financial and programming support provided by the São Paulo State Secretariat for the Rights of Persons with Disabilities. The disabled activists present also occupied a prominent place in discussions during the conference, and often referred to each other by two native categories, separating veteran members of the disability movement from the "new activists": the "Jurassic" from the "baby sauros." These native categories were a loving and humorous way that the "older" and "newer" Brazilian independent living movement activists related to each other, aiming to recognize generational changes, find commonality in the current moment, and preserve precious memories. The activist-academic Anahi is framed in the latter category.

Another milestone in the consolidation of disability studies in Brazil was the creation, in March 2012, of a Disability and Accessibility Committee within the Brazilian Anthropological Association (ABA), coordinated by anthropologist Adriana Dias (Unicamp), and including Anahi Guedes de Mello (UFSC), Debora Diniz (UnB) and Luiz Gustavo P. S. Correia (UFS). This group's first official meeting took place in São Paulo on July 2, 2012, during the 28th Brazilian Anthropology Meeting (28th Reunião Brasileira de Antropologia, RBA) held at the Pontifical Catholic University of São Paulo (PUC-SP). This initiative was in the in honor of two anthropologists with disabilities Rita Amaral[8] (USP), who died in January 2011, and Adriana Dias (Unicamp), both with *osteogenesis imperfecta*. The goal was to ensure that the Brazilian Anthropology Association provided accessibility to enable all people with disability to participate in their national meetings, just as at the Society for disability studies, which since 1984 tried to be a model of accessible conferencing. In Brazil it took four additional meetings before the organizers of the 2011–2012 Brazilian Anthropological Association, chaired by the anthropologist Bela Feldman-Bianco, officially created the organization's Disability and Accessibility Committee.

The Disability and Accessibility Committee began to consider not only the issues and demands related to accessibility in all its dimensions (architectural, communication, instrumental and methodological), but also the rights and the collective understandings that characterize ethnographic research on disability, and people with disabilities as research subjects. Thus, it was expected that the Brazilian

---

[8]Rita Amaral was also honored in the First National Meeting on the Politics for Women with Disabilities which took place during the XI International Technologies Fair for Rehabilitation, Inclusion, and Accessibility (XI Reatech) in São Paulo/SP, on April 14–15, 2012, through the memorial address given by Adriana Dias.

Anthropological Association triggered, much like the Society for disability studies, a vector of social change. This was especially true in its advocating greater participation of people with disabilities in academia, which included increasing the number of disabled students and teachers in higher education, and the need to teach their peer researchers how to make their work more universally accessible. With the practice of inclusive education guaranteed by Brazilian law, and with the increased presence of people with disabilities in universities across the country, the demand for accessibility would also grow and become an underlying assumption.

Another innovative Brazilian event that included critical perspectives on disability issues was the 10th International Seminar: "Doing Gender," the most important Women's Studies and Gender meeting in Brazil. It was held in Florianópolis, Santa Catarina, from September 16–20, 2013. Understanding that disability was mainstreamed implied the emergence of guidelines and demands for accessibility not only in governmental gender policies, but also in an effort to promote and entrench the principles of accessibility in Brazilian feminist theory.[9] Thus a commission was created, under the coordination of Anahi Guedes de Mello, and charged with the task of providing critical pedagogical perspectives on the implementation of accessibility for the full and effective participation of disabled students and researchers in the area of Women's Studies and gender in Brazil.[10] A well-timed initiative, given this was a moment when disability topics were beginning to appear as a category of analysis in Women's Studies and Gender, for example the recent work of Anahi and Adriano (2012), a review of national and international literatures on feminism and disability.

20.6 Disability and Intersectionality

As discussed earlier in this chapter, Brazilian researchers had much to contribute in the area of disability and intersectionality. There was well-developed scholarship in the areas of disability, gender and sexuality and much potential not yet fully realized to add race/ethnicity and social status to the scholarship of disability in Brazil. In particular, colonial and post-colonial, slavery and post-slavery experiences deeply influenced how Brazilians embody all these categories as shown by Brazilian critical race theorist Lilia Moritz Schwartz's emerging research on the racialized disability experiences of writer Lima Barreto (Schwartz 2013, 2014).

To circle back to Hecht's story, mentioned at the beginning of this discourse: Crab's desire to express his transgressive sexuality through the child prostitute was represented in Hecht's tale as a vulnerability that lead to his doom. The helpless

---

[9]One of the highlights of this event was a much-praised booklet entitled "Guide to Basic Guidelines on Gender, Disability and Accessibility," prepared by two members of the committee (Mello and Fernandes 2013).

[10]In Brazil the implementation of communication accessibility in 10th International Seminar "Doing Gender" was supported by the National Secretariat for the Rights of Persons with Disabilities (SNPD).

child prostitute now had power over Crab—the power to steal—and the power of life and death. This tale had a correlation to what Amaral and Coelho (2003) found in their research on the social self-image of people considered "disabled."

> Invisible "Defects" such as stuttering, color blindness, hemophilia, sterility, mastectomy, colostomy, AIDS, are those that, in the end allow what Goffman (1982: 16) calls "the manipulation of information" but which, in principle, are generally excluded from the category of disabled. The disabled themselves have also constructed a type of "gradation" of defects, placing some in superiority/inferiority with respect to each other. The main criterion for this classification seems to be how close it is (or can appear) to *normality*. Those who can pass as "normal" or have concealable disabilities generally occupy the "best places" in the classification system. This categorization is reinforced by family members and others with whom the disabled person lives. During the fieldwork, Roger, a deaf boy's mother, declared herself relieved because his deafness was seen as a lesser evil: "And what if he were blind? Or paralyzed? This [deafness] is [by comparison] no problem for us." Another mother of a deaf teenager says: "I went to visit a school for retarded children and left relieved."[11] (Amaral and Coelho 2003) (Translation by P. Block)

In an anthropological perspective, the more "deviant" and "deformed" the body, the more revulsion or fascination the "normals" felt about this body. There was a sexual dissidence[12] (Rubin 1998) to this, showing a unique form of vulnerability in the condition of disability, which, in turn, when crossed with power asymmetries present in the relations of gender, race/ethnicity, class, age, sexuality, etc., enhanced the appearance of other forms of inequality and violence against people with disabilities. The presence of disabled bodies revealed the enormous difficulty that people without disabilities had accepting human frailty. The teratological potential of disabled bodies showed how our humanity, set in the "able body," still had the germ of inhumanity (Gil 1994). Therefore, disability defined the wretchedness of materiality in its most radical sense. With his extraordinary body (Garland-Thomson 1997) Crab was profoundly disturbing to Conceição and Matuto because he represented one of the most totalizing experiences of corporal transgression.

20.7 Final Considerations

With this analysis of Hecht's story and preliminary review of key works and events highlighted here, we hoped to contribute to the record of the formation of the field of disability studies in Brazil. The field is still in the process of emerging. We note that the innovative conceptual perspective of disability studies in Brazil has not yet fully

---

[11] Free translation.

[12] The term "sexual dissidence" or "dissident sexuality" is a theoretical category of queer studies and was originally posted by Gayle Rubin in his seminal essay "Thinking Sex". Whereas that Gay and Lesbian Studies have focused their investigations on the issue of homosexuality being a "natural" or "unnatural" behavior, remaining within a binary logic, queer theory expands the investigative focus to encompass any kind of sexual practice or identity that are on border of normative categories or deviant. We consider the disabled bodies part of the list of dissident sexualities.

achieved a radical break from biomedical models–it appears in most cases to remain in some ways fused with medicalized notions from fields such as rehabilitation, psychology, and education. Even when inclusive principles are valued within these fields, it is still common to see implicit or explicit examples of the disabled body as having an inherent organic disadvantage—rather than a disadvantage produced by socio-cultural and environmental barriers.

Paradoxically, Brazil was one of the countries that most rapidly incorporated the Convention on the Rights of Persons with Disabilities, the well-known "UN Convention" into national policy. Thus, Brazilian public policy defined disability as the interaction of long-term physical, sensory, intellectual, mental and social barriers. Despite the relative ease with which the Convention was approved by the National Congress, the Executive Branch and the social movements, we cannot say yet that was used to leverage the field of Brazilian disability studies in proportion to its impact in other Brazilian social spheres.

Significant to the future of Brazilian disability studies, would be the need for more significant interdisciplinary scholarly participation in the epistemological foundations of the field, especially from feminist and queer perspectives. As Mello and Nuernberg (2012) argued, feminist theories touched the very core of assumptions about corporeality, interdependence, and the centering of disability in an intersectional framework, but they were not yet fully articulated in terms of the theoretical tensions and methodological implications. Without this epistemological concern, there will be no advancement in the understanding of the social and cultural barriers that not only serve as "influences" or "variables" of disability, but are central to constituting and determining the phenomenon. So what makes Brazilian disability studies different from disability studies in other countries? One of the challenges is to consider uniquely Brazilian approaches to the dimensions of gender, sexuality, race/ethnicity, class, etc., at the junction of disability experience and grounded in Brazilian realities.

Editors' Postscript If you liked this chapter by Mello et al., and are interesting in reading more about disability in Brazil, we recommend Chap. 19 "Crab and Yoghurt" by Tobias Hecht, which is discussed extensively in Chap. 20. Another chapter about disability and occupation in Brazil is "Artistic Therapeutic Treatment, Colonialism & Spectacle: A Brazilian Tale" by Marta Simões Peres, Francine Albiero de Camargo, José Otávio P. e Silva, and Pamela Block. If you are interested in intersections of disability, race, ethnicity, class, and violence consider Chap. 4: "Movements at War? Disability and Anti-Occupation Activism in Israel" by Liat Ben-Moshe and Chap. 21 "Black & Blue: Policing Disability & Poverty Beyond Occupy" by Leroy Franklin Moore Jr., Lisa 'Tiny' Garcia, and Emmitt Thrower. Other chapters that feature disability in the global south and legacies of colonialism include Michele Friedner: "Occupying Seats, Occupying Space, Occupying Time: Deaf Young Adults in Vocational Training Centers in Bangalore, India," Chap. 5 "Landings: Decolonizing Disability, Indigeneity and Poetic Methods" by Petra Kuppers, and Chap. 9: "A Situational Analysis of Persons with Disabilities in Jamaica and Trinidad and Tobago: Education and Employment Policy Imperatives," by Annicia Gayle-Geddes.

Acknowledgments The first author expresses her thanks to Capes for granting her the master's scholarship, and to CNPq for funding of the project "Feminist Theory, Queer Theory or Contemporary Social Theories?: the field of gender studies and sexuality in Brazil" (Process No. 402545/2010-9).

References

Amaral LA (2004) Resgatando o passado: deficiência como figura e vida como fundo. Casa do Psicólogo, São Paulo

Amaral R, Coelho AC (2003) Nem Santos nem Demônios: considerações sobre a imagem social e a auto-imagem das pessoas ditas deficientes. Os Urbanitas 1(0). http://www.osurbanitas.org/antropologia/osurbanitas/revista/deficientes.html. Accessed 3 Dec 2013

Bernardes LCG, Maior IMML, Spezia CH, Araujo TCCF (2009) Pessoas com Deficiência e Políticas de Saúde no Brasil: reflexões bioéticas. Ciên Saúde Colet 14(1):31–38

Block P (2007) Institutional utopias, eugenics, and intellectual disability in Brazil. Hist Anthropol 18(2):177–196

Bourdieu P (1986) The forms of capital. In: Richardson JG (ed) Handbook of theory and research for the sociology of education. Greenwood Press, New York, pp 241–258

Brasil (2010) História do Movimento Político das Pessoas com Deficiência no Brasil. Secretaria de Direitos Humanos; Secretaria Nacional de Promoção dos Direitos da Pessoa com Deficiência, Brasília

Clifford J, Marcus G (eds) (1986) Writing culture: the poetics and politics of ethnography. University of California Press, Berkeley

Diniz D (2003) Modelo social da Deficiência: a crítica feminista. Série Anis 28:1–8

Diniz D (2007) O Que É Deficiência? Brasiliense, São Paulo

Diniz D, Santos W (eds) (2010) Deficiência e Discriminação. Editora LetrasLivres, Editora Universidade de Brasília, Brasília

Diniz D, Medeiros M, Barbosa L (eds) (2010) Deficiência e Igualdade. Editora LetrasLivres, Editora Universidade de Brasília, Brasília

Foucault M (1983) The subject and power. In: Dreyfus H, Rabinow P (eds) Michel foucault: beyond structuralism and hermeneutics. The University of Chicago Press, Chicago, pp 208–226

Gardou C (2006) Quais São os Contributos da Antropologia para a Compreensão das Situações de Deficiência? Revista Lusófona de Educação 8:53–61

Garland-Thomson R (1997) Extraordinary bodies: figuring physical disability in American Culture and Literature. Columbia University Press, New York

Geertz C (1973) The interpretation of cultures. Basic Books, New York

Gesser M, Nuernberg AH, Toneli MJF (2012) A Contribuição do Modelo social da Deficiência à Psicologia Social. Psicol Soc 24(3):557–566

Giddens A (1990) The consequences of modernity. Polity Press, Cambridge

Gil J (1994) Monstros. Quetzal Editores, Lisboa

Glat R (1989) Somos Iguais a Vocês: depoimentos de mulheres com deficiência mental. AGIR, Rio de Janeiro

Goffman E (1963) Stigma: notes on the management of spoiled identity. Simon and Schuster, New York

Kittay EF (1999) Love's labor: essays on women, equality and dependency. Routledge, New York

Maluf SW (2001) Corpo e Corporalidade nas Culturas Contemporâneas: abordagens antropológicas. Revista Esboços 9(9):87–101

Marcus G (1998) Ethnography through thick and thin. Princeton University Press, Princeton

Mello AG (2010) A Construção da Pessoa na Experiência da Deficiência: corpo, gênero, sexualidade, subjetividade e saúde mental. In: Maluf SW, Tornquist CS (eds) Gênero, Saúde e Aflição: abordagens antropológicas. Letras Contemporâneas, Florianópolis

Mello AG, Fernandes FBM (2013) Guia de Orientações Básicas sobre Gênero, Deficiência e Acessibilidade no Seminário Internacional Fazendo Gênero 10. Florianópolis, 34 p. Cartilha da Comissão de Acessibilidade do Seminário Internacional Fazendo Gênero 10, Universidade Federal de Santa Catarina

Mello AG, Nuernberg AH (2012) Gênero e Deficiência: interseções e perspectivas. Revista Estudos Feministas 20(3):635–655

Nicolau SM, Schraiber LB, Ayres JRCM (2013) Mulheres com Deficiência e sua Dupla Vul-
nerabilidade: contribuições para a construção da integralidade em saúde. Ciên Saúde Colet
18(3):501–519
Nuernberg AH (2008) O processo de criação do Programa de Promoção de Acessibilidade da
Universidade do Sul de Santa Catarina (UNISUL). Ponto de Vista (UFSC) 10:97–106
Nuernberg AH (2009) Rompendo barreiras atitudinais no contexto do ensino superior. In: Conselho
Federal de Psicologia (ed) Educação Inclusiva: experiências profissionais em Psicologia, vol 1.
Conselho Federal de Psicologia, Brasília, pp 153–166
Nussbaum M (2010) Capacidades e Justiça Social. In: Diniz D, Medeiros M, Barbosa L (eds)
Deficiência e Igualdade. Editora LetrasLivres, Editora Universidade de Brasília, Brasília
Omote S (1994) Deficiência e Não Deficiência: recortes do mesmo tecido. Rev Bras Educ Espec
1(2):65–73
Omote S (2010) Caminhando com DIBS: uma trajetória de construção de conceitos em Educação
Especial. Rev Bras Educ Espec 16(3):331–342
Ortega F (2008) O Sujeito Cerebral e o Movimento da Neurodiversidade. Mana 14(2):477–509
Ortega F (2009) Deficiência, Autismo e Neurodiversidade. Ciên Saúde Colet 14(1):67–77
Piccolo GM, Moscardini SF, Costa VB (2010) A historiografia das produções em periódicos de
Sadao Omote. Rev Bras Educ Espec 16(1):107–126
Rubin G (1998 [1984]) Thinking sex: notes for a radical theory of the politics of sexuality. In: Nardi
PM, Schneider BE (eds) Social perspectives in lesbian and gay studies. Routledge, London/New
York, pp 100–127
Santos WR (2008) Pessoas com Deficiência: nossa maior minoria. Physis 18(3):501–519
Satow SH (2000) Paralisado Cerebral: construção da identidade na exclusão. Cabral Editora
Universitária, Taubaté
Schwartz LM (2013) Madness in the Brazil of the first republic. In: Aidoo L, Silva D (eds) Lima
Barreto: new critical perspectives. Lexington Books, New York
Schwartz LM (2014) Race and citizenship in turn of the century Brazil. Stony Brook University
Provost Lecture, February 26, 2014. Downloaded from youtube June 7, 2014: http://www.
youtube.com/watch?v=0H8SQwpwWTo&feature=youtube
Sen A (2010) Elementos de uma Teoria de Direitos Humanos. In: Diniz D, Santos W (eds)
Deficiência e Discriminação. Editora LetrasLivres, Editora Universidade de Brasília, Brasília
Torres EF, Mazzoni AA, Mello AG (2007) Nem toda pessoa cega lê em Braille nem toda pessoa
surda se comunica em língua de sinais. Educ Pesqui 33(2):369–386

Leroy F. Moore Jr., Tiny aka Lisa Gray-Garcia,
and Emmitt H. Thrower

Abstract

In this chapter three artists/activists of color with disabilities write about their lives, activism & cultural work around police brutality against poor people & people with disabilities before, during and beyond the occupy "movement." You will read the popular response after police brutality cases against people with disabilities and how this response has been repeated over and over again. The three authors will share their answers toward this issue and talk about the need for increasing cultural work from poetry to Hip-Hop to visual arts by not only disabled community but also from the artists arena. Lisa 'Tiny' Gray Garcia, Emmitt Thrower and Leroy Franklin Moore Jr. have come together to serve up another vision on the drastic real growth of police brutality against people with disabilities and poor people.

Keywords

Poor Magazine • Krip-Hop Nation • Where is Hope • Disability • People with disabilities • Police brutality • Police training • Occupy movement • Activism • People of color • Black people • Hip-Hop • Cultural work • Poor people • Poverty • Mental health • Autism • Autistic people • Media • Journalism • Wabi Sabi Productions Inc

L.F. Moore Jr. (✉)
National Black Disability Coalition, Sins Invalid, and Krip Hop Nation, Berkeley, CA
e-mail: blackkrip@gmail.com

T.L. Gray-Garcia
POOR Magazine, Oakland, CA

E.H. Thrower
Wabi Sabi Productions, Bronx, NY

© Springer Science+Business Media Dordrecht 2016
P. Block et al. (eds.), *Occupying Disability: Critical Approaches to Community, Justice, and Decolonizing Disability*, DOI 10.1007/978-94-017-9984-3_21

21.1   Introduction

As you will soon read this chapter has been written by three community journalists, artists and activists from San Francisco Bay Area and New York. The chapter starts out with Lisa 'Tiny' Garcia who is a poverty scholar, revolutionary journalist, lecturer, Indigenous mixed rave mama of Tiburcio, daughter of Dee and the co-founder of POOR Magazine and author of Criminal of Poverty: Growing Up Homeless in America. We discuss Poor Magazine recently published a handbook for the Occupy Movement entitled Decolonizers Guide to a Humble Revolution, then introduce Emmitt Thrower, who is a disabled retired NYC Police Officer and also a stroke survivor. He is the Founder and President of Wabi Sabi Productions Inc., a small community based nonprofit company founded in 2005 in New York City. The chapter ends with Leroy Moore who has been one of leading voices around police brutality against people with disabilities and has founded Krip-Hop Nation for Hip-Hop artists with disabilities.

Krip-Hop Nation, along with 5th Battalion, recently compiled and produced a Hip-Hop Mixtape on police brutality against people with disabilities. You will soon see that the chapter is from the authors above who are poor people and people with disabilities, explaining the realities of police brutality, polices, media misrepresentations, and "new Occupy activists" against them and their communities from San Francisco and New York before Occupy and now under Occupy and after Occupy. We laid out our pieces through our writings as cultural activists, street journalists, and poets, Poe poets, Krip-Hop songwriters etc. As you will read, each writer wrote about their life experiences/work/cultural work with people who are houseless, people with disabilities before, during and yes after occupy "movements." As community writers, artists, scholars and activists outside of the academic world and its way of writing, we like to thank our editor, another community artist, journalist, activist, Gioioa von Disterlo who shared her academic and street journalistic skills to get our chapter in an academic format without changing our messages. Are you ready to be challenged? We hope so!

> I am the.000 25- the smallest number u can think of in yer mind-
> Didn't even make it to the 99-
> love to all of yer awakening consciousnessness –
> but try to walk in mine . . .
> *tiny/Po Poets 2011*

21.2   Occupy Was Never for Me

Occupy was never for me. I'm Pour', I'm a mother, I'm disabled, I'm homeless, I'm indigenous, I am on welfare, I am not formerly educated, I have never had a house to be foreclosed on, I am a recycler, panhandler, I am broken, I am humble, I have been po'lice profiled and my mind is occupied with broken teeth, and a broken me. I am revolutionary who has fought every day to decolonize this already occupied indigenous land of Turtle Island in Amerikkka.

I do not hate. I am glad, like I said when it all first got started, that thousands more people got conscious. I am glad that folks woke up and began to get active. What I am not glad about is that in that waking up there was a weird tunnel vision by so many "occupiers" of the multiple struggles, revolutions, pain and deep struggle of so many who came before you, upon whose shoulders you are standing on. This is what I have now come to realize is a strange form of political gentrification.

Like any form of gentrification there is a belief by the gentrifyers/colonizers, that their movement is different, new form, that it has little or no historical contextual connection to the ones before it. And that it owes little or nothing to the movements and/or communities already there, creating, struggling, barely making it.

And yes, race, class and educational access matter. I have heard from elders that a similar thing happened in the 60s with the poor people of color movements raging on like Black panthers and Young Lords then suddenly the "anti-war movement" sprung up, driven by white middle-class college students and the political climate suddenly got large.

> I am The peoples on the corner
> the mamaz, daddys and baboes in the car –day laborers, in jaws of systems – living in
> SRO's, shelters, jails cells and houses made of cardboard
> The people u don't see, can't see or never want to be-
> I am a mental health diagnosis and your favorite academik research proposal.

Before going, on I must remind you what Poor Magazine is and our thinking about NO Po'Lice Calls EVER! POOR Magazine/Prensa POBRE is a poor people-led, indigenous people-led organization that follows our indigenous values of eldership, ancestor honoring, multi-cultural spirit, prayer and respect. We practice these values in everything we do. Including our dealing with any of the many very serious issues that come up in our family of poverty and indigenous skolaz. Which is why we have a no po'lice calls (engagement) policy in effect. When we have problems come up (which we do ALL the time as poor peoples in struggle) we convene Family Council based on a model taught by our ancient indigenous ancestors. The Family Council convenes for as long as it takes to resolve issues that requires self-accountability and ownership to the problem and a series of commitments to actions, change, healing, responsibility to the situation from each person who is responsible for the problem and as well requires commitment from the participants, elders, folks who are in community/family and extended with that person and POOR Magazine.

We are committed to this because we as peoples in struggle are occupied by Po'Lice, killed by police, profiled by police and forever in a struggle to liberate our mind and be truly free of the idea that an occupying army informed by white supremacy is the only way to ensure the safety and security of our children, elders, women and men. This is an ongoing and very difficult process of liberation because we live in a world with many oppressed and broken folks suffering from the PTSD of capitalism, imperialism and racism.

Now going back to my original point that this ironic disconnect was never clearer in the way that houseless people, people with psychological disabilities

existing outside, were treated, spoken about, problematized, and "dealt with" in the
occupations across the United Snakkkes this last year.

> "We are very excited because the police agreed to come every night and patrol... our
> "camp" because we have been having so many problems with the 'homeless people' coming
> into our camp," said an occupier from Atlanta, Georgia.
>
> "It took us awhile to forge a relationship with the police, but now that we did we feel
> "safe" from all the homeless people who are a problem in our camp," said an occupier in
> Oklahoma.
>
> "We have been able to do so much with occupy in this town, but we are having a real
> problem with "security," it's because of the large contingent of homeless people near our
> camp." (*Occupier from Wisconsin*)

City after city, occupation to occupation, in these so-called conscious and
political spaces which were allegedly challenging the use of public space and land
use and bank control over our resources and naming the struggle of the 99 % versus
the %1, were playing out the same dynamics of the increasingly po'liced urban and
suburban neighborhoods across the US.

The lie of "security," which it is for, the notion of "illegal" people and how some
people are supposed to be here and some are not. Our reliance on police as the
only way to ensure our community security and keep the overt and covert veneer of
racism and classism alive and well in every part of this United Snakkkes reared its
ugly head in all of these Occupations. In many cases the "occupiers" gentrified the
outside locations of the houseless people in these cities.

Taking away the "sort of" safe places where houseless people were dwelling outside. And yet no accountability to that was ever even considered by the "occupiers."

Perhaps it's because the majority of the "occupiers" were from the police using
neighborhoods, and/or currently or recently had those homes and student debt and
credit and cars and mortgages and stocks and bonds and jobs. Perhaps it's because
Occupy was never for me or people like me.

I walk thru addiction; racism and poverty- scared of CPS, the INS, the Po'lice,
and me

I am occupied with broken teeth, broken promises a broken heart, bench
warrants, deportation threats, and my own thoughts

In Oakland and San Francisco, the alleged "bastions" of consciousness there was
a slightly different perspective. Many of the houseless people were in fact part of
the organizing and then eventually, due to deep class and race differences, were
intentionally left out or self-segregated themselves from the main "occupy" groups
and began their own revolutions or groups or cliques, or just defeated huddles.

Several of the large and well-funded non-profit organizations in the Bay Area
re-harnessed Occupy into their own agendas and helped to launch some of the
huge general strikes and marches to support labor movements, migrant/immigrant
struggles, prison abolitionist movements and economic justice.

In the case of the poor, indigenous, I'm/migrant and indigenous skolaz at POOR
Magazine we felt we could perhaps insert some education, herstory and information
into this very homogenous, very white, and very ahistorical narrative and to the
empirical notion of occupation itself, so we created the Decolonizers Guide to a

Humble Revolution. With this guide and our poverty scholarship and cultural art we supported other indigenous and conscious peoples of color in Oakland who began to frame this entire movement as Decolonize Oakland, challenging the political gentrifying aspects of Occupy itself.

My land, body, babies, and mind has been long ago lost to case manglers, poverty pimps, philanthropimps and the never-ending war on the poor.

Never even got a credit card, much-less a mortgage—but I did catch a case—a marshal and jail term for stealing food from a store.

POOR Magazine in an attempt to harness some of the energy and minds of this time towards the very real issues of poverty and criminalization and racism in the US, created The Poor Peoples Decolonization (Occupation), traveling from both sides of the Bay (Oakland to SF) to the welfare offices where so many of us po' folks get criminalized for the meager crumbs we sometimes get, public housing where we are on 8–9 year long wait-lists for so-called affordable housing, the po'lice dept. where all of us black, brown and po folks get incarcerated, profiled and harassed every day not just when we "occupy" and Immigration, Customs Enforcement where any of us who had to cross these false borders, get increasingly criminalized, hated and incarcerated for just trying to work and support our families.

But in the end a small turnout showed up for our march, I guess our poor people-led occupations weren't as "sexy" as other 99 % issues.

Finally, in Oakland there was a powerful push to re-think the arrogant notion of "Occupy" itself on already stolen and occupied native lands, becoming one of the clearest examples of the hypocritical irony of occupy.

After at least a 5 h testimony from indigenous leaders and people of color supporters at a herstoric Oakland General Assembly, to officially change the name of Occupy Oakland to Decolonize Oakland, with first nations warriors like Corrina Gould and Morning Star, Krea Gomez, artists Jesus Barraza and Melanie Cervantez and so many more powerful peoples of color supporters presenting testifying and reading a beautiful statement on decolonization and occupation, it was still voted on that Oakland, the stolen and occupied territory of Ohlone peoples would remain Occupy Oakland.

So as the "Occupy" people celebrate 1 year of existence, I feel nothing. One year after Occupy was launched, lots of exciting media was generated, massive resources were spent, a great number of people were supposedly politicized and the world started to listen to the concept of the %99, the same number of black, brown, poor, disabled and migrant folks are incarcerated, policed, and deported in the US. The racist and classist Sit-lie laws, gang injunctions and Stop and Frisk ordinances still rage on and we are still being pushed out of our communities of color by the forces of gentriFUKation and poverty. So, I wonder, how have these political gentrifyers changed things for black and brown and poor people? Not at all, actually, but then again, Occupy was never really for me.

I am the 000.25 the smallest number u can think of in yer mind…
Didn't even make it to the 99.
Once on the inside looking out
Now on the outside looking in

I could not see
Though I was not blind
I could not hear
Though I was not deaf

I could not understand
Though I had a clear head
why the demeaning actions
that turned your face red?

Was this awful treatment because of something I said?
I ponder this enigma as I lay in my bed
Maybe it's because of how you are lead
Or maybe it's because of what your mind is being fed?

does my being disabled
affect you a certain way
your arrogant inhumanity
means that I have to pay

Does the color of my skin
cut you like a razor
That your automatic response
is to hit me with your Taser

What my eyes see now
My heart disbelieves
raking us away
as if we were leaves

my nose pressed up against the window
watching the pain
as one by one
Law keepers go insane

You took an oath
And so did I
But you abandoned your commitment
So now you're living a lie

you use authority
as your protective buffer
your brutal actions
causing mothers to suffer.

Did you not hear
that they were deaf?
Did you not see
that they were Blind?

Could you not stand
that they could not walk?
you made a cowards choice
and it wasn't to talk!

We cry out for justice
and we get tears of pain
We petition the media
But they still play their game

All Talk and No action
It is always the same
no one stands up
no one accepts the blame

We look to each other
in this time of rough weather
Only to discover
that even we are not together

You once enforced the law
To protect and serve
And now you victimize us
It's how you get your swerve

All across this great country
in the land of the abled
A community is targeted
because of being mis-labled

you ignore our needs
but expect us to smile
as you enforce your evil will
on the disabled profiled.

21.3   Part 2

My experience as a New York City Police Officer was one of the most rewarding times of my life. Working in the communities where I grew up. Places where I shared so much in common with the other residents. It was a time when I actually believed in the fairness of our law-enforcement system. A time when I believed that if you needed help you could call a cop and be confident that you would be protected and served. Now it seems all that happens is that we get served—served the indignity and brutality of a system gone badly. They have become traitors to the people they serve and especially for the community of people with disabilities.

The integrity and commitment I observed from the Police Officers I had the pleasure of working with in NY, is in sharp contrast to what I see in today's cruel reality. My experience working with a multitude of Police Officers of different races and cultures was really a very positive experience. That was the foundation that helped to re-shape and develop my renewed faith in the old broken corrupt law enforcement system from the 1960s and 1970s that I had come to know and hate.

Incidents of Police Officers committing brutal and horrible acts against law-abiding people with disabilities were for me, back then, a rare occurrence. There were many horrific years of very poor relations between the Police and the New York City Community of mostly poor, Black and Latino residents. These were the murderous and violent times in the 1960s and early 1970s when we were still proclaiming that we shall overcome. These days seems so much like the 1960s as it seems that we are still trying to overcome what we thought we had overcame.

A certain level of abuse by the police was the norm back in Bed-Stuy Brooklyn during my youthful days of the 1960s and 1970s. But it was also tempered with genuine offers of help and encouragement to young people from some of the more dedicated police officers. Many who grew up in or still lived in the community they served. When I became a Police Officer at the age of 20 years old in 1973 things were slowly beginning to turn around and change. And it did slightly change to a point. Fewer cops were being killed and fewer riots were engulfing the community. No it wasn't perfect harmony, but it was not in the critical state of inhumane turmoil like it is today. I'm not saying that Police Officers had all become angels, because surely they were not. The influx of Police officers of color and residing in the community was slowly changing the dynamics of what had been an oppressive, corrupt, abusive, disconnected and chaotic law enforcement system.

Back in the 1970s, I never observed the amount of routine abuse and brutality committed against citizens and people with disabilities, like what is happening in 2012. Known Incidents had dwindled down somewhat, or at least that is what we perceived. So, I seldom saw or heard of incidents of offending law enforcement officers committing brutal wanton acts against people with disabilities. There were some major news worthy incidents, however, that were reported of these type of incidents. But they were not connected to a general trend of abusive behavior by police officers, at least we knew of no trends. Those widely publicized incidents were attributed to a few badly trained or racist Police Officers. They had acted upon their emotions and not their good judgment as they had been trained. So the Police Department promised to quickly "Fix It." So the story goes. Of course nothing ever really got fixed but was continually recycled year after year.

Unfortunately, there are no reliable records of the numbers of incidents involving people with disabilities. So, it was impossible to determine exactly what was going on. Because no statistics were properly recorded, there was no effort to identify people with disabilities on standard report forms by law enforcement agencies. That was not a requirement on official government forms. So the incidents were just lumped together with all the other general police abuse cases. Even in today's modern Police Departments there is a lack of documentation related specifically to incidents of brutality, profiling and police abuse against people with disabilities. That is one of the major problems hindering efforts to have authorities to even recognize that there is a problem. They respond to the numbers game. No numbers equal no problem in their eyes and the eyes of the political Lords. They see only what they want to see. We all know their eyesight is biased and can't be trusted.

We, as a community, can clearly see the inequities and are well aware of what is really going on. Technology has leveled the playing field somewhat. Street surveillance and digital camera recordings by citizens using phones has unveiled the truth and frequency of the police assaults. The increasing number of newspaper and video accounts of this form of brutality against minorities, the poor and people with disabilities slaps us in our face every single day. It may be difficult to get stats, but make no mistake about it, the incidents are occurring at an alarming rate. Check out video sharing sites like youtube to get a small idea of what is being reported by victims, communities as well as newspaper accounts. That number represents just a small tip of this brutal iceberg.

Most Law Enforcement Agencies still do not organize or record their statistics in a way that would be useful in revealing this growing trend. So there remains no clear-cut method to identify victims who also have disabilities. It is nearly impossible to get accurate comprehensive numbers of the enormity of this epidemic even today. The authorities remain in a state of willing denial, as if no problem exists, because they have no stats to back them up. No stats equals no problem in their eyes. When they do make a halfhearted attempt to appease the community, they offer to give their officers more sensitivity training. The problem is, this does not alone resolve the issue.

Truth, is that they have yet to really become sensitive to the needs of the community of people with disabilities. What's needed is real community oversight, creative solutions and hands on involvement when the Police respond to known encounters with people with disabilities. Not becoming involved after the fact! Solutions involving more direct involvement by the affected community seem to be frowned upon by law enforcement and government officials, as if community residents are not intellectually equipped to determine better and safer ways of addressing potentially dangerous situations involving people with disabilities. Surely the community can offer possible solutions that are not based on just approaching these incidents as if they are military operations and targets. These incidents are not military operations, but human encounters with live people, that require taking into consideration the individual's disabling conditions.

Nice world if you can live in it. But we don't! And that is not what happens obviously in most cases. Why? Maybe they don't want us to really see what is going on inside their sacred patrol guide of procedures and simple guide to complex human encounters. Based on something other than what's in our best interest. Or maybe they really are not concerned about resolving the issues but only placating an agitated community for the benefit of the current political lords. Knowing, as soon as the fire dies down, it will be business as usual. Just my theory.

When I retired from the NYC Police Department in 1988 with a disability, life took on a new direction as well as a new perspective. I was now an outsider, detached from the law enforcement system that I literally grew up in. The time was ripe to explore a different path because of the new physical challenges I had to face. That path put me smack dab on a collision course with my dormant creative side. I found love when I embraced the creative arts and theater in particular. I had written poetry since before my teens. Not because I wanted to, but because these damn words and thoughts would bounce around in my mind keeping me awaken until I got up and wrote them down. So, I became a reluctant young poet so I could get some bleeping sleep.

But now, in 1988, I was all grown up. As a shy recently retired police officer in his 30s newly adorned with a physical disability, I began reaching for new tools to express myself. I began doing standup comedy, not that well, which then led me to doing theater. Theater seemed to be what I did well according to my teacher. So this was where I stiffened up and made my stand. I was to become an actor. Acting on stage allowed me to do anything I wanted to do. I was able to do some of the very things on stage that I was afraid to do in real life. That was so cool, I thought. Eventually my stage grew so large it covered the entire planet and beyond. Now I had a huge arena from which to operate. There had always been something burning deep down inside my quiet, conservative manner that wanted me to break out and start living "life out loud." So that is exactly what I did. I unleashed the activist trapped inside my disabled body and challenged the world to clean up its act or face … or face … well I wasn't sure what they would face, but it was gonna be something.

That something was born in 2005. It evolved and eventually emerged into what would become my Not- For -Profit Production company called Wabi Sabi Production Inc. The seeds had been planted years before, and now they were in bloom. I had an itching to see that ordinary people were treated fairly and humanely. It was one of the reasons I enjoyed being a Police Officer, other than the money and health insurance, and the fact that women seemed to adore men in uniform (that was nice). I grew up in Bed-Stuy Brooklyn, NYC during a time when Police Officers would routinely snatch up people from the neighborhood, and disappeared with them for a while. They would later return them to the block showing off their fresh tattoos of police brutality carved upon their bodies. Their red swollen faces, black eyes, broken noses, and bloodied sagging lips were a reminder who was still in charge in the hood. That was my experience with police back in the 1960–1970s.

I was very fortunate not to get involved or become a victim of their abuse at the time. Part was luck; part was because I kept much distance from them but mostly because I was blessed with blazing fast foot speed, and above average fence leaping abilities. When I became a Police Officer in 1973 at the age of 20, it was a time when Police Officers were being routinely shot. There was a poisonous divide between a deeply corrupt and racist Police force and the mostly poor African American and Latino communities. Police corruption was out of control. Drug use and economic distress were at epidemic proportions in minority communities. It was a time when police abuse was almost an accepted consequence of place and times. This was 10 years after Martin Luther King Jr. had declared, "I have a Dream" on the steps of the Lincoln Memorial. That dream was becoming a nightmare. As a young police officer my dream was to change a community in route to saving the world. I'm still working on that dream. During that time in the mid to late 70s things began to slowly change for the better. Or so it seemed, at least temporarily.

At some point in time, things soured and began to go terribly wrong again with the police and the community. In short it stunk again only worse! Fast forward to 2006. Now a retired disabled Police Officer, seasoned Actor, Producer and Director, and with my newly formed Not For Profit production company, Wabi Sabi Productions Inc. I was busy being busy. I met Leroy Moore of the Krip Hop Nation around that time. I was in NY and he was in California, but thanks to the Internet we were able to cross paths.

Leroy got wind of me doing a play I had written about Hurricane Katrina from a press release I had sent out. In it I stated that I was using a wheelchair user who herself was an actual survivor from the hurricane. She had endured the evacuation and horrors of the unsafe and filthy shelters. Survived the lengthy bus rides in her wheelchair with her young son and parents. I re-wrote the play "Katrina: A Whole Lotta Water" which had been performed successfully in NYC. Now I incorporated her struggle and made her one of the lead characters in the multimedia hip hop musical stage play. Leroy wrote articles in San Francisco Newspapers about the Hurricane Katrina play. The play and tour was also funded, directed and produced by me mainly because nobody else would do it. We opened the play on the 1-year anniversary of Hurricane Katrina in NYC.

I performed in the play as a character named Rufus. He represented the people fired upon by the police as they attempted to cross the bridge to safety. How ironic I thought at the time. The play was conceived from the actual stories of unknown survivors who told their experiences on the internet in obscure web forums as voices without names. Hundreds of Katrina survivors who had been relocated around the NYC-NJ tri- state area attended the opening that was an exclusive free performance event and party just for Katrina survivors and their family members. They were the first to see the dramatization of what were their voices and their stories. It was my gift to them. Sunshine, the wheelchair user who was living in Baltimore at the time and had heard about the play, attended the NY show with her mother. She was our special guest. This was my first meeting with her and her mother. After discovering she had been a dancer, and was a real Katrina survivor I asked her if she would dance in the show for me if I brought it to Baltimore. She said yes. This young talented wheelchair user, who was a graduate of the Baltimore Dance Academy was indeed Sunshine. She was the shining star that lit up this new version of the play.

Leroy and I were talking on the phone several years after our first meeting in 2006. It was now 2011 and Leroy had begun working on a CD project with artists with disabilities around the issues of Police Brutality and Profiling of People of Color with disabilities. I remember saying to him that we needed to expand on this even more. I myself was not even aware that there was a problem. Yea, even if you think you know what's going on, maybe you really don't. I didn't have a clue. But if this was true, more people needed to be made aware of that fact. For me when Leroy presented it to me I knew it was founded in truth. So I decided to take on the task to begin producing a Documentary film around the issues and around the artists who were creating the CD on Police Brutality and Profiling against people with disabilities. The project main purpose is to bring greater awareness to this rising epidemic of brutality happening in a very vulnerable community.

Currently in 2012 we are still working on the project and always looking for assistance as well as other stories or interview to add. We have interviewed survivors of Police brutality and Profiling in Richmond and Stafford County, Virginia, where we engaged in a protest rally and at the Richmond capitol building, advocating for Neli Latson a youth with autism who was wrongly incarcerated and victimized by the system. We interviewed victims and families of victims in Oakland California and San Francisco. Our journey so far also has taken us to Syracuse University in Upstate New York for a Forum led by Leroy Moore. I had the opportunity to interview and meet some of the activists with disabilities who are at the forefront of the fight against Police Brutality and Police Profiling against people of color with disabilities—like Leroy Moore of course. But also artists who are part of the CD project, like New Jersey artist Richard Gaskin, who also created a Rap music video and song based on a Washington, DC case of brutality against a wheelchair user. I also had the opportunity to meet other activists with disabilities, such as La Mesha Irizarry and Keith Jones, who have personal stories about Profiling and Police murders of their loved ones.

But during this process one thing has really stood out in my mind. That has been the lack of support from other organizations and groups engaged in the same fight as we are. They, for the most part, have been unwilling to work in collaboration with us, though when speaking they say they will. But nothing ever materializes, and they are never heard from again. Even after attending and supporting their events, and getting commitments from core members of the group that they will work together with us to get the Documentary done, it yields the same sad results. They disappear into the dead of night and fall off the face of the earth. Or maybe they no longer have cell phone or internet service. I just don't have answers to this. Though it appears as if many organizations only support their organization, and so goes the glory. Some are even national groups. Some who were contacted by email never even bothered to reply. This to me is the most shocking and unexpected response to our cry for solidarity and unification of all these individual group efforts to tackle these issues. But alas, it seems as if almost every group or organization claiming to be fighting the good fight for the cause is slave to his or her own agendas. But we, as activists and artists, persist nevertheless, with those who chose to join with us. Like the title of our documentary, I ask the question: "Where Is Hope?"

The police stopped me on my three-wheel bicycle as I was coming down the sidewalk. They stopped me as I entered a hotel to visit a friend. I was stopped in a bookstore by a security guard. Then my friend, another Black disabled man and co-Founder of Krip-Hop Nation, Keith Jones, was almost kicked out of his hotel by police. As a Black disabled activist/cultural worker these experiences that Keith Jones and I have experienced, tells me that once again people of color with disabilities experience discrimination that comes from being Black and disabled, and society is still not aware of the "isms" that are thrown upon people of color with disabilities, from police, to teachers, to a complete stranger. After all of these incidents of police profiling happened in a 2 months span in 2010 in four major US cities, Keith Jones and I put together a song called "Disabled Profiled."

Disabled Profiled (Song Keith & Leroy)

Leroy:
Yeah I'm a Black man
Known about racially profiled
Two Black hotel workers
Same race but in my face
Disabled profiled
Making assumptions upon appearances
Blocking the entrance
Can't be race because we are both Black

Black Disabled Man
Must be a drunk
Slur speech dragging feet
Must be begging for money

Disabled profiled
Making assumptions upon appearances
Blocking the entrance
Can't be race because we are both Black

Must protect others from this bum
Got to do my job
I summed him up from across the street
Poor cripple homeless beggar

Confused, disabled and black
The fear builds
As he approaches
Looking at him like he's a roach
Firing out questions upon questions
No not racially but disabled profiled
Here in the home of ED Roberts

Disabled profiled
Making assumptions upon appearances
Blocking the entrance
Can't be race because we are both Black
Mocking my walk
Didn't read my tense body talk
Friends saw my anger,
"Mr. We're together!"

Disabled Profiled
And I'm tired
Twice in one week
It's not race it happened from Black & White

Disabled Profiled
And I'm tired
Twice in one week
It's not race it happened from Black & White

Disabled Profiled
And I'm tired

Disabled Profiled
And I'm tired

I'm so tired

Keith:
The wheelchair got no diamond in da back and no sun roof top
but I still run da scene wit a disability lean nah what I mean and
every day dat im speakin and try to reach 'em cause they be lookin at me tryin to profile the
    black man
talking bout what happen to you damn see there was not no gun shot matter of fact I have
    my own kind of plot

I have to run dablock shut down because ya tryin to hold me down laughin at the way that I
   talk the way that I walk the way that I speak
but ya girl likes da way that I freak ya betta get it right man understand
cp is only part of da man I got something for the rest of yall listen something for the best of
   y'all
ya betta sit back and try to contemplate can you really demonstrate what it takes to create
   somehin kinda great in the face of hate ....

Leroy:
Hey Keith just like you
I was triggered last week
Memories floating back
Makes this grown man weep

Paul Dunbar's mask didn't hold up
Felt like I was shot no bulletproof vest
Two days ago & I still can't rest

Memories coming back
Woowooowoo "up against the wall
Hahaha are you drunk can't walk?"

"No officer I'm disabled
Just coming home from work!"
"What what can't understand?"

I was triggered last week
Memories floating back
Makes this grown man weep

Beep beep
"Mr. You is out late
Can I see your I'd?"

Why me
Don't feel like being a teacher
Please just let me be

Black man in a uniform
Sees me as a threat
Or a charity case

Can't look at me in my face
His mind is made up
Looking for my tin cup

I was triggered last week
Memories floating back
Makes this grown man weep

By Leroy Moore & Keith Jones. Yes this is a true story!

These incidents of police brutality and profiling against people with disabilities
didn't start with the so called occupy movement! Since my teenage years, I have
been extremely active in the movement to end police brutality against people with
disabilities. From New York, NY to San Francisco, CA I have worked with families,
protested, been a representative at hearings, written for numerous publications, spo-

ken out on the radio, appeared on television, and held workshops on police brutality against people living with disabilities. I have been involved in some of the most high profile police brutality cases against people living with disabilities and have worked side by side with some of the most well-known police brutality organizations including the Idriss Stelley Foundation, Cop Watch, Poor Magazine and many others.

As a street advocate, before I completely transferred my work around this issue of police brutality against people with disabilities into cultural work, I was involved with many cases, but two major cases stick out for me, in the San Francisco Bay area, that changed policy and perception on this issue. On June 12th, 2001, Idriss Stelley, a Black young man with a mental health disability was shot by San Francisco police officers, while his girlfriend at the time called Idriss's mother, Masha in the Sony Meteron Theater. Idriss was in a mental health crisis at the time. Short version, is many police officers empty the theater leaving Idriss, and as Idriss walked towards the officers, they filled the theater with bullets killing Idriss.

Mesha and many advocates demanded policies on how police deal with people with mental health disabilities, and demanded a change of location where the police commission met, and to open their meeting to have more public control, and the public demanded that they should have some control on who would serve on this commission. For almost 2 years Mesha, friends of Idriss, Poor Magazine, Ella Baker Center, the Coalition on Homeless, mental health advocates in San Francisco advocated for special training for police officers on mental health and other disabilities. Although we got the police training on mental health and other disabilities, it was a fight to get it implemented, and we had to get city's board of supervisors on our side. We did a radio program about police brutality against people with disabilities back in 2005.

The next case that I was involved in, was a physically Black disabled young man, Cameron Boyd, who had two prosthetic legs. After Boyd got pulled over by San Francisco police on May 5th 2004, police shouted orders to Boyd to get out the car and lay on the ground. Boyd tried to explain to the officers that he couldn't follow their rapid orders of getting on the ground, because he was disabled and needed to get his prosthetic legs from the back seat, but as he reached for his legs shouting, "I'm disabled," police shot Boyd, killing him. Months after this case, I lead one of the first open forum in the San Francisco area on the issue of police brutality and people with disabilities, that took place on July 14th 2001 with mothers who lost their disabled love ones, like Idriss mother Mesha and Cammerin Boyd's mother, with mental health advocates, Poor Magazine staff, a state coalition at that time on crimes against people with disabilities and many more.

The third turning point in the issue of police brutality against people with disabilities is that finally the general public and the cultural arenas are slowly writing, making art and speaking on the issue of police brutality against people with disabilities. The results are slow but since the shooting of Idriss Stelley in 2001 universities, October 22nd chapters, some mainstream and grassroots media, and parents have begun to speak up about this issue, and have reached out to me for support and cultural expressions locally and nationally. Read how cultural expression by Hip-Hop artists with disabilities came together to make the first ever Hip-Hop/Spoken Word CD around cases of police brutality/profiling. (Copy the link, click the link, and put it in your web browser http://poormagazine.org/node/ 4337).

I started to feel the age in my disabled body about 4 years ago, even earlier, like my late 30s. It moved me to shift my focus away from street action and towards cultural activism. I combined my love of poetry, journalism and music with my commitment to the struggle against police brutality against people living with disabilities, and other social justice issues such as homelessness and poverty. I continue to work with other disabled poets, musicians and activists. I deepened the relationships I had with organizations that I was already working in solidarity with, and I began to form relationships with new organizations, like Cop Watch Chapters, Disabled People Outside head up by Dan McMullan in Berkeley, California and Disability Rights California formerly Protection & Advocacy, Inc. and activists like Mary Kate Connor and so many more.

For years, I collaborated with other activists and artists fighting police brutality against people with disabilities in the street war and the culture war. For countless hours, I listened to Hip Hop artists with disabilities speak out against brutality against our communities. By 2006, I was motivated to use my years of activism and love of hip hop to create a cultural home for Hip Hop artists with disabilities. This was the beginning of what is now Krip-Hop Nation (Hip-Hop artists and other musicians with disabilities).

In the beginning, Krip Hop Nation had only an on-line presence, but it lived up to its byline: "Krip-Hop is more than music!" It was clear from the beginning that Krip-Hop Nation is about social justice. Artists flocked to it, For example in the first month back in 2006 after I put up a message for Hip-Hop artists, and all musicians with disabilities on MySpace, I received over 100 responses from all over the world, like Binki Woi in Germany, who pushed Krip-Hop internationally, so much that we started Mcees With Disabilities, MWD, under Krip-Hop Nation, and one of our first women to join Krip-Hop Nation and MWD was Lady MJ of the UK, who organized the first Krip-Hop party/get together in London, England. After the first year, artists started emailing me from Africa, like Ronnie Ronnie from Uganda, King Montana in New Mexico, Rob Da' Noize Temple from New York and the list continues to grow every day. From the beginning and today, Krip-Hop Nation tries to live by the following standards that we corrected, and they are as follows:

1. Use politically correct lyrics.
2. Do not put down other minorities.
3. Use our music to advocate and teach not only about ourselves, but also about the system we live under.
4. Challenge mainstream & all media on the ways they frame disability.
5. Increase the inclusion of voices that are missing from within the popular culture.
6. Recognize our disabled ancestors, knowing that we are built on what they left us, and nothing is new, just borrowed.
7. Know that sometimes we fail to meet the above standards but we are trying.

Krip Hop Nation implemented street activism and cultural activism in a way that makes real strides with and for the disabled community. When I founded Illin-N-Chillin through Poor Magazine in the 1990s, it was one of the first columns on race, justice and disability written from the perspective of the disabled community. My first article told the story of Margaret L. Mitchell. Mitchell was a Black woman with a mental health disability who was shot to death by the Los Angeles Police Department (LAPD.) Now over 12 years later, I am still producing media about police brutality against the disabled community, but the message has evolved.

Krip-Hop Nation picks up where Illin-N-Chillin left off—with a Black youth living with autism, named Neli Latson. He was physically, verbally and emotionally abused by police and wrongly incarcerated. Krip hop's pen turned into microphones when Krip-Hop Nation reached out to Neli's mother and started to put together Police Brutality Profiling, PBP CD. This collaboration was made in conjunction with another music project, 5th Battalion, led by 'DJ Quad' Jesse Morin of Los Angeles (LA), who is a wheelchair user. Microphones then turned into video cameras when, through Krip Hop, I also teamed up with Emmitt Thrower. Emmitt, a filmmaker and poet who is a retired police officer in New York, is now working on the upcoming film documentary on the process of putting the Police Brutality Profiling, PBP CD together and exposing cases of police brutality against people with disabilities. Then Krip Hop grew wings. In addition to music production and distribution, Krip-Hop Nation also travels to colleges, universities and local organizations to hold workshops and lectures using audio stories from families, the new CD and our on-going curriculum around police brutality against people with disabilities. Although these accomplishments are exciting, there is still much to overcome.

The lack of collaboration with organizations, artists, cultural workers, the Occupy movement and others who always want exposure, sometimes work in the field of against police brutality, and almost never include Krip-Hop Nation and other disabled activists, is a great source of pain for myself and the movement. We have spilled blood on this same battleground for generations. We have been creating cultural activism around the same issue since before many of them were even introduced to activism. We have been struggling against overwhelming odds of create networks of solidarity, but they have divided themselves from this history and these networks. Who are they? The Occupy movement!

For example, the Occupy movement calls for many of the same responses to police brutality as mainstream America: more police training. This might seem like a logical response if you're from a community that doesn't know that it's a strategy that has historically done us more harm than good. When someone from our community is victimized by the police, the mainstream and the occupy movement have both called for increase of police training. For example on KCB in Oakland reported on April 23rd 2012 under the title, "OPD Training Staff To Better Handle Occupy-Style Protests" that protesters of Occupy Oakland demanded Oakland Police Department to change how they respond to crowd control demanding more training. In some states, this is referred to as Police Crisis Intervention Training, but no matter what you call it, this strategy has a long history.

Communities all over the US demanded police Crisis Training after the increased rates of police shooting people with mental health disabilities and other disabilities. The model of Police Crisis Training came originally from Memphis, Tennessee. From the website of the Memphis police department under crisis intervention team (CIT) it explains the overview of the training as follows:

> In 1988, the Memphis Police Department joined in partnership with the Memphis Chapter of the National Alliance on Mental Illness (NAMI), mental health providers, and two local universities (the University of Memphis and the University of Tennessee) in organizing, training, and implementing a specialized unit. This unique and creative alliance was established for the purpose of developing a more intelligent, understandable, and safe approach to mental crisis events. This community effort was the genesis of the Memphis Police Department's Crisis Intervention Team. The CIT is made up of volunteer officers from each Uniform Patrol Precinct. CIT officers are called upon to respond to crisis calls that present officers face-to-face with complex issues relating to mental illness. CIT officers also perform their regular duty assignment as patrol officers. (http://www.cit.memphis.edu/resources/step%205/NAMI%20Memphis%20CIT%20Awards%20Banquet.pdf, Accessed 6/12/2014)

Most states have implemented these trainings at one time or another. Clearly it has not produced the desired result.

It has been in my experience that Police Crisis Training is more of a stall tactic than an effective counter-response to police brutality. In many cases the Police Crisis Training is on a voluntary basis, which means that police officers that need it most, can avoid it if they wish. Trainings are usually minimally funded, so they are always in danger of being cut when the economy is down. Additionally, in some states there is no oversight, and there are very few to no individuals with disabilities are on these oversight boards. While community members with and without disabilities have developed solutions to prevent police brutality, in general, and specifically against people living with disabilities, these solutions have largely been ignored in favor of more "popular" solutions.

A wonderful and recent example of police crisis training being cut, and at the same time police are asking for more toys to harm people, including people with disabilities, is the latest campaign by the San Francisco police department for a green light to buy taser guns, as an "non-life threatening" device, to protect the community, their selves and to get a person "in control." In San Francisco, there have been ongoing hearings with the community about the police demands of Tasers. After San Francisco police shot of Mesha Monge-Irizarry's son with mental health disability, Idriss Stelley, 48 times, to understand what her bereaved victims' client families suffered, Irizarry underwent tasering at her Idriss Stelley Foundation counseling office. She collapsed, immobilized by "unbelievable pain" and nerve damage. Now she walks with a cane. Also Mesha have told me that the police crisis training in San Francisco, that was implemented in 2005 after her son was shot, has been watered down and almost completely defunded. Has there been an elevation of the police crisis trainings throughout this country since the implementation of the model in Memphis, Tennessee back in 1988? There is no numbers locally or nationally on how many people with disabilities serve on the boards of police commissions or other boards that serve as an oversight boards when it comes to police crisis trainings.

For example, autism has become a hot button issue in the mainstream media and in the community. For example Michael Buckholtz, the founder of one of the only organization that makes the connection and work hands on with people in poverty dealing with autism, Aid for Autistic Children Foundation, Inc. and is a Black man living and thriving with autism, calls the recent media's attention on autism and I quote, "a mad "gold rush" to capitalize on all things autism, started quite organically." There also have been many more public cases of police brutality on children and adults with autism in the last 10 years. For example in the 90s I used to keep a running sheet of police brutality cases against people with disabilities, and when I started there were no high profile cases involving people with autism compared to now, that most of police brutality cases I write about involve youth and adults with autism, for example once again Neli Latson's case in Virginia, and so many more.

With the recent attention people with autism have received in the mainstream media and elsewhere, many experts have emerged that have shed light on the relationship between police abuse and people with autism. One of the people doing great work in the field is Dennis Debbaudt. Dennis was the first person to formally address the abusive interactions between law enforcement and people with autism in his 1994 report, Avoiding Unfortunate Situations. He has since authored a full length book, published over 30 reports, written numerous book chapters and produced innovative and acclaimed training videos for law enforcement and first responders such as paramedics, fire rescue, police, and hospital staff who may respond to an autism emergency. Dennis is also a father of a son with autism.

Today I see why these reports, combined with disability activism, writing and journalism, are extremely important. For one reason, it helps to bring awareness on this issue and it forces not only cities and states to start reporting on this issue, but it also wakes up activists' organizations like October 22nd coalition, to start reporting on cases of police brutality under different disabilities. More reports like Dennis and activists showing up to police commission meetings to make sure disability i.e. autism is highlighted throughout the activist community, makes it easier to keep police, policy makers, researchers, journalists on a paper trail that sometimes leads to legislation, community forums and other public awareness.

There are others in the community that have also developed response techniques for people living with mental health, developmental disabilities, autism and so on that do not require police intervention. Unfortunately, these cases are rarely given attention in the mainstream media. For example, on July 5th 2003 in Denver a young teen with a developmental disability, was shot by a Denver police officer. As a result of the shooting of Paul Childs, the Black community and disability community did call for increased police training, but the Black community went beyond police training. In fact, it removed the need for police intervention altogether. A group of Black ministers in Denver forced the city to implement a community response program that would educate people in Denver about their neighbors living with mental health and developmental disabilities, and how to respond to their needs in case of an emergency.

The group/non-profit organization called FACE IT in Denver was inspired by Paul Childs' death; Pastor Reginald Holmes of New Covenant Christian Church envisioned a nonprofit organization that would provide a Family Advocacy and Crisis Education Intervention Team (FACE IT) to work together for change in the Denver community. FACE IT was established to build, inform, support and help communities and people in times of crisis. A six-crisis intervention member team was brought together to work in building the organization with Director Bob Sattler. This community-centered model eliminates the need to call the police and protects people living with disabilities from the threat of police abuse and incarceration. Their conclusion was that the community had a lack of knowledge of people with disabilities, so the Black ministers of that community tried to implement more community awareness on disability through community forms. And on the legal side, there was a proposal to pass what was called Paul's Law named after 15-year old Paul Childs III. The law would of require all law enforcement officers and dispatchers in Colorado to undergo crisis-intervention training along with special instruction on how to deal with suspects who have mental illness and developmental disabilities such as autism.

Another example of not turning to police and police training is Critical Resistance of Oakland new project the Oakland Power Projects (OPP). From their website it says, "The Oakland Power Projects build the capacity for Oakland residents to reject police and policing as the default response to harm and to highlight or create alternatives that actually work by identifying current harms, amplifying existing resources, and developing new practices that do not rely on policing solutions. It goes on to say organized into short, medium and long-term steps, the Oakland Power Projects work to make our families and neighborhoods stable and healthy without relying on the cops. CR members spent the last year talking with allies, friends, neighbors, and community members." More info at their website http:// criticalresistance.org/chapters/cr-oakland/the-oakland-power-projects/

On May 29th, 2005 I and others held a radio show under Pushing Limits on KPFA 94.1 FM in Berkeley, California, that talked about police brutality against people with disabilities with many advocates and mothers in this field, including Allegra "Happy" Haynes, City Liaison of Denver who talked about the community response. It's not clear today in 2012–2013 how these responses to Childs shooting were funded, and if they are still ongoing. Usually years after police shootings of any victim including those with disabilities, the community pressure for changes gets weaker, thus implementations of training or other solutions falls from the implantation/funding table. In 2013 FACE IT and Paul Law has not been in mainstream news thus, I don't know any updates, and if they are still operating or on the law books in Denver, Colorado.

I hope we are not so divided that somebody else will conquer us!

As Lisa Gray Garcia aka Tiny laid out, Poor Magazine, unlike other media outlet, keeps the spotlight on many cases of police brutality and has their own practice about calling police. Poor Magazine is a poor people led/indigenous people led, grassroots non-profit, arts organization dedicated to providing revolutionary media access, art, education and advocacy to silenced youth, adults and elders in poverty across the globe. All of POOR's programs are focused on providing non-colonizing, community-based and community-led media, art and education with the goals of creating access for silenced voices, preserving and degentrifying rooted communities of color and re-framing the debate on poverty, landlessness, indigenous resistance, disability and race locally and globally. Lisa Gray Garcia with her mother Dee, founders of Poor Magazine, set a practice at Poor Magazine to never call the police, thus working out conflicts in what is called Family Council, where all parties come together to resolve problems. This is not easy and as you read in Lisa's section early in this chapter, that this practice is ongoing and takes thinking out of the box and commitment on all parties involved.

Building blocks are stacked to reach this ultimate goal, as Poor Magazine has laid out, we, as a society must be open to diverse tactics to communicate with each other. I argue that further, we must develop tactics with the explicit goal of eliminating police brutality against people with disabilities. In order to do this, society as a whole, the police specifically and outsider activists such as those from the Occupy Movement must tackle their own biases. Individualism, institutionalism, and the replacement of community authorities by outside "experts," with excess amounts of letters following their names, like PhDs, and the bling bling to close their eyes from the needs of the communities they supposedly represent, must be stopped in its tracks. Only then will we be open to diverse solutions that will both recognize people on the frontlines and give us the power to reflect, revise and reinforce these solutions to create sustainable solutions that truly protect the community, especially people living with disabilities, from police brutality.

As the dominant drivers of dialogue at the community level, music and cultural activism can and does play important roles in designing, implementing and sustaining these solutions. How? Most importantly, artists can and must recognize ableism in the cultural arena and in programs that come out of it. For example, community music projects that slam the door in the face of artists/musicians with disabilities, in general, must be called out and confronted. As stated previously, there were many Hip-Hop artists (and other musicians and artists) living with disabilities, but it was not until February 2012, when Krip-Hop Nation put out an entire CD, Broken Bodies PBP—Police Brutality & Profiling Mixtape dedicated to the issue of police brutality in the disability community was released, that disabled artist/cultural workers and their community had their cultural expression on this issue of police brutality! Next, promoters, agents and radio DJs that occupy the musical arena must be open and active in creating, raising funds, and promoting not only Krip-Hop Nation's media and cultural projects around police brutality cases, but they must start seeking out and including the numbers of other pieces, projects and visual arts produced by generations of disabled activists and culture warriors.

Although some radio stations like KPFA in Berkeley, California, WBIA in New York and KPFK in Los Angeles and KPOO in San Francisco showed their support by playing Krip-Hop Nation & 5th Battalion CD, artists from the disability community are still, far more often than not, locked out of the media and the activist dialogue by ableism from others. Krip Hop Nation/5th Battalion is working to kick down these doors of exclusion, but there is still much work to be done. Free yourself from I and turfism by connecting to your local disabled artists/activists, make programs, projects and organizations diverse and so much more.

One example of that support was on Sept 19th/2013 KPFA 94.1 FM Letters and Politics in Berkeley, CA Host Mitch Jeserich. I talked about police brutality against people with disabilities. Here are some of important points that go beyond training.

- Broken promises of decreasing cases of police shootings of people with disabilities by introducing more training. This answer has been around since the late 80s when I began to get involved in this issue. There has to be more answers, but if we have to only deal with training and be force to live with this broken record, then lets tweak the evaluation of these trainings. How?
- Have an independent board of people with all kinds of disabilities that would go from state to state, city to city, not only evaluate the training, but collect data of these cases for a national report. Remember there is not one report, data or anything on cases of police brutality against people with disabilities nationally that is publicly accessible to activists. There might be many reports in National organizations or in academia, but they are hard to get a hold of.
- Disabled orgs/activists can learn from the Malcolm X Grassroots Center in NY who did a report on police brutality against Black people (http://mxgm.org/wp-content/uploads/2012/07/07_24_Report_all_rev_protected.pdf), on pg. 7 of the report it talks about Black people with mental health disabilities. The disabled community/orgs must take on this issue nationally and locally. We live in a country based on numbers, for example we do the US Census every 10 years, non-profits keeps numbers to get more funding. So the same with this issue, we need to keep records, data, reports and numbers.
- Add race and class to police brutality against PWD. There was a recent case of a white young man with developmental disability roughed up at a movie theater and passed away in custody. Now the National Down Syndrome Congress is discussing, with media coverage, their efforts to develop a nationwide-training program for law enforcement and first responders on how to handle individuals with developmental disabilities. For people of color with disabilities, at this time, there are very few local organizations, and on the national level the picture is even bleaker. The disabled rights movement hasn't dealt with their racism, and because of that, many national disabled organizations lack strong voices of POC with disabilities. National organizations of people of color need to work with people of color with disabilities and the National Black Disability Coalition etc..
- As we all know, the majority of cases of police brutality against people with disabilities don't come under training, but just blunt discrimination, profiling and not listening.
- One thing has been common in some cases is parents, providers and others call police for help, but end up deadly. Can we have an alternative phone number?

* Tap into local orgs that have been on the front line on this issue like Idriss Stelley Foundation, Poor Magazine, Critical Resistance. 9 times out of 10, when funding/solutions are created, it is in the hands of the "Other" from above and not with community advocates on the ground. For example, in 2013 the DOJ gave a $400,000 grant to the national office of the Arc to create the first ever center dealing with police violence against people with developmental disabilities, but I don't know what they are doing, & community experts are not at the table . . . . .
* Increase cultural work on this issue into the broader arts/media arena like Krip-Hop Nation/5th Battalion Mixtape Hip-Hop CD by artists with disabilities with solid support and foundation through not only fudging but access to media on a local and national level.

Editors' Postscript If you liked reading this chapter by Moore, Garcia, and Thrower, and are interested in reading more about disability community's participation and response to the Occupy Wall Street Movement, we recommend Chap. 2 "Krips, Cops and Occupy: Reflections from Oscar Grant Plaza" by Sunaura Taylor with Marg Hall, Jessica Lehman, Rachel Liebert, Akemi Nishida, and Jean Stewart and Chap. 15 "My World, My Experiences with Occupy Wall Street and How We can go Further" by Nick Dupree. If you are interested in reading institutional ableism and responses and resistance from disability communities, we recommend Chap. 10 "Neoliberal Academia and a Critique from Disability Studies" by Akemi Nishida.

Great Articles to Read on This Issue

BILLYJAM. Latest Krip-Hop Compilation Addresses Police Brutality Against People with Disabilities. AMOEBLOG. http://www.amoeba.com/blog/2012/06/jamoeblog/latest-krip-hop-compilation-addresses-police-brutality-against-people-with-disabilities.html

Critical Resistance website. Fight the cops! The Oakland power projects and cr's 2014 policing year in review, 26 March 2015. http://criticalresistance.org/fight-the-cops-the-oakland-power-projects-and-crs-2014-policing-year-in-review/

David M. Perry. When disability and race intersect. http://www.cnn.com/2014/12/04/opinion/perry-garner-disability-race-intersection/

D Center, SDC host police brutality workshop http://dailyuw.com/archive/2013/05/12/news/d-center-sdc-host-police-brutality-workshop#.Ujuy-SSoXOt

Darwin BondGraham @Darwinbondgraha. Making Black Lives Matter. A group of Bay Area families has been fighting back by building a network of those directly affected by police violence. East Bay Express, NEWS & OPINION » FEATURE, 13 MAY 2015. http://www.eastbayexpress.com/oakland/making-black-lives-matter/Content?oid=4278747

Emmitt Thrower. Does the disability community need a documentary on police brutality from a retired disabled Black cop? San Francisco Bayview Newspaper, 27 March 2015

IDRISS STELLEY FOUNDATION. http://mysite.verizon.net/vzeo9ewi/idrissstelleyfoundation/

Latest Krip-Hop Compilation Addresses Police Brutality Against People with disabilities. http://www.amoeba.com/blog/2012/06/jamoeblog/latest-krip-hop-compilation-addresses-police-brutality-against-people-with-disabilities.html

Leroy F Moore Jr. The National Center of Criminal Justice & Disability, The Arc, DOJ, Police & The Community with Kathryn Walker, L A Davis, Program Manager of Justice Initiatives. POOR Magazine. http://poormagazine.org/node/5302

Leroy Moore. Community protector Bo Frierson tipped from wheelchair for protesting SFPD's assault on his cousin. San Francisco Bayview Newspaper, 27 January 2015
Link: Audio interview Leroy Moore on Letters & Politics on KPFA 94.1FM About Police Brutality Against People W/disabilities. http://poormagazine.org/node/4908
Malcolm X Grassroots Center, Report on the Extrajudicial Killing of 120 Black People. http://mxgm.org/against-and-beyond-police-brutality/
National Black Disability Coalition. A National Campaign for Minority Disability Legislation. http://www.blackdisability.org/content/news-alert
Police use Taser on deaf crime victim. http://www.kirotv.com/news/news/crime-law/police-use-taser-deaf-crime-victim/nP9mZ/
Police Violence and People with disabilities. Author: Thomas C. Weiss. Disabled World—Sep 01, 2013 | Updated: Sep 01, 2013. http://www.disabled-world.com/editorials/cops.php
Rochester, NY Police officers Assault Disabled Man in Motorized Wheelchair. http://www.copblock.org/31222/rochester-ny-police-officers-assault-disabled-man-in-motorized-wheelchair/
San Francisco Bayveiw Newspaper. How can I prepare my 13-year-old Black autistic son for encounters with police? 21 December 2014. http://sfbayview.com/2014/12/dear-nadir-how-can-i-prepare-my-13-year-old-black-autistic-son-for-encounters-with-police/?replytocom=177175#respond
Sunjay Tojuhwa Smith his work on police brutality against people with disabilities A video of those wronged by the police. http://pwdapv.org/
Toshio Meronek. Cops shouldn't be above the Americans with Disabilities Act. Fusion.net. 27 March 2015. http://fusion.net/story/107664/police-shouldnt-be-above-the-americans-with-disabilities-act/?utm_source=facebook&utm_medium=social&utm_campaign=socialshare&utm_content=desktop+top
When Cops Criminalize the Disabled. http://www.thenation.com/article/175561/when-cops-criminalize-disabled#
Zosia Zaks, Towson. Why no talk of Gray's disabilities? Baltimore Sun Newspaper, 4 May 2015. http://www.baltimoresun.com/news/opinion/readersrespond/bs-ed-gray-disabled-letter-20150502-story.html

Additional Readings

Dennis Debbaudt http://www.debbaudtlegacy.com/autism_law_enforcement_roll_call_briefing.cfm
http://sfbayview.com/2011/why-did-sfpd-shoot-randal-dunklin-in-his-wheelchair/. (by Carol Harvey, about the SFPD Shooting of Randal Dunklin)
http://poormagazine.org/node/726.(AboutSFDAMO)
http://www.abovetopsecret.com/forum/thread754073/pg1. (Trend of Police Violence against the Disabled)
http://5newsonline.com/2013/05/17/video-police-brutality-lawsuit-filed-by-95-pound-disabled-woman/
Leroy Moore article: http://disabilityrightnow.wordpress.com/tag/police-brutality/
spaami: stop police abuse against mentally ill!—Yahoo! Groups. groups.yahoo.com/group/SPAAMI/. As noted in a 1996 Amnesty International report: (PD) Excessive force has been routinely used against mentally ill (This is a group administered by Idriss Stelley Foundation). http://groups.yahoo.com/group/BBDB_LEROY/. (Broken Bones Disabled Brown Bodies)

Blindness and Occupation: Personal Observations and Reflections

22

Rikki Chaplin

Abstract

This chapter will explore the various types of occupation in which I engage in as a person with a dual sensory disability. I will discuss three levels of occupation that I have observed myself engaging with different intensity throughout my life thus far. I will also explore the interaction between my emotional state and my ability to engage in the three different levels of occupation.

Keywords

Blindness • Adaptation • Occupation • Deaf/blind

22.1 Introduction

What is it that I do as a person who is blind and has a hearing impairment that is unique to this situation into which I was born. It is as though people imagine that we, as people who are blind and who may have other disabilities are occupied differently to those people who do not experience disability. I therefore want to explore whether or not this is the case, and if it is that I am differently occupied to my non-disabled peers, why this might be so. The things with which we each find ourselves being occupied are as much dependent on our daily requirements and our personality differences as they are on being blind or having any type of disability at all. Yet there are layers of occupation that I suggest that people with disability

R. Chaplin (✉)
National Policy and Advocacy Officer, Blind Citizens Australia, Melbourne, VIC, Australia

Norrie Disease Association Borad, PO Box 3244, Munster, IN 46321, USA
e-mail: Rikkichaplin@gmail.com

© Springer Science+Business Media Dordrecht 2016
P. Block et al. (eds.), *Occupying Disability: Critical Approaches to Community, Justice, and Decolonizing Disability*, DOI 10.1007/978-94-017-9984-3_22

share. This layered occupation may be unique to people with disability insofar as the combination and interaction of those layers is concerned. So let's consider some examples.

22.2   Examples and Discussion

For me, employment and voluntary activity could not be further apart in terms of meaning and purpose. I have experienced employment in which a great deal of meaning could be found through the rewards of watching the lives of clients I worked with change for the better. I have also experienced meaningless work, the futility and humiliation of which was heightened by certain managers whose attitudes towards people with disabilities were somewhat misinformed, despite working in the disability sector themselves.

On the voluntary front however, I find a great deal of meaning in my activities. My qualification as a social worker has permitted me to develop knowledge and skills which I contribute to Blind Citizens Australia, the peak advocacy body of people who are blind or vision impaired in Australia, as a member of two committees. My skills in the audio and music field allow me to provide a high quality publication which disseminates information to others who are blind or vision impaired in our local area and who do not readily access the internet or other computer related applications to get a sense of what's going on in the world. I am a father of two children, and this occupies me in terms of play, and guidance throughout their lives. Like anybody else, I wash up, cook, fix the family computers if problems are within my limited technological expertise, and act as a sounding board for my friends and hopefully, for my children as they grow up.

There are three layers of occupation for people who are blind which I perceive, and indeed which could be generalized to people experiencing other types of disability. Here it would be good to name the three layers of types of occupation. These occupations, I will refer to as:

- the occupation of adaptive learning, (layer 1), the occupation of learning life and living skills;
- the occupation of contributing and providing, (layer 2), the occupation of living, contributing, sharing, leading, and of functioning as an active member of society;
- and the occupation of education and advocacy, (layer 3): the impact which the combining of the first two layers of occupation in order to live a fulfilling life has on those around us.

22.2.1 Layer 1: The Occupation of Adaptive Learning

For me, and most likely for other people with disabilities, there is a layer of occupation which is shared by people who must master alternative ways to complete everyday tasks. I will refer specifically to blindness in providing examples of how this adaptive learning layer applies. Reading braille to access the written word, or using a screen reader to access the internet and other functions of a computer, are activities unique to blindness. They might be better described as unique ways of interacting with the printed word, the online shopping mall or bank, or the children's story at bedtime. Specific knowledge of how to interact with this technology and with braille as a medium is required. A computer is operated using an almost endless combination of keyboard shortcuts as opposed to the use of the mouse for example. Words in braille are abbreviated by the use of specific contractions or groups of commonly used letters combined in just one or two cells. These are sub-occupations which at some point in our lives, we were fully occupied with because it was necessary to learn the intricacies of these unique methods of interaction with the written word and the virtual community.

There are also less technological skills to master, such as the way to cook dinner without burning oneself on the hotplate or grill, how to match clothing, make the bed, do the dishes, and other skills which must be learned using tactile methods to achieve the desired outcome of a clean plate or a well-made bed. This first layer of occupation is necessary to be involved in if one is to reach the second layer of occupation, which might be considered to be the most commonly experienced level of occupation when we take into account the perceived differences between people who are blind and our sighted peers.

22.2.2 Layer 2: The Occupation of Contributing and Providing

The second layer of occupation is the occupation of living, contributing, sharing, leading, and of functioning as an active member of society. The first layer of occupation becomes a sub-occupation as I referred to earlier, as we apply the skills which have been learned to tasks which almost everyone needs to complete to contribute to their environment at all levels. The sub-occupation functions in the background as we enhance the skills we have learned, or we identify new skills that we need to develop. A good example of this is the changing of technology and our need to keep abreast of these developments and learn new ways of interacting with evolving technology. It is a level of occupation which never ceases, but which out of necessity, must remain behind the scenes if we are to make a difference to the lives of others around us and not to become preoccupied solely with the means which are supposed to lead us to productive and worthwhile ends.

22.2.3 Layer 3: The Occupation of Advocacy and Education

The third layer of occupation is one which can be subconscious. This is the impact that combining the first two layers of occupation in order to live a fulfilling life has on those around us. People who do not have disabilities often observe us and express admiration for what most of us consider to be just normal, everyday activity. People who are blind or vision impaired and who may still be adjusting to their own situation may look to those of us who have lived with our disability for a long time and feel comfortable with it for guidance, inspiration, or assistance with learning the practicalities of life in what might be a new or more unfamiliar situation to them. Often I receive unsolicited comments from people I meet in the community or in my recreational pursuits expressing admiration for how I cope with life. Some become offended at these sorts of comments because they feel they are patronizing. I have made a decision not to do so for two reasons. Firstly, people gain inspiration and a sense of confidence that they might cope in a similar situation if they can observe me living a productive life, and surely that is valuable for them. Secondly, it is important that I am available to talk to both people with and without disability to educate them about how we as people who are blind function so that our community and society can improve our access to all aspects of life based on education from people who have lived experience of disability. It is my belief that one cannot make demands of people who have the power to change things without a willingness to engage in dialogue with them. Therefore, whether we feel comfortable with it or not, education, advocacy and role modeling become integral in our occupational experiences, and can be identified as a third and sometimes unappreciated layer of occupation for all of us as individuals.

A recent example which will impact on all of us as people who experience disability in my home state of Queensland is the Liberal government's decision in 2012 to attempt to drastically reduce the amount of money spent on providing subsidised taxi fares. Due to numerous circumstances, people who are blind or have dual disability use taxis on a very regular basis to make transport more efficient, for safety reasons and to go about both professional and recreational activities more easily. The State government's proposal was to reduce the subsidy from an unlimited cap, under which it is currently possible for any one taxi trip to be subsidised at half the original cost for all trips up to $50.00, to a cap of $400 per year. For work alone at that time, I made 8 taxi trips per week at approximately $18.00 (full fare) per trip. At that rate, I would use up a $400.00 cap in the space of approximately 7 weeks. While I may still have been able to afford to go to work, the impact of the doubling of my transport costs just to be employed would have, for the majority of the year, have a profound impact on my ability to attend other community activities I was involved in, and to purchase things I might want or need, thereby reducing my capacity to contribute to the economy. Thankfully the initial $400.00 limit which was proposed was overturned after considerable outrage from a variety of groups experiencing disadvantage. The proposal to review the sustainability of the Taxi Subsidy Scheme was upheld, and a panel consisting of advocacy groups representing various disability types was formed. It became essential that as people who are blind or vision impaired along with other people with disabilities, we unite, combine, and seek a strong position in the stakeholder panel which reviewed the scheme. Advocacy on behalf of our specific group, and collaborative advocacy efforts with other stakeholders was critical in achieving a positive outcome. It was necessary at individual and collective levels so that it could have the greatest impact on the attitudes of decision-makers. This is an instance in which as individuals, we could not afford to assume that organizations acting on our behalf would do the advocacy for us. If those organizations are going to have the greatest impact, it is necessary for advocacy to become a part of our individual occupational experiences so that their efforts are supplemented by a passionate response from the community of people such a decision was going to affect. As a result of this combined effort, it was decided that the subsidy would not be altered.

This example of the need for collaboration in advocacy leads us to a philosophy which underpins my approach to occupation. I have made a point of focusing on interdependence. That is, I realize that I have strengths, but also I have needs. It is imperative for me that I use my strengths or gifts to assist others, and I will seek assistance for the areas in which I have limited skills or capacity. This philosophy runs contrary to individualism, which emphasizes self-sufficiency and competence in all areas. I have stressed the importance of interdependence within the blindness community in order to avoid a situation where a part of the third layer of occupation I mentioned, (particularly peer support and genuine acceptance of the lack of confidence or skills which some people may have), could be undermined. The philosophy upon which one bases an occupational approach may be the most essential element of that approach, and indeed the way we go about advocating for inclusion and accessibility can be influenced by a chosen philosophy.

Often, it is the occupations which people who are blind share in common with our non-disabled peers which have required the attention of blindness organizations, through advocacy and the demonstration that via the unique methods of interaction which I outlined earlier, a person who is blind can participate fully in the occupations which are most often taken for granted. It is the assumption that people who are blind cannot participate in these everyday occupations which has needed to be quashed. It is a tendency towards exclusivity, either through the medium via which one accesses these occupations, or through paternalistic sheltering by making people who are blind subject to draconian service models, which has required advocacy to overcome. Blind Citizens Australia (BCA), the peak advocacy body of and for people who are blind or vision impaired in Australia, is the united voice of blind and vision-impaired Australians. BCA's mission is to achieve equity and equality via empowerment, by promoting positive community attitudes, and by striving for high quality and accessible services which meet the needs of all people who are blind or vision impaired.

Objectives D and E in Blind Citizens' Australia's mission statement are particularly relevant to this article about blindness and occupation. They are:

> D. To work for the progressive improvement and modernization throughout Australia of public policies and practices governing the education, health, welfare, rehabilitation, employment and recreation of blind people.
>   E. To promote or engage in any activities or programs designed to enhance the education, health, welfare, rehabilitation, employment or recreation of blind people of other countries, in furtherance of the organization's Objects and of the aims of the World Blind Union. (http://wordpress.bca.org.au/about/history/)

These objectives appear to be based on the assumption that people who are blind or vision-impaired do not participate fully and/or equally in occupations of all types that their sighted peers take for granted. This is a view shared by other blindness advocacy and consumer groups, such as the National Federation of the Blind in America. To demonstrate the pertinence of this approach, it will be useful to look at the sorts of changes which Blind Citizens' Australia has been successful in advocating for, and those which are still being pursued today. It should be noted here that a key strategy for advocacy, assuming that one adopts the philosophy of interdependence, could be that people who are blind or vision impaired will be better able to contribute to their communities if the built environment is more accessible, or if technology or websites are developed with accessibility in mind. The notion of contribution becomes important as opposed to the emphasis on self-sufficiency.

One of the earliest successes achieved by BCA's tireless advocacy was the installation of audio tactile traffic signals at most major intersections in capital cities. While members are still advocating for particular signals to be installed in specific areas, it is acknowledged throughout the country that audio tactile traffic signals are a mechanism which assist people who are blind or vision impaired to go about the business of travelling around their community to participate in any given occupation. The fact that these traffic signals are readily provided give the individual who is blind or vision impaired a greater sense of freedom to move about their community safely, and hence, a greater sense of autonomy and achievement as they accomplish tasks which may otherwise have been more difficult, or perhaps not achievable at all without significant assistance. Autonomy is not necessarily synonymous with independence. Rather, autonomy gives us the ability to choose to contribute. A lack of autonomy removes choice.

On a more recreational note, BCA is currently engaged in a campaign to introduce audio description to movie cinemas, live theatre, and television broadcasts throughout the country (http://wordpress.bca.org.au/accessible-dvds-blu-rays-released-in-october/). They have been largely successful in their efforts thus far, but there is still work to be done to achieve the same universality enjoyed in other countries. Audio description refers to a separate audio track which accompanies a movie or performance that describes the scenery, actions of characters and the more subtle nuances in each character such as dress, facial expressions and demeanor. The presence of such contextual knowledge allows a person who is blind to enjoy a movie, television show or theatre performance equally as much as people with sight. It eliminates those moments where everyone else is laughing and the blind person asks "what happened," and laughs belatedly, if they receive a description of events at all.

It would be accurate to say that advocacy for people with many types of disability, has necessarily been an historical occupation. It is an approach which has become necessary as people struggle for the right to participate in everyday occupations which they fight to convince their non-disabled peers that they can contribute to. At this point now that three levels of occupation as I perceive them have been explained.

It is also important to consider and reflect on how dual disability affects my occupational experience. I wear high quality hearing aids and I have done a considerable amount of research to allow me to make the best use of them, and also to maximize the usefulness of my existing hearing. Learning to cope with hearing loss as a person who is blind has been an exercise in patience, information gathering, experimentation and at times frustration. As a musician, discovering that

I had developed significant hearing loss was devastating as I learned that I could no longer pitch accurately when I sang or process music automatically as I once did so that I could know what key a given song was in. I learned how to process sound again using good quality headphones and perseverance. Now that I have achieved this goal, I have aspirations of re-entering the music industry professionally. These events however, have led to the loss of income from an activity which I loved. Employment in the music industry, whether it is in a recording studio or on stage, did align more compatibly with my sense of meaningful occupation. One might argue that for a time, I was occupied with dealing with the emotions of knowing that I could not work professionally.

In order to develop the ability to work professionally again in the music industry, it has been necessary for me to return to a concentrated engagement in the first layer of occupation, the occupation of adaptive learning. That is, I went through a process of information gathering, exposing my ears to sound through headphones, learning what my limitations were, and learning new strategies to deal with difficult listening environments. I also used existing knowledge about music and sound frequencies to inform my experimentation and to communicate with my consulting audiologist in order to achieve the best result from my hearing aids. I am now reasonably knowledgeable in the art of coping with hearing loss, and I can function well even as a musician once again. While I am continuously striving to improve my skills and knowledge in the area of hearing loss, this process has become more of a background function as I move to the second layer of occupation, which involves applying my new skills and knowledge to my everyday life. For example, I learned about the use of telecoils in hearing aids to make talking on the phone easier. For a time, One of my primary responsibilities at work was to answer the main phone line, and although I don't have a perfect record by any means, I can fulfill this responsibility adequately if I accept my limitations (that is, not always getting the name of a person on the other end of the phone right), and I am honest with my colleagues about those limitations. I have learned how to cope in meetings at work by having someone sitting next to me to relay any information I may miss at close range so I can record meeting minutes accurately. I can make use of different mediums of communication after the meeting if I am unsure about certain aspects of the information.

It is ironic that following my hearing loss, I was asked to take on the editing of an audio magazine. I have done so, learning how to use an audio editor successfully, and using a combination of my knowledge gained in the recording studio and radio stations with my skills at making speech as clear as possible via the use of software and other techniques to enhance a speaker's clarity. Through this process, I learned new skills and realized that I had talents that I had no idea I possessed. I have taken on additional interviewing and editing activities for Blind Citizens Australia, and I have continued to play for local community events. This voluntary musical activity indeed acted as the vehicle through which I was forced to develop new ways of processing sound, and gave me the opportunity to continue playing even when I was struggling to comprehend what I was hearing.

This last example highlights the tendency for layers of occupation to be interwoven. They are not necessarily mutually exclusive, and the interaction between layers of occupation can encourage or even force people to develop skills they may not otherwise have felt they could learn. I find more and more that I am even entering the third layer of occupation, (education and advocacy), in the area of hearing loss. I recently attended a conference about Norrie's disease, (my genetic condition), at which I participated in a panel of men who all experience the condition. We took questions from the audience, many of whom were parents of young children with the condition and who wanted to know about how we experience and cope with many aspects of life, including our hearing loss. Many people at the church I attend and at work ask me about all sorts of situations and issues regarding both blindness and hearing loss. In this way, all three layers of occupation can interact as I might gather information for people when I am uncertain about the answer to a question, or refer them to people with more appropriate knowledge and skills than I might have. Without participating in the second layer of occupation, (the layer of contribution and provision), these opportunities could not arise. The first layer of occupation is about learning, while the third is educational, but the second layer provides the experiential aspect of life necessary to make one's educational and advocacy efforts based on accurate information and observation.

It is important to note also the interaction between occupational and personal experiences. For example, for a long time when I was a teenager and young adult, I refused to become involved with the advocacy efforts of Blind Citizens Australia. This decision was due to a values base that I had developed as a result of the lack of exposure to people experiencing life in ways which were far removed from my own life experience. I grew up in a middle class family where my father came from a tough background as a child and applied his incredibly strong work ethic and belief in looking after himself and his possessions to be a wonderful provider for his wife and children. I gleaned from his example, that despite the disadvantage that I experienced, it was up to me to make my way in the world. I generalized this belief to include everybody in this responsibility, ignoring the contextual nuances that prevent many people from being able to pursue their goals. I viewed the work of Blind Citizens Australia as "causing trouble."

As I was made aware of the shortcomings of my values and my discriminatory attitudes, my attitude towards advocacy and the educating of the public began to change. In my final year of university, I completed a supervised placement at an organization by the name of Queensland Advocacy Inc. This was an organization focused on systems advocacy for the most vulnerable members of society. As I worked alongside other people with disabilities different to my own, I gained an appreciation of the concept of interdependence, and came to understand how people who were not afforded interdependence often experienced both direct and subtle discrimination which prevented them from contributing to society at the level they were capable of if the right supports were in place.

Due to personal circumstances affecting me at different times, I found that I did not always have the energy or even the interest in advocating for issues which I felt were irrelevant to me. It is undeniable, at least for me personally, that the combination of my own value base with my emotional state at any given time, influences my ability to interact with the occupation of education and advocacy, (layer 3), as fully as I perhaps could have.

To remain engaged at the third occupational level is a challenge for all of us, as it often requires a spirit of selflessness, particularly when advocating on issues which do not necessarily affect us personally or even interest us at all, but which profoundly impact upon the lives of others. What may assist us in remaining engaged at this level is a strong sense of social justice, and a value base which emphasizes the importance of all members of society and their unique contributions. Advocacy in a practical sense however has been dependent for me on whether I am coping emotionally with the stresses that come with daily contribution and provision, (layer 2), and even the first layer, (adaptive learning), at times.

When people approach me with those unsolicited comments of admiration, or with questions about how I cope, it would be untrue to say that I have never felt as though I'd rather be left alone at the times when I am struggling emotionally to cope with life events.

I would like to elaborate on my statement that even the layer of adaptive learning (layer 1), can be difficult to interact with if one is experiencing difficulty in coping emotionally. Learning new skills requires energy and enthusiasm over functioning, to (1) be a person, to (2) be a disabled person, to (3) be a disabled teacher and advocate, if they are to be learned thoroughly and ingrained into daily practice. This is a common challenge for people who experience the loss of vision later in life, as they wade through the natural grieving process that accompanies any type of loss. It would be difficult for example, to learn how to use a computer in a different way, or to learn how to cook using tactile and other adaptive methods, if one is experiencing anger that they were placed in such a situation at all. Denial may cause someone to assert that they have no need of adaptive technology or new skills, and they may continue to try and operate in the same way they always have.

Attitudinal factors can also influence one's willingness to engage in the learning of these skills. A good example from my own life is the fact that for many years, I deliberately paid no attention to learning how to use a standard computer effectively. I believed that adaptive technology such as the note-taker apps specifically designed for users who are blind that I was using could meet all my needs, and I saw no reason to engage with new technologies of the time such as the internet. Coupled with this was my belief that my profession of social work relied primarily on my communication with people about their emotions and practical situations. I therefore felt that to concentrate too hard on learning about computers and technology would direct my energy away from what was really important. For the first few jobs I held, I suffered no obvious consequences for adopting this mindset. When I finally did experience a situation which could have been largely avoided if I had possessed greater technological skill, it was devastating. I had failed to take into account the importance of paperwork in my professional work, and the realization of the emphasis on file management and the concerns all human service agencies have about being able to demonstrate publicly that they have acted with integrity. My refusal to become familiar with standard computer applications had left me unprepared for being able to carry out these responsibilities.

Since I experienced these difficulties, I have become gradually more able to work with standard Microsoft applications. There will always be databases and websites which are not designed with accessibility for blind computer users in mind, but it is nevertheless important that one develops the skills and knowledge to be able to inform others of how and why such applications are inaccessible. Intrinsic to my refusal to concentrate too heavily on technology was my beliefs about what social work should be, rather than a willingness to accept what it is in reality in a culture which emphasises outcomes which are financially viable. These challenges are not unique to social work. Every profession in the human services field is beset with requirements which inevitably divert us from our real purpose. However, for a professional who is blind, a willingness to constantly engage with the occupational layer of adaptive learning, (layer 1), is essential if one is to succeed at the second level of occupation, the layer of contribution and provision.

The key to such a willingness to engage is the acceptance that there are cultural and attitudinal characteristics of the broader society and the workplace that one cannot change single-handedly.

From a more domestic perspective, a lack of ability or willingness to engage in the occupational layer of adaptive learning may mean that one begins to struggle with accomplishing tasks which many of us take for granted. Chores at home may begin to be left undone, bills may not be paid on time, or participation in social events may be diminished. Yet all of us, at one time or another, experience emotional upheaval and consequently cannot engage in such practical tasks or in learning the skills we require to participate fully in everyday life. This is not unique to blindness or disability, but it may have a greater impact on people with disabilities because in order to participate in valued occupation, there is first an interaction between learning to cope emotionally with one's situation and accepting that it is necessary to be fully occupied for a time in learning the foundational skills that lead to those valued occupations.

22.3 Conclusion

I have demonstrated that there are three levels of occupation that I have observed myself engaging in as a person with a dual disability. These are: layer 1, (adaptive learning), layer 2, (*contribution and provision), and layer 3, (education and advocacy). I have also explored the interaction between one's emotional state and the ability to engage with all three levels of occupation discussed. This interaction* I believe warrants further exploration in order to better understand what people with disabilities experience in an everyday context, and how they might be better assisted to manage this complex interaction. The ideal scenario might be a situation in which I can engage with all three levels of occupation simultaneously, with a healthy balance between each level. However, this appears to be an almost impossible goal to achieve in a consistent manner, often due to circumstances out of one's control. It is certainly a goal which could be kept in mind however as we seek to assist people achieve ongoing and fulfilling life occupations.

Editors' Postscript If you liked this chapter by Rikki Chaplin, and are interested in reading more about sensory aspects of disability, we recommend Chap. 14 "Occupying Seats, Occupying Space, Occupying Time: Deaf Young Adults in Vocational Training Centers in Bangalore, India", by Michele Friedner. If you are interested in reading more about decolonizing Australian perspectives of disability and occupation, we recommend Chap. 5 "Landings: Decolonizing Disability, Indigeneity and Poetic Methods" by Petra Kuppers.

Surviving Stevenage

23

Roy Birch, Ann Copeland, Geoff Clarke, Neil Hopkins, Rosie Berry, Richard J.N. Copeland, STL, Bruce James, CYNTH, Paul Evans, Darren Messenger, Lucia Birch, and Andrew H. Smith

Abstract

Surviving Stevenage is a brief history of Stevenage Survivors Poetry group. The group was created in 2000 by Darren Messenger and Roy Birch, to, as the group's mission statement says, "employ poetry in all its forms to assist survivors of mental distress to survive more adequately." The chapter tells the story of the group's evolution; its successes and failures; gives examples of the work of group members past and present, and expresses what they feel about the group and its effect upon the canon of survivor literature and its therapeutic use locally.

Keywords

Stevenage • Survivors • Poetry • Group • Writing • Sharing • Together • Therapeutic

23.1   The Story of Stevenage Survivors

On April 19th, 2000, six members of Stevenage-based performing arts group Parnassus Performance met in one of the band practice rooms at Bowes Lyon House, the town's Youth and Community Centre. We (for I was one of the six) did not however, meet as Parnassus Performance, but as the newly-formed Stevenage Survivors. We had a few months earlier performed, as Parnassus, at the Somers Town Blues Night, at the Somers Town Community Centre in North London, at that time the venue for the Survivors' Poetry monthly performance event. This, our first visit to a Survivors' Poetry evening, had inspired us to want to use our own artistic

R. Birch (✉) • A. Copeland • G. Clarke • N. Hopkins • R. Berry • R.J.N. Copeland • STL
B. James • CYNTH • P. Evans • D. Messenger • L. Birch • A.H. Smith
Stevenage Survivors, 156, Gonville Crescent, Stevenage, Hertfordshire, SG2 9LY, UK
e-mail: roybirch42@gmail.com; luciaebirch@gmail.com; info@survivorspoetry.org

© Springer Science+Business Media Dordrecht 2016
P. Block et al. (eds.), *Occupying Disability: Critical Approaches to Community, Justice, and Decolonizing Disability*, DOI 10.1007/978-94-017-9984-3_23

abilities to help in the alleviation of mental distress. At this point it may be worth pointing out to anyone who isn't aware (most of you) that Survivors' Poetry was, and still is, nominally at least, a National charity whose mission statement claims it, 'promotes and publishes poetry by and for survivors of mental distress.' I say nominally because it no longer serves the wider survivor poetry writing community, being these days interested almost exclusively in poetry which has "quality" in the mainstream publishing sense. It may also be worth pointing out that at this particular time Parnassus was in steep decline. There were crippling tensions within the group which had brought it almost to a standstill, socially and creatively. The upshot of this state of affairs was that following our visit to Somers Town we defected and became Stevenage Survivors.

That Stevenage Survivors became a reality rather than simply an ideal was largely due to local drugs counsellor and psychotherapist Darren Messenger, whose experience at Somers Town inspired him to want to set up a local mental-health oriented creative writing group. As I had connections with Survivors' Poetry he asked me for help and advice and between us we created Stevenage Survivors. Why Stevenage Survivors you may well ask. The reason was that a part of the Survivors' Poetry canon of activity was a national network of affiliated local creative writing groups and Darren was keen to set up a group which could be a part of that network.

Our first year was hardly the most auspicious. With few friends and almost no money our principal achievement was survival itself, achieved largely through donations by group members, not least among them the very fine (and since published) local poet Bruce James, who almost single-handedly kept us financially afloat. And there were lights in the performance darkness too, the first coming in September, when, after four months of persistent phoning, we were finally granted permission to hold a workshop and poetry reading in the Mental Health Unit of the town's Lister Hospital.

We sat in a large circle, some 30 of us, a mixture of staff, patients, and Stevenage Survivors poets. I spoke briefly about the group and its antecedent history then read a poem and we took it from there. The session was enjoyable and successful, so much so that with almost one voice patients and staff asked us to return and hold further sessions. Unfortunately, NHS (National Health Service) bureaucracy intervened and after another 4 months of letter-writing and telephone-calls we were informed that the Lister was amalgamating with the QE2 (Queen Elizabeth 2nd) Hospital in Welwyn-Garden-City and all projects were on hold for at least a year. In spite of our best efforts, that was the group's last contact with Lister Hospital until July 2004.

In October 2000 we received a grant of £100 from the Heartlands project, an area-based community arts endeavor funded by the Single Regeneration Budget. This grant enabled us to organize our first Network Evening.

The Network Evening had a dual purpose. Firstly is to put survivor and non-survivor poets on stage in front of a survivor and non-survivor audience. Secondly to get representatives of the local mental health voluntary sector together under the same roof at the same time and actually talking to each other. And it worked. The evening was both enjoyable and informative and the representatives of the local mental health voluntary sector actually did meet and communicate; something they tend to do only at seminars – and even then somewhat grudgingly. Let me say at this point that in a life of three-score years and ten, the most striking difference I have noticed between *survivor* and *non-survivor* artists is their official status; *survivors* generally being defined as persons having at some point been in receipt of some form of mental health treatment.

In November we were invited to give a reading for the University of the Third Age (U3A). A 70-strong audience received us enthusiastically, listened attentively, enjoyed what they heard and insisted that we return, which we did in March 2001.

During our first year the group acquired a new member; a recovering alcoholic who, 7 years earlier, had been part of the very first intake of patients at Vale House, East Hertfordshire's only major residential drug and alcohol treatment center. He suggested contacting rehab as he felt we could be of service there. Contact was made and we were given permission to hold a poetry evening. The session took place in April 2001, approximately a year after the group's inaugural meeting and it was not only a huge success leading to Stevenage Survivors holding a fortnightly group at Vale House it also marked the beginning of our acceptance into the wider world of recovery and the therapeutic use of poetry.

Our second year consisted mainly of our regular meetings and the Vale House sessions. We gave a third reading to the University of the Third Age (U3A) in October and in November we received a grant of £300 from the co-operative Partnerships Award Scheme. We were in fact the last group to be funded from this particular scheme.

In January 2002 Stevenage Survivors became the first poetry group to be on the bill at the Diorama Blues Night, the Survivors' Poetry monthly performance session at its new home in the Diorama Arts Centre. This was a real achievement for us as the Diorama sessions tended to showcase individual poets.

In February we became part of the FWWCP (Federation of Worker Writers and Community publishers). We continued to hold sessions at Vale House and in July spent half our £300 to produce *The House that Hope Built*, a collection of poems written by residents of Vale House.

2003 began with a grant of £1200 from the Hertfordshire Community Foundation, for which we have to thank John Pye, External Funding Officer of Stevenage Borough Council, and Barbara Follett, at that time the MP (Member of Parliament) for Stevenage. The grant was to enable Stevenage Survivors to hold four network evenings, and produce two poetry anthologies and a quarterly newsletter. The grant was followed closely by *The Space Between*, our second anthology and the first by members of the group. This in turn was followed closely by a grant of £3300 from the Hertfordshire Foundation Key Fund, for the purpose of running 20 creative writing workshops culminating in the production of an anthology/workbook of writings from the sessions. A generous but somewhat complicated grant, The Key Fund was created to dispense European Social Fund monies to voluntary sector groups to enable them to run projects which improve the employability of the marginalized and excluded. We accepted the grant while feeling somewhat fraudulent. There is no way in which 20 creative writing workshops and an anthology can make anyone employable who wasn't before the project began. Though, as was pointed out to me, success in one area can often lead to success in other areas, leading eventually to the desired result.

From this point our activities rationalized themselves into our regular workshop sessions; our sessions at Vale House; University of the Third Age (U3A) readings; visits to London and the Fedfest (the annual gathering of the FWWCP); our publications; our Network Evenings. In September 2004 we held our most successful Network Evening, with attendance from David Royall the mayor-apparent of Stevenage and MP Barbara Follett who turned up as a civilian rather than a member of parliament and supported the event as a human being who understands suffering (her first husband, a prominent anti-apartheid activist, was assassinated, and she and her family were forced to flee South Africa). Her attendance helped raise the levels of understanding of the whole group.

We made links with Parentline Plus, a help-line for troubled parents in Hatfield and briefly ran a session in the Mental Health Unit at the Lister Hospital until staff unhelpfulness made it impossible to continue. Several members of the group represented Survivors Poetry at major Literature and Arts festivals. In 2006 staffing difficulties at Vale House forced us to withdraw the poetry group.

With regard to the creative writing workshops, the Hertfordshire community foundation wanted us to employ a qualified Poetry Workshop Facilitator. We were aware that because of the way in which we worked, such would not be viable and might even lead to the collapse of the group. I was, happily, able to explain this to the funders, and obtained their sanction to use the group members themselves as facilitators; which was a huge success. For many of the participants it was the first time they had ever been given that level of responsibility and authority, much less payment for their efforts, and for others it was a precursor of their return to the world of paid employment.

The history of the workshops was collected in 'Workbooks,' a kind of interactive anthology series. The details of each workshop – date; facilitator's name; explanation of the exercise; attendance figures; number of pieces offered for the Workbook – were followed by the writing itself; some of the pieces printed, some hand-written without any editing, some a combination of the two. A combination which created a very live collection of poetry.

The Workbooks themselves were formatted in a deliberately unusual way for a specific reason. Firstly, between each exercise and the one following it there was a blank page. This was for anyone reading the workbooks who wished to make notes of any kind about the workshops. The workbook pages were A4 in size and the work was only printed on one side of each page. The reason this was done was to encourage people to create their own Workbooks by turning the book upside down and using the blank side of each page. Although it did not prove hugely popular, it was nonetheless a good idea.

Since the ending of the funded workshop program, the group has been funded mainly by The Co-operative (Formerly the Co-operative Society, a company created for public benefit and owned by its shareholders) and the NHS Hertfordshire Health and Wellbeing Partnership. This funding has enabled the group's latest venture –

The Stevenage Survivors Annual Creative Therapy Day. A day of workshops including: Creative Writing; Art; Music; Yoga; Meditation; Reiki; Healthy eating; EFT (Emotional Freedom Technique); reflexology; auricular acupuncture; Tarot Reading; and an open mike session to round the event off. We have so far held three therapy days and we are hoping to eventually expand it into the Stevenage Creative Therapy Day across the whole town. The major obstacle to its even continuing in its present form is of course funding. Always money for bombs, bankers' bonuses, and politicians' expenses. Seldom any for an improved quality of life for the poor and the marginalized. But we hope.

Stevenage Survivors was created to – in the words of its mission statement – 'use poetry in all its forms to enable survivors of mental distress survive more adequately.' And it does. And one of the main reasons it is able to do so is the realization that life itself is the best poetry there is. Although first and foremost a poetry group, it recognizes the value of, nay, the need for, tea, biscuits and chat as part of the process in which it is engaged. Also it runs as an unofficial collective. By unofficial I mean that there is a recognizable leadership structure in place but it only evidences itself at need. I am the official coordinator of the group and in fairness people defer to me when all else fails. The rest of the time the group operates as a co-operative, with the appropriate person doing the appropriate thing at the appropriate moment. I believe it is known as the model of co-operation. No-one is put under pressure to do anything but each of us does what we are called to do. And it works extremely well. People coming to the group for the first time have often asked the question 'Is anyone in charge? The group seems to run itself.'

Stevenage Survivors operates a humanistic system which allows everyone an equal voice. And the beauty of the way in which that equality is offered and received is the fact that very few people choose to abuse it. People who come to Stevenage Survivors hardly able to relate to life in any meaningful way are quite soon playing a full part in the group. And often writing breath-takingly powerful poetry. While poetry in the literary sense is obviously the life-blood of the group, it is the poetry of our humanity that enables the group to create its best work – the re-uniting of disassociated and marginalized people with their true personalities.

If I have dealt at some length with the history and basic philosophical perspective of Stevenage Survivors it is because it was felt important to give readers a feel for the group as a living entity. But, when all is said and done, we are a poetry group and a selection of our work is essential. It will be all too short a selection, in part because of shortage of space and in part because it is so very difficult to choose adequately from so much good work. This is my selection and I make no apologies for it. I hope, however, that it meets with your approval. And most of all, I hope you enjoy it.

Roy Birch

23.2   Untitled

Surrender fully to the Light
and you'll become the greatest knight
who ever walked upon Life's land
for you will truly understand
the classic need of Chivalry
-to shine the Light unceasingly
on all souls exiled by their pain
and bring them safely home again
                                    Roy Birch

23.3   To My Son

It is not
thrift prevents my
gushing hot suds over you. Nor
merely that
you would be
embarrassed. It is that
soap would rot your skin, hot water
melt your bones. You are
allergic to warmth and fragrance. I maintain
a tepid bath for you, free from any taint of
sweetness. And that
is love even though it
feels like indifference.

I know I
should love you for what you
are. But I
hate what you are. I love
who you were, and what you
might have been. I run your baths tor
duty's sake; and for
pity's sake. And that is
love even though it feels like
indifference.
                                    Ann Copeland

23.4   Push the Whoosh

Amber shards ignite
Sparks of electric
Blue laser brainform
Channel splice fractures
Transform faultline yellow
Spectrum greyblown matter

Im plodding ultra optical
Fibre piercing raygun
Fuses orgasmic mindmeld chaotic
Geoff Clarke

23.5   The Moment of Reflection

It comes, and your whole world seems to shift,
a turning of that safe, familiar landscape

into somewhere unknown – hard, alien ground.

Certainties held for years quickly evaporate.
The heat of new thought draws them up,
creates a humid atmosphere, heavy on the mind.

The parched soil yields little meaning.
Cracks appear that tantalize, offer clues
but, when studied closer, reveal only darkness.

Clouds form, then a faint sound of thunder;
The horizon quivers in the electric haze:
Hopes hang on replenishment, the distant rain.
Neil Hopkins

23.6   Bipolar Lament

I stand at the edge of my desire
Daring to choose which way to take
Why is Life so opaque?
A touch of olanzapine will give me
New balance.
Shivering on the brink of my mania
Dark despairing depths
Call me to plummet to the plunge pool
Of misery.
I want my life to cascade into
Elemental freedom
Not wavering between two worlds
Flecked with uncertainty.
I am who I am in the waterfall of life.
Rosie Berry

23.7 The Jacket

It was old, or, put another way, not new,
yet something happened when I put it on.
It made me a poet.

People scoffed, wondering how
an old coat might affect
the stringing together of words,

the structure of language, metre and rhythm,
all these and sundry things that make up verse.
The jacket ignored them and carried on.

Perhaps it was the cut or the colour
that first drew me to it, or else some charm
bound into its threads –

spell-woven cloth that made it feel so right.
Who knows? The arcane English doctor tells me that
these things don't happen. I don't know.

As far as I'm concerned the jacket works –
makes me feel good, so I shall wear it
till its word-stitched threads run bare.
                    Richard J.N. Copeland

23.8 The Ocean's Magic

Ocean waves reaching their way into land,
cool evening breeze, as the tide starts to rise,
smelling sea air listening to the sea as music,
an act of freedom is born again.
No rules or city smells, rushing cars, screaming youths.

Running through incoming waves,
walking on the sand, not a care in the world,
living as One with nature.

The sky darkens as you sit peacefully,
enjoying the magic of a priceless wonder
the ocean
            STL

23.9   Christchild

I see
the flat landscape
of the open palm
of his right hand
stretched straight out
so that the light and the rain and the snow
in our expanding universe
falls safely on his skin
and when he folds his fingers
into a clenched fist
will he close all life as he does so
to a crushed inarticulation
or fling us free
as he opens his palm again
into his fraternal eternities?

Bruce James

Sadly there is no space for more examples of the groups work. There is, however, space for some appraisals of Stevenage Survivors by members of the group. I thank you for this opportunity to write about Stevenage Survivors. I hope the words you are reading here will give you a flavor of the group and what makes it so special.

Roy Birch

23.10   Stevenage Survivors Poetry Group

Every other Friday evening we meet; a group of friends who write poetry, we sketch a poem and read it out, during the next fortnight hone and perfect the work.

I have seen people with low self-esteem who could only sit miserable and listen to us, slowly a short poem would be written and someone, probably Roy would be asked to read it; the person now writes lovely poetry and takes pride in reading it out to all of us. More than one poet has emerged in this way.

I find it an enjoyable evening to chat with like-minded people; I have always loved poetry and book reading and find the chance to expand my knowledge of poets and the lovely use of words, a very satisfying way to end the week.

About once a year we meet with the Fed (TheFED, the writers' organization which grew out of the sad demise of the FWWCP) and other groups and workshops are experienced, this is a great day where familiar faces are recognized from the year before and new friends made all with the same love of words.

In this age of fast communication, with shortened words on the mobile phone and strange ways of communicating over the Internet, it is good to know that language is still alive and very healthy thank you.

Roy Birch

23.11 My Poem

Sometimes the words I cannot find
Sometimes I sit and think
All sorts of things go round my mind
Its hard to find a link

Other times it comes to me
I rush and grab my pen
I sit and drink a cup of tea
Or these words will go again

Here is my masterpiece you see
The poem of the year
I really hope you will agree
And hold these words most dear

CYNTH 28/09/2012

23.12 My Name is Paul Evans

I'm a member of Stevenage Survivors poetry group.
I run and maintain the creative writing group at MIND in Stevenage
I'm an organizing force on "creative therapy day."
I have attended the last three fedfests at Syracuse University.
I perform poetry to music.

Stevenage survivors is a wonderful, uplifting poetry group. I have been attending for about four years.

I really love the people who run Survivors poetry group. They are Intelligent, hardworking, kind and caring. They are the main reason I keep coming back.

Since my early days. Stevenage survivors has increased my confidence to such a degree that I now have the ability to take on tougher tasks, sometimes without support but with a firm belief that I can do it.

Rosie Berry was the original workshop facilitator of creative writing at MIND. She is a kind and caring tutor with a wonderful ability to inspire and raise imagination. I really like Rosy. She introduced me to Roy and Lucia and by doing so created a wonderful friendship with two lovely people.

I now run creative writing at MIND. I do my best to maintain the link between survivors and writing at MIND.

Long live writers.

Paul Evans

23.13 Any Day

Fathers day, Mothers day, Birthday,
Christmas day, Soul recognition day.

With the sun rising in the east
Following a dawn chorus
The sound of someone tampering
With the frequency dial on the radio set
Getting static interference

The mist rising from dampened ground
Which lifts hearts and souls from all around
Walking barefoot feeling the flush dew
and the morning ritual to bathe, wash and clean

We look on this day not like any other day
With warmth and love. Feeling the presence
Of greater powers add support and love
Which are all around.

The change of location and an embrace with nature
Is where my spirit has been
Away from concrete slabs and mobile telephone masts
Instead a contact with mother nature

The awesome power of love and gratitude
Has put me here now
I feel today, living in the now
Not in the past or pondering the future.

I am happy, my heart is smiling
My mind is spinning feeling great
Happy to be here with you all
Right here and now.
                    Paul Evans 25/6/2012

23.14 Passage for Survivors

Stevenage survivors grew out of a shared and growing dissatisfaction that Roy and I had with the performance poetry group in Stevenage at that time, called: Parnassus Poetry.

My own connection with Parnassus poetry, with writing and performing poetry, had become integral to my emergence into a community of others. What do I mean by this?

I had commenced a psychological and spiritual journey that had entailed having extremely strange and difficult experiences and which I would now describe as a form of 'spiritual emergence.' I had become extremely isolated because some of these experiences had no words to describe them but I had found some solace from the literature of poetry and philosophy. *I would prefer to say that: "I was consoled rather by other people who were also poets and philosophers and by the fact that other people could have such experiences of despair, timelessness, beauty, Inter connection of meaning and synchronicity."*

I learned through my readings that these (experiences) were 'okay' experiences and 'not' experiences that were revealing of some underlying mental health disorder. However: By speaking poetry at Parnassus poetry readings I experienced a way of languaging this world view in a shared world with others. This perspective (informed by philosophy) and it's therapeutic effect upon me (finding a fellow poet community in a town that merely seemed to offer the ideologies of consumerism and materialism) was truly much more of an experience than just joining a poetry or writing group.

The original founder of Parnassus, Margaret Pickersgill, had (I think) intuitively known this – that sharing and performing poetry was itself therapy. However; both Roy and I were becoming dissatisfied by the increasing dominance of a less inclusive and less therapeutic tendency within the Parnassus group of that time.

Roy had made connections with the Survivors organization in London and there had been some poets from Parnassus who had contributed to these events and who, naturally, felt more of an affinity with the philosophy of Survivors Poetry.

Hence we hatched: *Stevenage Survivors.*

The poets that followed us into this group were truly Survivors. We had survived angst (in the Kirkegaardian sense; not the Freudian), we had survived Thatcherism (Rampant individualism, consumerism and materialism) and many of us had survived psychiatry and the medicalization of our problems. We had survived with a poetic vision intact.

Most of what followed was down to Roy's continued efforts: for instance the work at Rehabs and in Psychiatric wards.

My own interest in 'languaging' as a form of 'Existential Therapeutics' led to my own journey into the professional worlds of philosophical psychotherapies but I still would describe myself, foremost, as a poet and see poetics as central to an illuminated psychotherapy approach.

Darren Messenger

23.15 Raw

If I could show you the singing of words
I wouldn't be telling it like this
we'd be howling or shooting or
squawking like birds.

If I could say it like it is
I wouldn't ruminate, pen poised
but sidle up to you
and let being speak

We might not sit dumb & transfixed
plainly succumbed by the remote controlled pix,
the soft cotton, the elevated boredom of our
armchair living room theatres

Our solitary threesome & foursomes
glazed, mesmerized, TV eaters

If I could show you the singing of words
I would cut off my head and let my heart speak.

Then perhaps we'd sing together
hug-dance, argue, struggle

And then breathe the ether

My pen is poised on the edge
of the unsayable.
When I cry
please
look into my eyes
                    Darren Messenger

23.16 Write Around

I came to Stevenage Survivors as a musician and singer whose original song words were written by my husband, and I had never considered myself as a writer, so it was with some trepidation that I joined in our very first writing exercise among poets and writers whose skills I really admired. Unbelievingly, I found my pen actually created something on the page and it wasn't too bad. Writing together, sharing and listening has proved to be a truly fulfilling experience for me and everyone who has ever attended our sessions. We have all learned so much from each other and the mutual enthusiasm for such diversity of writing is constantly amazing and deeply profound. Everyone takes a turn at setting the exercise, everyone participates and everyone is heard. I now confidently add to my list of skills: 'Writing Workshop Facilitator,' and I can describe myself as a 'Singer-Songwriter,' all thanks to Stevenage Survivors.

Improvisation
The guitar sings to me
my fingers stumble
the melody catches me
my fingers fly
away among the winds of time
and long forgotten pathways
away across the ocean
blue and wandering
deep and still
beyond sound and sense

and through the crashing waves of light
to tremble on a distant shore
to walk and seek
and ask for more
time to dance and
time to play
and search for you and me
to say I love you now
loved you before
love you for ever
infinity calls the tune
the rhythm is in the falling leaves
in sunlight gleaming on morning dew
in winter frosts
the soft scent of spring
in every soul that's ever been
and all the moments of creation's dream
my fingers stumble
the guitar sings
and love is in the air.
                                                    Lucia Birch

23.17 My Time with Stevenage Survivors Poetry (SSP)

I first went along to SSP in 2005. I had been in recovery from alcoholism & psychotic illness since 1989 and although I had successfully avoided alcohol for 16 years my recovery journey had recently stalled, In fact I had starting to go backwards and a broken marriage had left me homeless and back in a hostel. Once again!

I had already spent almost 8 years homeless so this reoccurrence was a bitter blow; I also had physical difficulties; a frozen shoulder and a chronic back problem. My mental health consequently began to plummet and a return to mental health services led to me being diagnosed with a 'personality disorder.' My first thought after this totally unhelpful therapeutic intervention was to seriously contemplate hanging myself and I felt more isolated than ever.

The group at SSP accepted me immediately. My first writing attempts were quite stilted and clichéd. Over time I developed and began to get in touch with the buried emotions that lay under the anger that I carried. The more I engaged with the 'processes' of writing – the more of my inner life I began to reveal to myself. I had found the creative outlet I desperately needed to re-launch my recovery journey.

As I began to find a range of emotional language and enjoy the companionship of the group I was able to even start supporting new members. Over time my poetry really improved (I started to like it,) through using the workshop method employed by SSP; writing for half an hour and then all sharing our efforts with the group.

SSP is an amazing organization which was able to support me when statutory services had failed me. Working with people often on the margins of society their work is vital and I would commend my local group to any would be poet, writer or 'funder' looking to support a community venture which consistently produces excellent outcomes for people who engage with them.

Andrew Henry Smith 26/10/2012

23.18 Numerology – This I Date: 10.10.10

18..19..20
Counting out time
Marking the processional movements
Quantifying experience
Telling the stories of the more than one
Small parts of the all

A drunk has a gun
Fifty-nine officers
One hundred weapons
Till the thunder comes

23.7.666
Pleasing on the page
The accountant a mage
The drunk driver kills three
For two years and a day
They send him away

John 3:16

A hand unseen
One tyrant
Two-hundred thousand bombs
Laming, maiming,
Mystic measures of the heart
Occult counts
Dead body amounts

Scientology
8 – 8008
An owner's manual
Brushes against the spaniel
Three hairs on the fabric of the universe
An augury
Of the future

1066
Four point five billion years
One-hundred & eighty six thousand miles of light
For the cheetah moves at seventy
Numerology continues
And the artist sees the sacred numbers
And calls them to order
For the scientists attention

In the tomb of nineteen
The universal soldier
Guarding the truth
Of the world
A triple helix
Three strands of life
A man and the wife

Mystic measures
Occult counts
Which end
In the time of the reign of the holly king
    Andrew Henry Smith 23/12/2013

Thank you
Stevenage Survivors

Editors' Postscript If you liked this by Stevenage Survivors, and are interested in reading more about arts and performance, we recommend we recommend Chap. 7 "Scenes and Encounters, Bodies and Abilities: Devising Performance with Cyrff Ystwyth" by Margaret Ames and Chap. 8, "Artistic Therapeutic Treatment, Colonialism & Spectacle: A Brazilian Tale" by Marta Simões Peres, Francine Albiero de Camargo, José Otávio P. e Silva, and Pamela Block. If you are interested in reading more about survivor action for psychiatric rights and policy, we recommend Chap. 16 "Beyond Policy – A Real Life Journey of Engagement and Involvement" by Stephanie de la Haye.

If Disability Is a Dance, Who Is the Choreographer? A Conversation About Life Occupations, Art, Movement

24

Neil Marcus, Devva Kasnitz, and Pamela Block

> Someone said 'It is great to see people with disability a part of
> our community.' I would rather say, people with disability
> should be part of THE community, it's not 'our' community, we
> are not a separate group of people. We are the ONE community
> and we are all part of it.
> (Maurice Gleeson Australian/Advocate/Elder Statesman)

Abstract

What does it mean to occupy disability? Or, does disability occupy us? To be read like a performance script, this chapter explores our experiences of communication impairment and communication triumphs in the lives of three friends. It is a conversation about intention. It is a conversation about conversation and riffs on all kinds of occupation. What you read below is a transcript of several long Skype chat sessions in twos and threes that we then added to and edited. We can be academic, but did not choose that route here. We skirt around our lives as artists and thinkers and teachers, but most of all, doers. We occupy time, space, power, and we hope, hearts.

N. Marcus (✉)
Disabled Country, Berkeley, California
e-mail: Storm@well.com

D. Kasnitz
Disability Studies, School of Professional Studies, The City University of New York,
New York, NY, USA
e-mail: devva@earthlink.net

P. Block
Disability Studies, Health and Rehabilitation Sciences, School of Health Technology and
Management, Stony Brook University, Stony Brook, NY, USA
e-mail: pamela.block@stonybrook.edu

© Springer Science+Business Media Dordrecht 2016
P. Block et al. (eds.), *Occupying Disability: Critical Approaches to Community,
Justice, and Decolonizing Disability*, DOI 10.1007/978-94-017-9984-3_24

347

Keywords
DISABILITY • Dance • Speech • Speech impairment • Friendship • Co-counseling

24.1   Setting the Scene

The play begins. What does it mean to occupy disability? Or, does disability occupy us? Where does occupational therapy fit into the mix? We are three friends with shared passions for disability rights, arts, and scholarship—two with significant speech impairments and one whose sister does as well—explore virtual conversation. Neil and Devva have idiopathic familial torsion dystonia with a childhood onset. People usually think we have Cerebral Palsy (CP). The substantive and counter intuitive differences between CP and dystonia are that although our form of dystonia is genetic, it does not show up until well after birth (9 for Devva, 8 for Neil), whereas CP is not genetic and does show up by definition around birth. In addition, dystonia changes; it can get worse or better and move around the body. CP usually stays put.

Pam's big sister Hope is autistic and does not speak. She is a spicy, smart woman who gained a voice by supported typing, the disputed kind of facilitated communication (FC). Hope does not type with Pam. Hope types with non-family members in order to communicate in English with Pam. Hope has been known to (lovingly) rake Pam over the proverbial coals by telling stories about her that no one else knows. She delights in doing this at disability studies meetings where we all gather and present. Pam turns a lovely shade of pink and any doubts about the legitimacy of Hope's use of FC melts in the warmth of Pam's characteristic embarrassment.

Neil is a professional artist. He writes, acts, and is a stunning and positive observer. Devva and Pam are both anthropologists interested in disability studies theory and communicative performance. We both teach disability studies, often to budding occupational therapists and other human services professionals in training. Here follows our conversation—the intertwining paths we create by our own occupy disability work group in Berkeley, Eureka, and Setauket. We weave our turns "talking" with our fingers as we edit together our real-time chat transcripts with unreal-time reflections. Read it like a performance script. Imagine the dance.

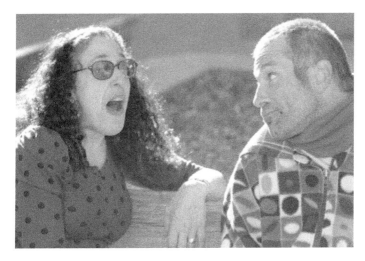

Neil and Devva Talking: Taken on the quad at UCB, Devva and Neil are sitting on a bench leaning slightly toward each other, face to face. The image shows Devva, with dark curly hair, tinted glasses and a pink shirt with black polka dots. Her mouth is wide open as she is caught in the act of speaking. Her arm, with bracelet and ring, is resting on the top of the bench. Neil, with short-cropped salt and pepper hair and face rather unshaven, looks at Devva with a knowing look (as if something is about to pop out of her mouth at him). His eyebrows are raised, his brow furrowed and he looks like he may be about to smile. He is wearing a colorfully patterned shirt with circles, squares and ovals in various shades of blue, purple, green and white. Though the picture is a close-up, the viewer can see a branching sidewalk in the background. (Photograph by Gary Ivanek)

Pamela and Devva Selfie: Our two faces, face forward and touching at the top. We both wear glasses and we are dappled with sunlight. (Photograph by Pamela Block)

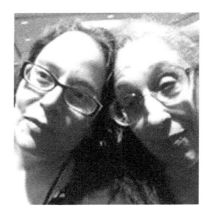

24.2 Occupying Disability

Devva: What does the phrase "occupy disability" mean anyway? Yes, disability can be an occupation—all those "activities of daily living"—and it takes most of your time to manage societal "benefits" for the ungainfully occupied. Unfortunately, the only paid occupation many disabled artists and scholars can get is in the disability industry, or, now in disability arts. How does the disabled movement relate to the "occupy" movement? Does it? Does disability have anything to offer "occupy?" I think so.

Neil: I do not occupy in protest. My occupation is a gesture of belonging, and perhaps, even more important, *knowing* that I belong.

I hesitate to eat in public sometimes, a very good reason to occupy disability.

Devva: I hesitate to talk in public. If people are not focusing on all of me, I feel they won't understand. I watch a lot. I try to occupy what I want to communicate so we are not so speech dependent. And then if they don't look at me and just cock an ear towards me, I gently turn their head to face me with a finger under their chin, and I smile.

Neil: Yes, I want to think of the occupation of the world in this new way.

Devva: Occupation as taking over?

Neil: I don't want to take over, only influence, for all our benefit.

Devva: We "occupy" time/space. We also "occupy" ourselves. We embody ourselves. I think Occupational Therapy (OT) is after the latter.

Neil: Like when you helped me dance those first times for instance... in public. OT's should be helping us or we them.

Devva: It is mutual. Having you there, encouraging you to dance, helped me dance in turn. My dancing improved.

Neil: Mutuality is occupation then?

Devva: Or occupation is mutuality? We do help OTs—they earn money helping us, good money too. But the money goes one way. Politics interferes.

Neil: Help still goes both ways.

Devva: Ok, you are always the optimist, more than me. A generous one too. I still have trouble getting past the economic inequity of disability.

24.3 Dance, Poetry and Art

Pamela: How long have you been dancing?

Neil: All of this is in my oral history (Marcus 2004), but Devva and I were dance-jamming in the early 1980s. It all has all to do with body pride.

Pamela: Context of performance?

Neil: The kiss?

Pamela: Sexuality.

Pamela: This makes me think of your partner Petra's Chap. 5 where she discusses how the two of you presented that poem in the self-advocacy conference. You were unsure of how it would be received, but the participants with intellectual disability loved it, felt connected by it, felt both heard and understood by you.

Neil: Romance = Poetry = Pride.

Pamela: And Love.

Neil: Touch as well saved my life.

Pamela: How so?

Neil: It brought me to my own beauty/power.

Pamela: What are you working on now?

Neil: An audio poem and video for the Smithsonian website on disability: Every-Body: An Artifact History of Disability in America (see http://everybody.si.edu/place). Also, in a recent disability book by Kim Neilson (2014), I am on the first page, with the introductory poem to the book.

Pamela: What else? What do you think about museums consuming disability? Or creating or recreating disability for consumption?

Neil: There was a curated show created by UC Berkeley museum "Create." It went all over the peninsula to Oakland and Richmond. They had a glossy book, but the curator did not involve the artists in the actual show, even when the artwork was being discussed, even though I brought it up. The curator thought it would be too much trouble. It was actually quite awful. The curator wanted the art to be passive—didn't want the art to talk back. Just the message: "look at what these special people have done." Petra wrote a review of the show, published in Disability Studies Quarterly (Kuppers 2012, http://dsq-sds.org/article/view/1733/3041). She quoted my letter to the curator.

End segregation
Refuse diagnosis
Hear/listen to the artist voice
Identity politics
Nothing about us without us
Educate humanity
Acknowledge the revolution
Acknowledge the protest
Acknowledge the prisoners chains
Seek integration
Separate art from any medicalization
Acknowledge unpleasant histories of institutions
Create fair speech
Marcus in Kuppers (2012, n. p.)

Devva (reading): I would have gone on the attack!

Neil: I talk back real good = love. It's powerful.

Pamela: And the impact is limited when it doesn't happen.

Neil: Self is powerful.

   Some people suffer from a lack of touch. They need hugs. Petra and I have Helping Dances. We dance in the park near my apartment. We collaborate in movement as their bodies and the way they dance is changing. Out in public. Really lovely. There has been a series of them, both locally and on the road.

I am tactile and visual, not just a talking head.
The Importance of Art in Reaching People
Art on the walls. Art in the trees. Art in the gaze. Art in the clay.
Art in the flesh. Art in the move. Art in the stoke.
Text from a video made Nov. 2007 in Michigan.

The stage is a studio at the university. I am doing my criptography—the painting of brush stroke simple figures that, in my mind, are all representations of disabled people moving—the view of the view of the view of the view of the view.

Neil Calligraphy Self Portrait: This striking painting in bold black, red, and yellow is a brushwork abstraction self portrait of the artist, Neil Marcus, in a wheelchair seen in profile. The painting is playful and uses calligraphy-style technique so that the image looks variously like an abstract Chinese character and a human figure. (Drawing by Neil Marcus 2001)

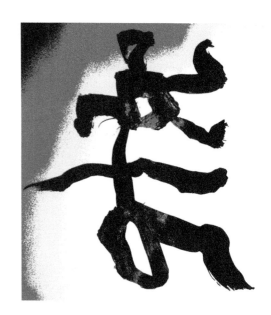

24.4 Communication

Neil (to Devva): I was thinking how the occupy movement reinstated the human microphone method of speaking with assistance from others. That assistance is useful and pretty basic. One person speaks and others pass the message on chain-like from one to another. (A possible solution to phone company desire to make access?)

Devva: "Human Microphone!" Love it. I've been thinking of Moses and Aaron, his revoicer microphone. For most of human society the only microphone was human, the town crier professionalized it. When I first started having people "revoice" for me others thought it was easy. They thought of it as interpreting, like from sign language. But it is NOT. It is a repetition. My echo.

I don't need my words "interpreted" in English, nor in French, Spanish, or Italian thank you. Russell Shuttleworth and I insisted it be called revoicing. The phone company calls it "Speech to Speech (STS)" after its best advocate, Dr. Bob Segalman (see Hanson, 2014, http://www.nchpad.org/1012/5305/Dr~~Bob~Segalman~~President~~~Founder~~Speech-to-Speech retrieved 6/8/2014). You and Petra have really focused on the performance aspect.

Neil: Communication is like Jazz improvisation and opinion "preaching throughout the necessity of improvising one's own graces and divisions on the spot in performances" (from *Observations on the Florid Song*, no date, no page). DISABILITY IN SONG AND SPEECH. (See *James Ellis is ... James Zealous,* http://www.youtube.com/watch?v=urKkrqXeUbQ, retrieved 6.8.2014)

Pamela: I was thinking about what you said about jazz improvisation and vibration and thinking how my sister vocalizes selectively and privately and how this is also matched with stimming movement. She does not do this in public with strangers or acquaintances. It is with her intimates and loved ones where she will relax and hum her feelings. Happy, excited, pissed off, frustrated, angry . . . Actually her staff probably do hear the pissed off, angry, frustrated ones, but I doubt they interpret it as music and calming movements—some staff see it as a sign of escalating behaviors that need to be managed, redirected and controlled.

She hums her feelings but also used to hum whole songs, but she doesn't do this anymore. Actually her hums are more compositions than improvisations. Particular hums consistently represent particular feelings. I can think of about 4 or 5 separate hums that she uses all the time. Some of them have been put to words by family members or else always represented words and family members guessed what they were. "Hopie is a good big girl" (content/groovy) and "ASSHOLE!" (most often heard while in the car during traffic jam or at red lights). Some don't have words attributed to them but the meaning is so obvious anyway; Disappointment, Deliciously Excited Anticipation.

Neil: I was influenced heavily by the counseling movement. CO COUNSELING. It's an international practice of semi-structured exchanges of listening and speaking roles with a peer. (See http://www.cci-usa.org/.)

Pamela: Tell me how it influenced you? Co-counseling missed me, I am just a little too young, and what I learned about it from other people did not make a good impression.

Neil: Love self/pride/much contact with people. I helped THEM!

Pamela: Got you. Were there other disabled people involved in the co-counseling movement? I can see how it breaks down paternalistic distinctions between client/patient and counselor/health professional.

Neil: Yes. Marsha Saxton, Laurie Summers: We were some of the leaders.

Neil: *Complete Elegance* was our journal; I was the editor/founder.

Pamela: And earlier? What emerged first in terms of poetry, art, dance, essays, plays? Did you have periods where you focused on one form then move on to others, or did it all evolve simultaneously?

Neil: High School. Love Letters. Bucky Fuller—Buckminster Fuller geo dome inventor. I began co-counseling at age 14 and met Harvey Jackins.

Art = Love = Art. Self-hate doesn't belong in art?

Pamela: So what was the role of supportive community in generating art?

Neil: They looked to me for help.

Pamela: So you were no longer focused internally. Resisting self-hate may be an important part of the generative impulse.

Neil: I knew I was important.

Pamela: You were helping people; you made a difference, and were also being heard. There was dual cultivation of listening and expressing.

Neil: And that just grew and grew and continues....

Pamela: Did your different ways of expressing yourself emerge simultaneously? Or how did you come to use so many different forms?

Neil: Writing . . . led to public speaking . . . etc. etc.

24.5 Technology

Devva: Next big point is technology. My new technology is the early exhale. My speech therapist taught me to start exhaling before I start talking, so the sound is supported. I always used to wait to exhale. Waiting to Exhale, I need to learn not to do it. Hard, when you have my critical eye. I had to learn to not rush to speak no matter how much I had to say. It's a kind of technology.

Neil: It's never spoken of.

Devva: Why not? Using phone/computer/whatever. Is it money? With all the "services" that go to us, we support a lot of people. For example the California Deaf and Disabled Telecommunications Program (DDTP, http://ddtp.cpuc.ca. gov/). They spend millions a year for not enough people on the relay service. Give that money directly to the "approved" users and bingo . . .

Neil: Our strength isn't acknowledged. We are seen as weak and pitiful. System allows no mutuality.

Devva: Strength, and our CREATIVITY is not acknowledged. Current systems don't allow mutuality, absolutely. It can happen despite but not because of services.

Neil: It's an oversight that we are humannnnnnn . . . oops.

Devva: Like the telephone program is limited to land lines by law or habit. We are in danger of being frozen out of the future unless we can bypass the government benefits' that cannot keep up with what real independent mutuality needs. Transitions in communicative technology could be behavioral/emotional/intellectual and let us demonstrate how to best occupy disability to all those aging and yet-to-be sick or injured—people who are destined to experience true disability.

Neil: Like there was a guy advocating as to cell phones in late 1990s. He was so hip.

Devva: Yep, yet the one cell phone that the California deaf and disabled telephone access program gives out is so minimal we would not want it. The system is about

20 years behind the forefront of technology. I guess that's why they wanted me on the committee. I do have to routinely ask myself are we being bought off?

Neil: And we must not forget to visit the person we called on the cell phone and break bread with them.

Devva: Pretty hard. VERY IMPORTANT. Cell phones / texting creates SO many new kinds of relationships at a distance. Can we break bread virtually?

Neil: Poetic XO's. Good question. Yes I have my 1st TTY conversation in print. I saved it. It is a beautiful explosion of repressed thought learning to flow.

Devva: If our lives at home are a balance with "in situ" and "virtual" human contact, what's wrong with some relationships being all virtual? That's the power of different media too—just having the transcript changes what you talk about and what you remember.

Neil: That seems a good thought. I need to ponder it. Wow!

Devva: You made me think of all the people who were assumed to be "dumb" like non-speaking, autistic, or with CP, who, given a keyboard, can communicate. Like Pam's sister Hope.

Neil: Exactly. I was one of them. Never used a phone till I was 21.

Devva: Like Matthew Wangeman who talks about how some in his family never read his board, even today. It seems that most of the folks that never talked or wrote until adult age or at least as older children, once they have a means to communicate, they know the meaning of words, can read and write. It's not that they have whole ideas for the first time at adult ages—no one thought they understood more than a dog does—and yet they are literate!

Pamela: Well, some people are deeply invested in refusing to believe this is the case (Block et al. 2012; Kasnitz and Block 2012). Careers are on the line. But technologies are changing, improving and people are able to communicate who were never able to in the past.

For my sister Hope the iPad has been liberating. She actually gave a presentation about communicating with the iPad at a conference in October 2013. I remember when she presented at the Society for Disability Studies (SDS) in 2010 and her Dynavox (older communication technology) froze. It was always doing that. She was so upset! Her fiancé read her presentation and I captioned it for the audience. She was able to answer questions using a borrowed computer but—you know how it is in a presentation when your technology fails. At SDS a whole group of conference participants volunteered to try to help fix the problem and find solutions. But she was beside herself. The iPad does not do this sort of thing, and is a fraction of the cost of the older communication technologies.

Devva: I accept Hope's typed voice and her hums as her voice, as speech. Does she? Does she identify typing as her speech?

Pamela: I would say yes, it is her speech but very contested speech, and she seems to mostly want to use speech in performance contexts. She doesn't want to use it to choose food in restaurants. She wants to use it at conferences, in front of an audience.

24.6   Occupying Disability Again

Neil: So I say the world needs disability? It's one of the lost arts.

Devva: I didn't notice it was lost. As my dystonia improves I want MORE help from OTs to capitalize on the improvements. But that's when they cut me off—insurance requires that it look like a new or worsening condition to pay for it. Catch 22. We have plenty of disability; we just don't apply the label the same way. So, isn't it a matter of calling it what it is? A problem of recognition?

Pamela: There are also scope of practice issues. OTs are told they can't poach into areas "owned" by speech language pathologists—such as computer-mediated communication.

Neil: It's not looked upon well. But that is changing. We are changing very fast.

Devva: And when people meet me now they assume my disability is new or progressive. But in reality, some of the progress is in all different directions, sideways and backwards. ***The only true reality is change***. We may change faster because of disability—we must just to keep up.

I'm making a note about the worsening / improving / change issues . . . People assume I'm new to this disability thing with aging. Reality is the opposite. I'm not as disabled now as I was. First, the dystonia changes, second—everyone else is catching up with us—disability is all around us. Expectations change. For example, my peers used to consider me plump. Now they tell me I'm slim. I haven't changed size, they have. So here we are. Stronger, in better physical shape than ever, occupying disability so well people lose track of how old we are getting. In our 60s we outshine our norm friends in their 40s and 50s as they try so hard to NOT occupy disability.

Pamela: What does occupying disability mean to you?

Devva: To me it means that I embody it. I occupy myself with disability and am occupied by it. I can't shake it so I embrace it. The only way to have relationships that get past disability is to fully claim it, as Simi Linton (1998) would say. Once you make the effort to fully occupy it, then it can disappear.

Pamela: What does occupying disability mean to you?

Neil: Means knowing oneself, ones position in the world. Means freedom.

Pamela: What is your position in the world? And what "means freedom"?

Neil: A poem.

> a reduction a synthesis word/letters/that's falling from the sky [this guy]
> raining art
> text rain
> my life
> in pictures
> my philosophy
> i was so lucky to get interested in dance early on in my liberation practices i saw the
> 'disabled' body become free
> become Art Full

Pamela: So you occupy yourself with art, text, dance? And this is occupying self. If the "disabled" body becomes free. Is this occupying disability?

Neil: I'm an artist. I love. I create. I speak out to "power."

Pamela: This is how you occupy yourself, through your art and other ways too?

Neil: Yes and thru battling my own demons, loneliness etc . . .

Pamela: Can you give me an example of this?

Neil: That speaks to power, it affronts it/confronts/pauses it.

Pamela: Neil provides some examples below of his writings and short films written and created between 1987 and 2012.

    Special Effects (1987) was written at the very beginning of disability studies and still rather early phase of the disability rights movement.

Neil: It made me aware how to approach the oppression love = art = love. See video in the list.

Pamela: It was a way of occupying disability—moving it away from purely medical frames: a cultural approach and political approach. I love the way it is interactive. It still lives and evolves through how people react to it online. It breathes.

    Do you have anything you want to tell the OT community about how disability should be occupied?

Neil: Wrestle with us. Touch. Be touched. Eat alfalfa sprouts.

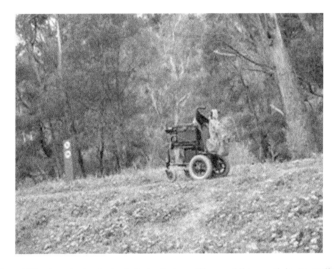

Wheelchair on Hike: A motorized wheel chair sits in profile on a hiking path in Australia Park, near Canberra. There are trees in the background and in front of the chair the flower covered ground slopes down toward the viewer. There is a big full pink backpack handing on the back of the chair. The chair is unoccupied. (Photograph by Neil Marcus)

Editors' Postscript If you enjoyed this chapter there are several others that discuss art and performance including: Chap. 5 "Landings: Decolonizing Disability, Indigeneity and Poetic Methods" by Petra Kuppers; "Scenes and Encounters, Bodies and Abilities: Devising Performance with Cyrff Ystwyth" by Margaret Ames; and Chap. 8, "Artistic Therapeutic Treatment, Colonialism and Spectacle: A Brazilian Tale" by Marta Simões Peres, Francine Albiero de Camargo, José Otávio P. e Silva, and Pamela Block. There are also others that discuss communication such as Chap. 13 "Why Bother Talking? On Having Cerebral Palsy and Speech Impairment: Preserving and Promoting Oral Communication Through Occupational Community and Communities of Practice" by Rick Stoddart and David Turnbull. Like this chapter, others also play with the idea of occupation and social justice like Chap. 11 "Soul searching occupations: Critical reflections on Occupational Therapy's Commitment to Social Justice, Disability Rights, and Participation" by Mansha Mirza, Susan Magasi and Joy Hammel.

References

Block P, Shuttleworth R, Pratt J, Block H, Rammler L (2012) Sexuality, dating and intimacy. In: Pollard N, Sakellariou D (eds) Politics of occupation-centered practice: reflections on occupational engagement across cultures. Elsevier Churchill Livingstone, Oxford, pp 162–179

Co-Counseling International: Are You Ready? http://www.cci-usa.org/. Retrieved 3 July 2014

Ellis J (n.d.) James Ellis is … James Zealous. http://www.youtube.com/watch?v=urKkrqXeUbQ. Accessed 6 Aug 2014

Hanson L (2014) Dr. Bob Segalman, President & Founder, Speech-to-Speech. http://www.nchpad.org/1012/5305/Dr~~Bob~Segalman~~President~~~Founder~~Speech-to-Speech. Retrieved 6 Aug 2014

Kasnitz D, Block P (2012) Participation, time, effort, and speech disability justice. In: Pollard N, Sakellariou D (eds) Politics of occupation-centered practice: reflections on occupational engagement across cultures. Elsevier Churchill Livingstone, Oxford, pp 197–216

Kuppers P (2012) Nothing about us without us: mounting a disability arts exhibit in Berkeley, California. Disabil Stud Q 32(1). http://dsq-sds.org/article/view/1733/3041. Accessed 18 Sept 2013

Kuppers P, Marcus N, Steichman L (2008) Cripple poetics, a love story. Homofactus Press, Ypsilanti

Linton S (1998) Claiming disability: knowledge and identity. NYU Press, New York

Marcus N (1993) Storm reading. Play. The New Sun. http://www.newsun.com/StormRead.html. Accessed 18 Sept 2013

Marcus N (2004) Oral history. http://digitalassets.lib.berkeley.edu/roho/ucb/text/marcus_neil.pdf. Retrieved 18 Sept 2013

Marcus N (2011) Special effects: advances in neurology. Publication Studio. www.publicationstudio.biz/books/93. Accessed 18 Sept 2013

Marcus N (2012) Special effects (performance). http://www.youtube.com/watch?v=jix-mY-W2d4&feature=youtube. Retrieved 18 Sept 2013

Olympias (2013) Olympias performance research projects. www.olimpias.org. Retrieved 18 Sept 2013

Tosi PF (1742) English translation: observations on the florid song (trans: Galliard JE). J. Wilcox, London (1742 or 1743)

Critical Approaches to Community, Justice and Decolonizing Disability: Editors' Summary

25

Pamela Block, Devva Kasnitz, Akemi Nishida, and Nick Pollard

Abstract

This chapter is a reflection on the whole book. It looks back to the themes from the introduction and forward to the conclusions. We reintroduce our themes, discuss how the sections and chapters approach the themes, and develop the ideas in the chapters in more depth. Taken together, Chaps. 1, 25, and 26 are an expression of our development of the not unproblematic ideas evoked by the phrases occupying disability and decolonizing disability.

Keywords

Occupation • Occupational • Occupying • Occupational therapy • Occupational science • Disability • Disability studies • Anthropology • Theory • Practice • Activism • Justice • Decolonize • Community • Movements

P. Block, PhD (✉)
Disability Studies, Health and Rehabilitation Sciences, School of Health Technology and Management, Stony Brook University, Stony Brook, NY, USA
e-mail: pamela.block@stonybrook.edu

D. Kasnitz
Disability Studies, School of Professional Studies, The City University of New York, New York, NY, USA
e-mail: devva@earthlink.net

A. Nishida
Disability and Human Development, Gender and Women's Studies, University of Illinois at Chicago, Chicago, IL, USA
e-mail: anishida922@gmail.com

N. Pollard
Occupational Therapy, Faculty of Health and Wellbeing, Sheffield Hallam University, Sheffield, UK
e-mail: N.Pollard@shu.ac.uk

© Springer Science+Business Media Dordrecht 2016
P. Block et al. (eds.), *Occupying Disability: Critical Approaches to Community, Justice, and Decolonizing Disability*, DOI 10.1007/978-94-017-9984-3_25

25.1 Decolonizing Disability

Disability is contested territory. In the Aramaic Hebrew bible while there is no collective word for "disability," it is a matter of fact—only sometimes noteworthy. Moses' speech impairment becomes a foil for God's voice, the irony very deliberate as Aaron becomes an example of revoicing as developed and used by Devva Kasnitz and her long-term anthropology colleagues Russell Shuttleworth and Pamela Block; an example of the human microphone as Neil Marcus coins it in this volume (Chap. 24). In the Christian bible disability is not a matter of fact but now it is a foil for Jesus to demonstrate divinity by making miraculous cures. Disability is observable, a sign of evil at worst and pity or powerlessness at best. While the Viking warrior's missing leg may be a sign of triumph over both enemy and death, in anyone else it is more likely a sign of punishment or a test of faith. If colonies exist for the benefit of the colonizers, disability exists for the benefit of and in contrast to the non-disabled. However wretched your life, you are "lucky" you are not one of us.

The metaphor of an identification between disability and colonialism emerges as a *strategy* when disability becomes more medicalized and medicine more ableist. As Ben-Moshe describes (Chap. 4), the use of "colonialism" as a metaphor is problematic. We acknowledge that while colonization and decolonization are not true metaphors, the lived experience of disability and the continuing struggle under ableism with intersecting social injustices interactively overlaps with colonialism. We contemplate how such settler colonialist mechanism is used on our disabled bodies, and some chapters do literally look at postcolonialist populations. Disability was/is the observable and incurable failure of medicine. Medicine continues to create disability as people survive with changes that were once not survivable. Medicine creates disability as more and more behavior becomes a sign of "something wrong." As the colonizers view the colonized as needing order, the medical industrial complexity needs the disabled to need medical order, starting with a diagnostic label. As anthropologists, disability studies scholars, and occupational therapists, all also activists, we as editors of this book, ardently hold "decolonizing disability" as our necessity and our goal. "Occupying disability" is our method.

We eschew exaggerated academic binary models. The medical/social model binary is oversimplified along with disabled/non-disabled, scholar/activist, and perhaps the most difficult illness/disability. We look broadly at the conceptual layers of disability scholarship from the bio-physical world to impairment to disability to community to participation to justice. We borrow from many disciplines and theoretical models shamelessly, we borrow from many disciplines and theoretical models shamelessly and apply them to our topic and goal. We seek to decolonize ourselves in order to occupy disability in many ways. Disability is an experience as is colonization. With the recognition of these experiences they become an attitude, a dance, our source of strength, a community. As Neil Marcus says "Disability is an ingenious way to live" (see Chap. 24).

Devva Kasnitz tells us "I knew from quite young that you may forget my name or my face, but you won't forget my body," but somehow she didn't "claim" disability until she was 20, after spending a year in the 1970 student strike resistance to the 4/30/1970 invasion of Cambodia. She truly "came out" vocally as disabled in 1981 after 10 years of gestating her anti-war activism. She had designed costumes for her first 25 years and then owned a clothing store for 15 years. She costumed herself, she realized. "If people were going to stare at me, I might as well give them something to stare at." Quite amazingly "people gave me hundreds of thousands of dollars to dress them!" Crip style trumped cookie-cutter mass-market style. Coming out disabled is not easy. But, once you realize the alternative, change happens.

To refresh the progression of the book, we remind you here of the themes from our introduction (Chap. 1) and then review the other chapters, a second introduction! We start with Sunaura Taylor et al. (Chap. 2) who demonstrates the radicalizing, strengthening process so well and so started us off. Describing process is important. We put Mami Aoyama's work on Minamata Disease next (Chap. 3). We almost didn't include this chapter. We struggled with was it about justice for disabled people or environmental justice? Was it about disease or disability? Did it focus too much on suffering rather than resistance, a focus on death instead of living with disability? Environmental injustice creates disability all around it, human and otherwise. And this was a case of conscious and criminal disablement. We present it in that context.

Liat Ben-Moshe (Chap. 4) untangles intricate anti-occupation struggles and disability activism: from the hierarchy of disability to diversity within these movements. Thus, Ben-Moshe depicts the limits of disability rights and peace activism in the context of the Israeli military occupation. As she states, "[d]isability is always inherent in anti-occupation and anti-war and vice versa," (p. 56); disability and occupation take on particular and ominous meanings in this context of Israeli-Palestinian struggles. This chapter carries a particularly devastating power for us, since missiles were falling in Gaza and Israel when we were writing this in July 2014.

We next take you to Australia to Petra Kuppers' (Chap. 5) beautifully optimistic meditation on decolonization via art and trained listening. Here she honors the experience of hundreds of years of colonization. She turns her method internally— not unlike the best ethnography—and learns about others by studying herself in others' places, in interaction. Other chapters use her same method but more often unconsciously. It is paradoxical that this deep ethnography comes from a non-anthropologist in a book rich with anthropologists. She reflects on truth in knowledge upon which we all need to reflect. Use her example.

Melanie Yergeau (Chap. 6) similarly gives voice to people deemed voiceless. She clearly describes a group of people whose difference—autism—has just recently, but thoroughly, been claimed and appropriated, if not colonized, by others from family services, to the educational sector, to medicine. She gives us an example of a growing body of autobiography of autism. This remarkable and accessible literature is a perfect example of Petra's decolonizing methodology of art and deep ethnography. It also prepares us to look at other examples of communication disability as is discussed later in the book (Chap. 13) by Turnbull and Stoddart and (Chap. 24) by Marcus, Kasnitz, and Block. To risk overstatement, communication impairments are some of the internally scariest, particularly when coupled with other impairments that make you dependent on instrumental help from other people. If we err, let's err on the side of assuming competence. Do *not* let protectionism focused on presumed incompetence allow colonization. Risk too is a human right.

Margaret Ames (Chap. 7) adds to this message. She too talks about liberation from colonization through art. She also works with a population of presumed incompetence—learning disabled in United Kingdom English—cognitive or intellectual disability in United States English usage. She also contends with another layer of colonialism, that of Welsh culture and language in the UK. She describes how claiming both disability and Welsh identity provides meaning if not escape from colonization. Art training is commonly deemed an appropriate occupation for people with "learning disability," but as a part of "therapy" or a holding pattern against other more instrumental and remunerative activities they "can't" do, not as a true occupation to be celebrated and shared in the larger art community and valued and compensated by the art-consuming public.

Marta Simões Peres et al. (Chap. 8) again looks at the role of art in disability, in this case as practiced in psychiatry in a total institution. Here the colonization of disabled art is even more explicit than in Wales. The Welsh program is mainstream, voluntary, community-based, respectful, and empowering compared to the Brazilian example. The institution-based art therapy approach in Brazil would be more acceptable if it were called therapy and left at the institution. However, the described endeavor points out how the international renown of the "therapists" is the true desired outcome, which could only be enhanced by its therapeutic efficacy if it led to improvement in the mental health of some patients, but does not require that outcome as a measure of the program's value. Here decolonization is explicitly dual: the colonization of Brazil by Europe and European "Art Therapy," and the colonization of psychiatric disability within Brazilian institutions. Here decolonization needs a local refocus.

Annicia Gayle-Geddes (Chap. 9) on Jamaica, Trinidad, and Tobago closes *Part I Decolonizing Disability*. Her work is a departure from a focus on art and autobiographical methods, but no stranger to the politics of colonization, both in its common political sense and as applied to disability experience as a colony within larger society. We need reminding that disability correlates with most of what is least admirable in modernity: strict notions of the value of labor; inequity in metrics such as wealth, health, longevity; barriers to participation; isolation and unhappiness. Disability has yet to be decolonized by development in most of the world.

These chapters raise issues about how we train for collaborative work. We need collaboration that is cross discipline and transformational. It needs to discuss data all people involved value and understand. Community organizers have their own problems being collaborative with their "community." As occupational therapists, anthropologists, and disability studies scholars we all have our professional machismo. As researchers, even as we participate, we watch the doers. Anthropology teaches us to triangulate. We look at what people say they do, what they say they should do, and what we see them doing—Petra's deep autoethnography (Chap. 5). Occupational therapy trains people to watch what and how people do what they do and to help them do it better. They study impairment—

they may or may not study disability. Anthropologists are careful to not only study "down," e.g., focusing on those with less social status. So studying "up" to study a statused clinical profession such as occupational therapy is an option, one that medical anthropology has embraced. Of course in the hierarchy of health service providers, occupational therapists don't perceive themselves as having high status in comparison to doctors, for example. Also, providers don't necessarily like being the object of study. Collaboration is key. Disability studies has a more problematic relationship with studying providers. It is a valuable approach. We need to study power. But, if you study the people who "take care of disabled people" from their point of view, is that disability studies, or is it the anthropology of work? If it is the latter, just as work on therapeutic approaches to impairment, it is rarely disability studies. Although, we do indeed agree that reappropriation of disability should follow the slogan: *Nothing about us without us!* So, medical work on impairment should include disabled clinicians. However, not everything about us, even with us, is disability studies. Question all labels.

25.2 Disability and Community

For a long time community has usually been perceived as a positive word (Williams 1976) but it is a term which often masks differences. People often belong to different groupings within the communities they inhabit and inhabit multiple communities. Such groupings frequently constitute differences concerning social identities and occupational activities. In order to identify themselves they may operate entry and exclusion criteria, so while communities might be about who is included in a group, they also concern rules about who is ineligible, or about facilities and spaces which might only be used by some but not all. The interpretation of group membership might be formal or informal, it might rely on criteria determined by the group in a narrow way, or accorded in some form of consensus amongst community members. All of this might be necessary to enable people to maintain their distinctive identities, develop their consciousness, knowledge, or skills, but it can often bring about injustices where many communities are also characterized by their diversity, or where distinctions are related to the occupation of territories and the maintenance of physical boundaries.

In the second set of chapters (Part II) authors explore the connections between disability and community, viewing them through the lenses of different impairment and disability experiences and intersecting identities such as race and gender. What disability makes evident is that there are many extra layers to the membranes which may form patterns of exclusion. The term disability was not explored by Williams (1976), and it has only been since the 1970s that the significance of the experience of disability has been pushed forward through bottom up encounters which occur in, or despite, or in the disputes about, access and rights to community settings. As the authors in *Part II* reveal, both the concepts of disability and of community are complex, but they are prone to being made too simple to be useful. Occupation is also a complex term in its relationship of activity to territory and place as well as the act of being physically present in a particular space. These complexities can produce obstructions and also provide creative and strategic opportunities that challenge disabling structures.

Akemi Nishida (Chap. 10) examines the impacts of neoliberal academia on those who participate in it—particularly through a disability studies lens. This chapter reveals physical and psychological consequences of various demands, such as hyper-productivity, under which scholars are often put. Thus, what does neoliberalization of academia (e.g., corporatization, individualization of responsibility, and increasing inter-colleagues, –departments, and -universities competitions) mean to disabled people, while academia is historically contested for its ableist and saneist foundation and practices. Finally, the chapter criticality discusses the accessible and more inclusive academic justice activism and significance of interdependent relationships as a micro resistance among those who work to change academia from inside-out.

Mansha Mirza, Susan Magasi and Joy Hammel (Chap. 11) look at the risks which may stem from an over simplistic understanding of participation and narrowed practice of occupational therapy. A clinical perspective which does not reflect the wider economic and social environment, the real context of disability, cannot expect to meet the needs of people who are more likely to be marginalized because of their multiple issues. They suggest the introduction of a more interdisciplinary approach to professional education to tackle and counter the reproduction of a middle class privileged normative culture in clinical assessment, and thence the perpetuation of disabling practices.

Denise M. Nepveux (Chap. 12) reveals the way that a normative culture impacts community facilities when it is combined with real estate interests in the gentrification of run-down neighborhoods. She charts the resistance organized by the members of a senior center to its relocation under the guise of a public-private partnership between the Syracuse city council and the Salvation Army. The members were the last people to find out about the plans for their center and through their actions have persuaded local politicians of the need for a more participatory approach to local decision making.

Rick Stoddart and David Turnbull (Chap. 13) take another look at these kinds of divisions in relation to the occupational communities of professionals and the occupational communities in the wider social environment. They chart Rick's history of trying to find a job and operate his life roles in ways which reflect his level of capacity rather than being forced into a position of being a person with disability who has to accept other people's operating practices and rules in his private space. Arguing from Rick's experiences in asserting his dignity, they critique the ethical underpinnings of professional care services.

Michele Friedner's (Chap. 14) account of deaf young adults in Bangalore is an ethnographic investigation of the ways in which vocational training programs offered by NGOs provide trainees with opportunities to develop social skills, networks, and share learning. These exchanges occur through the social relationships deaf people have worked out for themselves. The extramural outcomes are more valuable than the limited scope of the repetitive training, and as they inhabit the spaces of a world which is unheeded by the trainers and their employers Michele identifies alternative ways in which occupation figures in their lives.

Nick Dupree (Chap. 15) describes his adventures in taking his ventilator from Mobile, Alabama to New York City, getting out of Medicare to live with his partner and so to participate in the events around the Occupy Wall Street movement. Drawing on aspects of the protest movements across the globe at the end of the first decade of this century, his chapter asserts the position of disability activists in the current political struggle against corrupt and corporate power and its social and economic consequences.

Stephanie De La Haye (Chap. 16) explores ways in which the service user movement can address health policies, particularly with regard to asserting their inclusion in the development of research processes that influence them. She sets out examples of cultural change amongst professional groups initiated through service users which enable more inclusive practice, but warns against the loss of service user independence.

The concluding chapter in *Part II*, by Eva Rodriguez (Chap. 17) is on self-advocacy self-determination and access to the US education system for disabled students. She describes how some of the assessment processes are administered and experienced in ways that do not involve students or their families. As a result, parents may be unaware of how their children are denied opportunities because of the assumptions made by educational professionals.

These experiences reveal some of the disabling obstructions which range from the huge and obvious to the nuances of administrative prejudices to be uncovered in the negotiation of everyday life and the expression of the right to live in communities. There are practical things to implement, strategies to adapt and follow, questions to ask, both rules to break and to make, powers to seize and tools to use in the communities that we are about to develop.

25.3   Struggle, Creativity and Change

In Part III we continue our exploration of difference, meanings, and experiences related to disability, culture, and occupation by focusing on extremes and continuities of struggle, creativity, and change. As a species, we career into the future, as that which was once distinct becomes blurred, societies and peoples collide and intermingle, we find distinct forms of oppression as well as new ways to work together and enjoy each other. Technology provides us with toys for elite enjoyment, assistive technologies for those who can afford them, and opportunities for enhanced survival and quality of life. It also provides us with weapons of mass destruction, and, for many, the realities of oppression. In many ways we are under surveillance, observed and policed by militarized systems of control that regulate our bodies and behaviors in the context of (with the excuse of) administering bodies politic. These systems are amongst the prime means of generating new forms of disability either through the consequences of using them or having them used against us, being involved in manufacturing them, or through living amid the polluting wastes they produce.

Through the mechanisms of surveillance systems, regulation, control, and the use of militarized technologies, humans are distinguished into "us" and "them." These are powerful and seductive tools which encourage us to accept controls and even participate in our own surveillance, but our relationship with them is complicated, with positive elements as well as negative aspects. Also it is critical to note how usage of technologies is deeply related to the market force: creating demand for technologies and those concerned with surveillance are designed to protect the propertied from the property-less. Because we appear to benefit from the technologies and the marketing of them, we do not always recognize how much we are enslaved to them. It becomes unthinkable not to have these technologies, many of the industries and processes which support our society and at the same time endanger it. Despite the extent of these capacities for the abuse of power and the limitation of rights, disabled people's struggles against ableism and saneism demonstrate the inventiveness that comes with resiliency, and some of the strategies people have developed depend on the access provided by new technological environments and facilities. We explore opportunities for resistance and creative change, while recognizing that across the globe, and in our own communities, there are struggles for the most basic human rights and survival.

Disability communities' struggles for liberation and against ableism and saneism can take many forms. In the sociocultural context of Hecht (Chap. 19), we have a short story in which disability and ableism encounter racism, sexism, and classism as the disabled character, the Crab, solicits prostitution. In the eyes of the child prostitute Conceição, observing the Crab in the street and in his home, he has a freedom of physical and social movement as well as security of home and foods that she longs for. He has a certain freedom of movement, seeming to fly suspended just above the ground, but progressing with a smooth rapidity as if "possessed of an urge to move faster than they," (p. 274). At the same time, his physical differences and sexuality are heavily questioned and examined. To Conceição, the Crab's life is a life of privilege, even though the ending of the story takes a dramatic turn and complicates her observation. Who is on top is all a matter of perspective. While Conceição's perspective is fictional, the series of events depicted in this story are based on interview data collected by anthropologist Hecht while he was conducting ethnographic research in Northeastern Brazil.

Struggle can also involve advocating for life-saving or life-changing technologies and the use of virtual media such as the internet for building networks of protest. Surveillance can be a life-saver, as in the case of people on ventilators, who require constant monitoring to ensure breathing, or take life-threatening risks as Dupree recounts (Chap. 15). In contrast, Seelman (Chap. 18) complicates the notion that monitoring can be a form of unwanted surveillance and oppression. As robot care-givers, once the realm of science fiction, may soon be part of systems of disability management, Seelman poses questions on the advancement of technologies in relation to topics of bioethics and disability rights movement principles such as self-determination. Seelman explores the ever-blurring line between human and technology with the advancement of assistive technologies. Mello, Block and Nuernberg (Chap. 20) discuss the emergence of Brazilian disability studies with its unique intersectional opportunities. They use Hecht's short story to open discussion of some of the complexities of how disability intertwines with gender, race, class and sexuality in Brazil. Moore, Garcia, and Thrower (Chap. 21) describe violence enacted by police to disabled people at an intersection of disability, race, class, nationality, and more. Not only do these authors problematize surveillance by police, they also question uses of law enforcement by the Occupy Movements and lend critical analyses on mainstream activism movements from disability justice perspectives. Creative and powerful alternative ways to fight for various layers of justice are introduced by Moore, Garcia, and Thrower and are particularly important for us to consider in the wake the movements sparked by Fall 2014 rulings not to indict police officers who were responsible for the deaths of African American men in Ferguson, Missouri, and Staten Island New York. We are particularly haunted by the Staten Island death of Eric Garner, which was caught on audio and video. "I can't breathe" he cried 11 times, as his asthmatic struggle for breath was mistaken for resisting arrest (see Chap. 21). This becomes a new and tragic example supporting Moore, Garcia, and Thower's arguments. "I can't breathe," with hands held high, will become an iconic slogan of protest. Based on his personal experiences as a blind person with hearing impairment, Chaplin (Chap. 22) creatively engages in three layers of occupation. He describes how his daily energy interactively affects his functioning and the importance of interdependency. First, there is the occupational layer of learning life and living skills. Second, is the occupational layer of living, contributing, sharing, leading, and of functioning as an active member of society. Third, is the occupational layer of educating and advocating to advance disabled people's rights as we combine the first two layers of occupation in order to live a fulfilling life. The Stevenage Survivors (Chap. 23) explore the power of the collaborative and generative processes of creating art together and for each other in the community around their Hertfordshire town in the UK, but this is set against and framed by their continuing pursuit of funding to secure the group's survival through each project they develop. Their creativity depends on the hand to mouth process of identifying and applying for various grants, £100 here, and £1200 there. This precarious existence supports their bold mission: "use poetry in all its forms to enable survivors of mental distress to survive more adequately" (p. 335). They have survived their own inner struggles, the economic systems that surround them, and psychiatry's medicalized systems with an understanding that "life is the best poetry there is." Finally Marcus, Kasnitz, and Block (Chap. 24) discuss the occupations of communication, intimacy, dance and art. Who occupies disability? What might be the role of occupational therapists in the context of struggle, creativity and change? What is the role of technology?

    Change is an unstoppable force in all these chapters—some choices can never be taken back, and some of the authors depict extreme and violent choices enacted upon or on behalf of disabled people. In some cases, occupational change is the result of technological innovation, or simply aging bodies, or changing states of mind, or slow yet steady steps toward just society. Whether we are talking about changing

368 P. Block et al.

military regimes, economic systems that promote violence, ways that we interact with each other, or political, educational, and artistic interventions to pursue justice at different localities—contained in this book we see hints of dystopian nightmares and utopian possibilities.

25.4 Conclusion

We have come full circle. Whether you read this chapter right after our introduction (Chap. 1) or after reading the whole book, we brought you back to the themes that are the collection's glue: community, justice, decolonization, and of course occupation. This is where both aspects of the various strains of the international disability rights movements and the occupy movements now stand.

Our goal was and is to bring the tools of academic disability studies, anthropology, and occupational science to the service of future social growth by bringing the voices of non-academic activism into the choir. The next chapter, our last, is where we peek at futures both feared and desired.

Reference

Williams R (1976) Keywords. Fontana, London

Science (Fiction), Hope and Love: Conclusions

26

Pamela Block, Devva Kasnitz, Akemi Nishida, and Nick Pollard

Abstract

This final chapter considers the future directions of a connection between disability and occupation as they are framed in disability studies, occupational science and occupational therapy, and anthropology. Using examples from science fiction literature, the authors explore how this discussion can move beyond arguments around equality to addressing inequities, and at the same time remain grounded in human values.

Keywords

Occupational science • Science fiction • Disability • Disability studies • Anthropology

P. Block (✉)
Disability Studies, Health and Rehabilitation Sciences, School of Health Technology and Management, Stony Brook University, Stony Brook, NY, USA
e-mail: pamela.block@stonybrook.edu

D. Kasnitz
Disability Studies, School of Professional Studies, The City University of New York, New York, NY, USA
e-mail: devva@earthlink.net

A. Nishida
Disability and Human Development, Gender and Women's Studies, University of Illinois at Chicago, Chicago, IL, USA
e-mail: anishida922@gmail.com

N. Pollard
Occupational Therapy, Faculty of Health and Wellbeing, Sheffield Hallam University, Sheffield, UK
e-mail: N.Pollard@shu.ac.uk

© Springer Science+Business Media Dordrecht 2016
P. Block et al. (eds.), *Occupying Disability: Critical Approaches to Community, Justice, and Decolonizing Disability*, DOI 10.1007/978-94-017-9984-3_26

Magalhães (2012) has written a book chapter entitled: "What would Paulo Freire think of Occupational Science?" It is framed as a letter to Paulo Freire, author of *Pedagogy of the Oppressed* (2005) and numerous other books outlining participatory social theory and practice. Freire wrote *Pedagogy of the Oppressed* while in exile from Brazil's military dictatorship but he eventually returned, and Magalhães was fortunate to have studied with him in the 1980s. In her chapter she discusses the establishment of occupational "science," and quotes Yerxa's (2009) concerns about framing the study of occupation as an "evidence-based" science: "As an occupational scientist and occupational therapist, I have seen the *it* mentality gain prominence in the science and practice of our field as the profession emulates other sciences and responds to pressures to prove its efficacy," (p. 490, cited in Magahaes p. 12). Magalhães follows this by asking: "Is there a risk that by labelling this new field of study as a science, we lose control over its complex roots and come to embrace a soulless discipline? That would be the *it* science that worried Yerxa (2009). Is science always an oppressive social exchange?" (p. 12).

Duke cultural studies professor Fredric Jameson referred to anthropology as "Science Fiction" in *Archaeologies of the Future: The Desire Called Utopia and Other Science Fictions* (2005), a searing analysis of the relationship between anthropology and science fiction.

> The discipline of anthropology is in other words necessarily normative, and re-establishes the model of a norm even where it is unthinkable: only Colin Turnbull, in *The Mountain People* and Levi-Strauss himself, in *Triste Tropiques*, have reflected on the frustration involved in coming upon a society not merely in decline but in utter collapse. Still, anthropology (and SF itself) have a conventional context with which to domesticate such phenomena, and it is projected by the Second Law of Thermodynamics[1] and indeed by Wells' *Time Machine*[2] (if not by Spengler): namely the grand narrative of entropy and devolution. This then returns a meaning to the diseased symptoms and reconfers an order and kind of evolutionary or devolutional normative on the aberrant objects of study. (Jameson 2005 p. 123)

Yet we can also think about it from another direction: well-written science fiction is also a powerful form of cultural anthropology, consider the fiction of Ursula Kroeber Le Guin, (daughter of Alfred Kroeber a founder of American anthropology, student of Franz Boas, and founder of the University of California, Berkeley Anthropology program).

Actually anthropologists—some clearly influenced by cultural studies, others from materialist social science perspectives—have documented societies fundamentally transformed by colonial and postcolonial power structures (see Taussig 1991).

---

[1]The second law of thermodynamics explains that increasing the temperature in any material will produce other linked changes in the material, such as oxidisation, and that this will continue until maximum entropy occurs, i.e. the point at which all the material is consumed in the production of heat.

[2]In this story the protagonist is able to travel forward in time to the very end of the Earth and all life on it. It supposes an ultimate future of degeneration.

Kasnitz, who began her anthropology graduate study in 1971 at Michigan when and where Taussig first taught, blended emphasis on power and on the symbolic in the study of health and immigration and later in the study of disability. In the 1970s her fieldwork included "going native" and taking a job as the Research Officer of a new Australian multicultural community health center. By the 1990s Kasnitz had left academia and been the director of a rural, poor California independent living services center and then moved back to applied anthropology research to support the disability advocacy in which she participates. Kasnitz saw the anthropology/cultural studies fissure as an interesting bump in the road to understanding the underpinnings of inequality. We all believe that applied anthropologists, occupational therapists, and applied disability studies researchers have the potential in their professional lives to do more than document *inequalities*; we can directly address fundamental *inequities* in our practice. We see this in the *Occupational Therapy Without Borders* series (Kronenberg et al. 2005, 2010). We see this in the "Translational Research in Disability Studies and the Health Sciences" strand of the Society for Disability Studies (funded by National Institutes of Health/National Institute on Child Health and Disability 2012–2014). We see this in the endeavors of the Society for Applied Anthropology. Conscious of our connection to Paulo Freire (2005), we think about how professionals in these fields intervene by bridging theory to practice, engaging in community-based research and hands dirty program development, working at the grass roots and translating truth to power. The emphasis is on capacity-building through a dialogic participatory process, and includes a dedication to activism and social change. It also allows the space for unapologetically hybrid theories and practices that incorporate both disability studies and health sciences and clinical practice (see Mirza et al. Chap. 11).

We are avid science fiction fans. In Kasnitz and Block (2012) Kasnitz repeatedly used *Star Trek* to underline key points of the chapter. At the conclusion of this collection of works depicting historical and current ways that people *occupy disability*,[3] we have decided to discuss the imaginings of how disability might be occupied in the future. A small sub-genre of science fiction considers how new forms of disability may be produced by future technologies. We became interested in three works in particular; Bujold's *Falling Free* (1988), Butler's *Parable of the Sower* (1993), and Bacigalupi's *The Windup Girl* (2009) provide three different examples of this. Bujold's Quaddies were genetically engineered for a gravity-free environment—their bones are low-density and instead of legs and feet, they are born with an extra set of arms and hands. This works well for a zero-gravity environment, but renders them disabled should they ever travel to a location with gravity. Butler's character Lauren Olamina is an empath who responds to the physical pain of others by experiencing it herself, an "organic delusional syndrome" (p. 10) which has resulted from her mother's use of a new intelligence enhancing drug. Emiko, the windup girl has been genetically modified, bred as an office assistant/sexual toy

---

[3] We use this term to refer to how people creatively turn disability into strengths.

with an inbuilt conditioning which forces her to respond sexually and to walk in a stylized way that indicates her function.

These darkly themed novels offer critiques of corporate/capitalist control over bodies, the exploitation of and creation of disabled bodies for profit, and the intended and unintended consequences of this; they explore the sexualities flowing from this control and resistance to control; and contrast occupations (social roles and life qualities) imposed by corporations verses wishes of individuals and communities. They represent the ultimate biogenetic expression of the work ethic and the subjugation of the personal to a bioethical capitalist world order. Disability is presented as a key component in a critique of corporate and free-market capitalism and politics, including the enslavement of individuals and communities; explorations of forms of resistance and utopian alternatives. In summary, technology does not offer cures in the worlds presented by these texts, but is one of the accessories in the iatrogenic nature of society's ailments. Yet within the systemic constraints, space for resistance and counter-hegemonic life narratives remains possible in each of these fictional futures.

Bujold, Butler and Bacigalupi offer interesting contrasts. Bujold's Quaddies, a utopian community within a corporate petri dish, move from trusting the guidance of their corporate creators to a successfully orchestrated rebellion, with the help of able-bodied allies. Butler's protagonist Lauren Olamina lives in a near-future dystopia where the political and economic infrastructures have crumbled. She keeps herself and the people around her safe via good emergency planning. She sets out a moral creed which enables her to cope with the forces around her and the people with whom she lives; in a second book Butler (1998) challenges some of this by the pragmatic survival strategies of the character's brother and daughter. Bacigalupi's Emiko has to find her way in a society where many elements of community have totally vanished. Her harsh corporation dominated environment (of which she is literally a technological product) is one where every person has to look out for themselves: unlike Lauren Olamina, Emiko has no ideological formula. Bacigalupi's people are commodities with a limited shelf life, and Emiko's disability is an aspect of the utility which enables her to survive but at the same time threatens her existence.

The message of these stories for people who experience disability is perhaps that it is necessary to fight and play tough to survive. The difference between the three authors' perspectives concerns the motives for human co-operation. Bujold's Quaddies, finding they are enslaved when they are not granted the right to choose their own occupations, move about freely, or choose with whom they have children. They quickly learn community action strategies such as savvy use of social media protest (interesting since the book was written in 1987), passive resistance, and sabotage to make it unprofitable for their corporate creator to resist their demands for autonomy and a chance to profit from their own labor. Butler's Lauren strategically and intuitively finds the right buttons to get other people's co-operation and works patiently. Through the experience of various setbacks she models an example of how to act as a survivor, maintain principles, and work ethically and morally. In *The Windup Girl* none of these conditions are really present, instead the main value seems to be utility as the source of survival and a basis for co-operation. There is an absence of emotional connection between any of the people depicted, an expectation that life can be lost at any moment.

The protagonists of all three novels inhabit very dangerous and chaotic environments, and disability in them proves both a liability and an asset that the protagonists of the books learn to take advantage of, very creatively. This use of disability is legend in disability activists' circles. Turning disadvantage to strength is a deeply held tactic and part of self- and community-empowerment. From the outside, ableism may misguide the public to see this advantaging of disadvantage as "privilege," the coveted blue parking space, the reserved theater seats, for example. Fictionalizing this life strategy, as in these novels, is an effective social critique that could support improved social policy if properly couched. When Kasnitz, Marcus and Hope Block (see Chap. 24) occupy disability by speaking and typing they are aware of this process. Kasnitz frequently reminds that, because of her speech impairment, although she can enter few conversations, she can stop any conversation and take the floor. Her practice then is to eschew small talk and hone her oratorical skills. Speaking then is a serious, conscious occupation. It is work. Luckily, we can express hope and love without speech if you listen differently. It is this listening differently that might break through the darkness of our sample science fiction disability dystopias.

Magalhães fears that by conceptualizing the study of occupation as a science, "somehow we have been able to *sanitize* our work so that it is free of such contentious topics as *hope* and *love*, for example" (Magalhães 2012, original emphasis). This concern also peeks through the "cultural studies residing in humanities and anthropology residing in social *science*" fissure. Disability studies too started off in the 1980s with emphasis clearly in the social *sciences*, particularly in the UK. This seemed natural as medical science was our foil. So many scholars still use overly simplistic medical versus social models of disability as if they were all explanatory; while some began challenging the binary and engage with critique and expansion of the social model (Kafer 2013, for example). Like medical anthropology, disability studies vacillated between meeting the power of medicine on their territory and in their language, and resisting this temptation. This vacillation continues in medical anthropology and in too many medical anthropologists who adopt the word "disability" but do not truly engage in disability studies scholarship. Our work in all three fields, occupational therapy/science, anthropology, and disability studies now has turned the screw one revolution deeper. We may have resisted "science" to reclaim humanity but we are stronger now. We understand the possible dystopias that emerge from imbalance and carefully and strategically reclaim science by acknowledging that the dynamics of science are also socially constructed and politically influenced. We do not entirely share Magalhães' concern that occupational science will sanitize occupational therapy. On the one hand, Jameson's (2005) work that pejoratively sees anthropology as science fiction can backfire and thoroughly sanitize away even the clearly useful instrumental concepts of science. On the other hand, in each of the three science fiction novels described above, hope and love persist, even in situations of dire disaster. As they do in every chapter of this collection.

As perhaps H Beam Piper illustrated in his 'Little Fuzzy' stories (1962[2012]) human beings are a fuzzy species and the nature of human occupation is messy given our capacity for improvisation (see Dupree, Chap. 15). We use these differences and proclivities to create solutions. Each of the three dystopias presents a future which is not entirely incredible—whether locating industry in space, social crises, or drastic environmental change—all are being proposed as realistic and conceivable developments. However, these narratives hinge on the experiences of disability. The future and the past are part of a human continuum, and just as the people of the past can be understood and their dilemmas pose questions that we can learn from, so might these proposed futures. At the time of writing there are concerns that within the century there might be a mass extinction event, and significant climate change may contribute to that. Health and wealth inequalities are driving considerable unrest in parts of the world; in other areas elites are resorting to technological defense solutions such as the use of drones, surveillance, and even new currencies which might insulate them from some of the consequences of change. Corporations are preparing for the initial phases of commercial space travel. Changes such as these are part of the backdrop to human development through adjustment and adaptation, they are also the conditions which expose and challenge experiences of difference—another book we also considered for this chapter was Anne McCaffrey's (1972) *The Ship Who Sang* in which a cyborg spaceship is piloted by the brain of a woman born with a severe disability for whom this career has been presented to her parents as her only option for survival. There are many potential controversies about these representations of human futures. As witnesses to the present, the authors of these chapters are not starry eyed about the way human actions will be negotiated through and around people and disability in the coming years. We have, however, set out some places from which future dialogues can begin without sacrificing hope and love.

References

Bacigalupi P (2009) The windup girl. Nightshade, San Francisco
Bujold LM (1988) Falling free. Headline, London
Butler OE (1993) Parable of the sower. Aspect, New York
Butler OE (1998) Parable of the talents. Aspect, New York
Freire P (2005) Pedagogy of the oppressed: 30th anniversary edition. Continuum International Publishing, New York
Jameson F (2005) Archaeologies of the future: the desire called utopia and other science fictions. Verso, London
Kafer A (2013) Feminist, queer, crip. Indiana University Press, Bloomington
Kasnitz D, Block P (2012) Chapter 14: Participation, time, effort, and speech disability justice. In: Pollard N, Sakellariou D (eds) Politics of occupation-centered practice: reflections on occupational engagement across cultures. Elsevier Churchill Livingstone, Oxford, pp 195–217
Kronenberg F, Simo Algado S, Pollard N (2005) Occupational therapy without borders—learning from the spirit of survivors. Elsevier Science, Edinburgh
Kronenberg F, Pollard N, Sakellariou D (2010) Occupational therapies without borders, vol 2. Elsevier Science, Edinburgh

Magalhães L (2012) What would Paulo Freire think of occupational science? In: Whiteford GE, Hocking C (eds) Occupational science: society, inclusion, participation. Wiley-Blackwell, Hoboken, pp 8–19

McCaffrey A (1972) The ship who sang. Corgi, London

Piper HB (1962 [2012]) Little fuzzy.http://www.gutenberg.org/files/18137/18137-h/18137-h.htm. Retrieved 8 January 2015

Taussig M (1991) Shamanism, colonialism and the wild man. University of Chicago Press, Chicago

Yerxa E (2009) The infinite distance between the I and the it. Am J Occup Ther 63:490–497

Author Biographies

Margaret Ames, MA is a Senior Lecturer at Aberystwyth University. She was Artistic Director of the community dance project called *Dawns Dyfed* covering the three counties of the west of Wales in the UK. Founded in 1987 she worked with this small but influential company until its closure in 2007. *Cyrff Ystwyth*, the Dance-theatre company she continues to direct was originally part of *Dawns Dyfed* and was formed in 1988. The work of the company now forms the major part of her practice as research. She has performed in dance and physical theatre, notably with former Welsh company *Brith Gof* and also worked as a Dance Movement Therapist with children and in adult psychiatric settings. She is interested in how live performance work created by people with learning disabilities asserts challenges to mainstream theatre. She is particularly concerned with the culturally specific context of Wales and how such work might reveal embodied expert knowledge about place and identity that may be an alternative to the more stereotypical constructions of the rural and of disability.

Mami Aoyama, Ph.D., OTR (Japan) is Professor of Occupational Therapy at Nishikyushu University (University of West Kyushu) in Kanzaki, Japan. After training as an occupational therapist at Kawasaki Rehabilitation College, she obtained a BA in Japanese literature from Ritsumeikan University and a M.Sc. and Ph.D. in biological anthropology from Tōhoku University. Her recent publications include "Indigenous Ainu occupational identities and the natural environment in Hokkaido" in *The Politics of Occupation-Centered Practice: Reflections on Occupational Engagement Across Cultures*, edited by N. Pollard and D. Sakellariou (Wiley-Blackwell, 2012) and "Occupation mediates ecosystem services with human well-being," in the Journal of Occupational Science (2012). Her research interests include occupational justice, sustainability, and community development.

Liat Ben-Moshe, Ph.D., is an Assistant Professor of Disability Studies at the University of Toledo. She holds a PhD in Sociology with concentrations in women and gender studies and disability studies from Syracuse University. Ben-Moshe is the co-editor of *Disability Incarcerated: Imprisonment and Disability in the United States and Canada* (Palgrave McMillan 2014) and *Building Pedagogical*

© Springer Science+Business Media Dordrecht 2016
P. Block et al. (eds.), *Occupying Disability: Critical Approaches to Community,
Justice, and Decolonizing Disability*, DOI 10.1007/978-94-017-9984-3

Curb Cuts: Incorporating Disability in the University Classroom and Curriculum (Syracuse University Press 2005); as well as a special issue of *Disability Studies Quarterly* on disability in Israel/Palestine (Summer 2007) and an upcoming special issue of *Women, Gender and Families of Color* on race, gender and disability. She is the author of numerous articles and book chapters on such topics as deinstitutionalization and incarceration; the politics of abolition; disability, anti-capitalism and anarchism; queerness and disability; inclusive pedagogy; academic repression; representations of disability; the International Symbol of Access and critiques of the occupation of Palestine.

Roy Birch is 72 years old and officially retired. He is married (has been for 36 years), has five adult children and six (soon to be seven) grandchildren. He began writing age four, and has written and discarded a huge number of words. He has self-published a volume of poetry. The only thing that changes is the way it all stays the same and currently has a novel *The Gunfighter* available on Amazon. He has survived a checkered working life which has included clerk, shop assistant, grave digger, field worker, self-employed gardener, and Mentoring and Outreach coordinator for national literature charity Survivors Poetry. He is a reflexologist and a Reiki Master and was recently initiated into the Munay-Ki rites, a Peruvian shamanic technique only recently revealed to the west. A zennist since his twenties, he has always felt an affinity for the marginalized and the underprivileged. He is currently Chair of writers' organization TheFED.

Pamela Block, Ph.D. is Associate Dean for Research in the School of Health Technology and Management, Associate Professor in the Occupational Therapy Program, and Director of the Concentration in Disability Studies for the Ph.D. Program in Health and Rehabilitation Sciences at the State University of New York, Stony Brook. She is a Fellow of the Society for Applied Anthropology and was recently President of the Society for Disability Studies (2010–2011). Dr. Block received her PhD in cultural anthropology from Duke University in 1997. Her dissertation was entitled "Biology, Culture and Cognitive Disability: Twentieth Century Professional Discourse in Brazil and the United States." She researches disability experience on individual, organizational and community levels, focusing on socio-environmental barriers, empowerment/capacity-building, and health promotion. Her qualitative research combines historical analyses with community-based ethnographic and participatory approaches. Most recently, Dr. Block has been involved in supporting disability social entrepreneurship through organizations such as EmpowerSCI—a nonprofit providing independent living skills and secondary rehabilitation to individuals with recent spinal cord injury, and VENTure—a policy and technology think tank on issues of concern to people who use ventilators. She also studies autism in Brazil and the United States, and the emergence of Brazilian disability studies.

Francine Albiero de Camargo is a psychologist (UNESP), with a master's degree in Therapeutic Pschycoanalysis (Universidade de São Paulo) and in Planning,

Implementation and Management at Universidade Federal Fluminense. She works as a distance education instructor in different disciplines of public policy at the National School of Health (ENSP-FIOCRUZ) for the Bolsa Familia (family grant) program and the graduate program in Special Education at the Federal University of the State of Rio de Janeiro. She is director of ReAbilitArte Institute for Research and Rehabilitation of Neuro-locomotor System. She was a technical expert in the coordination of public policies for Health (SUS) and Social Services (SUAS) in the state of Sao Paulo.

Rikki Chaplin was born totally blind in the small town of Beaudesert, Queensland on April 23 1976. He grew up in Brisbane, first attending a special school for the blind and then mainstream schools with special education units attached. He completed a Bachelor of Social Work from the University of Queensland in 2000, and has worked professionally in a variety of roles. Rikki enjoyed success as a musician and singer, scoring a top 5 birth in the "Best New Talent" category of Australia's "Golden Guitar" awards in 2002. These awards, celebrating the nation's top country music artists, are held annually. Rikki was forced to abandon his singing career following the loss of his hearing, caused as a result of Norrie's disease. This is a rare genetic condition affecting only males, in which those experiencing symptoms are born totally blind, then progressively lose hearing in early childhood or young adulthood. Rikki has gone on to use his skills as a musician and record producer to compile and edit an audio magazine, and in his role as national presenter of Blind Citizens Australia's weekly radio program, "New Horizons." He is a board member of the Norrie Disease Association, and after 10 years living in regional Queensland, he has returned to his home town of Brisbane to pursue further career goals. Rikki has two sons aged 10 and 7, and lives with his partner Paula.

Stephanie de la Haye, MSc. BSc (hons). WMT (med) QTLS. Cert Ed. is the chair and co-founder of Business Boosters Network CIC, as well as a freelance trainer, consultant and researcher delivering in mental health and well-being with 27 years' of expert experience and as a health and social care professional. Stephanie delivers AHMP and mental health advocacy training within, social work and mental health nursing at Sheffield Hallam University. Stephanie is a member of the UCLAN national IMHA research team and is currently a member of the UCLAN IMHA implementation group and a p/t doctoral researcher at the University of Oxford. Stephanie also practices in Emergency Medicine (pre hospital care) and an Expedition medic within the NHS and the private sector. Stephanie's extensive profile includes being a practice assessor for a BA in Social Work, and a research associate and peer researcher in a number of academic establishments. Chair and Founder of S.O.D.I.T (a mental health charity for women) and she sits on the executive group of the Social Perspectives Network. A new venture for Stephanie is delivering mental health and resilience training to senior managers within global organizations across the UK and Europe, including the NHS.

Nick Dupree is an artist, activist and writer in New York City. He has been on different forms of mechanical ventilation since 1992, and is best known for his campaign in Alabama, "Nick's Crusade," which ended in a new Medicaid program to extend home care past age 21 for vent-dependent Alabamians. He studied at Spring Hill College, a Jesuit college in his hometown, Mobile, AL on the Gulf coast. He works to articulate and advocate for the interests of people on ventilators, and in addition to writing for VENTure Think Tank (www.stonybrook.edu/commcms/venture), he blogs about topics as varied as the constitution, Medicaid, and nineteenth century America, at www.nickscrusade.org. The collected Bloggings of Ventboy Alcatraz can be found at: http://www.nickscrusade.org/coler-chronicles-collected-bloggings-of-institutionalization/.

Gelya Frank is a founding contributor to occupational science and a leading scholar of life history and life story approaches. She received her BA, MA, and PhD degrees in Anthropology at the University of California, Los Angeles. Dr. Frank is a past president of the Society for Humanistic Anthropology, has served on the Board of Directors of the American Anthropological Association, and is on numerous editorial boards including Journal of Occupational Science. Her book, "Venus on Wheels: Two Decades of Dialogue on Disability, Biography, and Being Female in America," received the 2000 Eileen Basker Memorial Prize of the Society of Medical Anthropology. Dr. Frank is a two-time recipient of the Phi Kappa Phi Faculty Recognition Award. She was named a 2002–2003 National Endowment for the Humanities Resident Scholar at the School of American Research in Santa Fe, New Mexico, to author a book reconstructing the lived experience of a nineteenth-century Native Californian tribal community.

Michele Friedner, Ph.D. is an Assistant Professor of Health and Rehabilitation Sciences at the State University of New York, Stony Brook. A medical anthropologist, Michele has mostly worked in urban areas of India with sign language-using deaf young adults. Michele is interested in how changes in India's political economy have impacted deaf people and disabled people and how they engage in social, moral, and economic practices to create inhabitable worlds and better futures for themselves. More broadly, Michele is interested in the relationship between stigma and value and how disability is seen as possessing social, moral, political, and economic value in neo-liberal times. Michele has received funding for her work from the National Science Foundation, the American Institute for Indian Studies, and UC Berkeley. She is a former postdoctoral fellow in the Massachusetts Institute of Technology's Anthropology program.

Annicia Gayle-Geddes, Ph.D. is Visiting Scholar, at the Sir Arthur Lewis Institute of Social and Economic Studies, University of the West Indies, Mona and Program Manager of the National Poverty Reduction Coordination in Jamaica. She is a social policy and program development, monitoring and evaluation practitioner. Dr. Gayle-Geddes has conducted Caribbean research and related training in disability studies, poverty reduction, social protection, health, community development, public safety, agriculture, tourism and public sector management. She has served as member of the National Disability Advisory Board and the National Disability Act Committee as well as Chairperson of the National Consultation Committee for a National Disability Act in Jamaica.

Marg Hall was born in 1947 in Rochester, NY, the hometown of Susan B. Anthony. She has been a lifelong social justice activist. She stopped working in 2006 because of disability (chronic pain). When some street activists came into her neighborhood and set up tents, she was happily recruited into a community of disability rights activists. She used to be a nun, but now is a neo-pagan witch, practicing earth-based spirituality. She lives in Berkeley California with her wife, Elaine, and continues to be part of a lively community of troublemakers.

Joy Hammel, Ph.D., OTRL, FAOTA. is a Professor in Occupational Therapy and Disability Studies at the University of Illinois at Chicago. She also holds the Wade/Meyer Endowed Chair in Occupational Therapy. She received her PhD in Educational Psychology from the University of California at Berkeley. Her scholarship focuses on community-based participatory research related to community living and participation choice, control and societal opportunity with people who are aging with disabilities and disability and aging communities. This includes: (1) research to identify key environmental barriers and supports to least restrictive community living and full societal participation and their impact on health outcomes, (2) research to create and test new assessment tools and item banks to evaluate participation disparities, and (3) participatory intervention research to effect systems change and social justice, action plan environmental and policy issues, and build community capacity related to community living and participation. She has served as Principal Investigator on grants from NIDRR, NIH and the Retirement Research Foundation, and has served as Chair of the NCMRR Advisory Board and Executive Director of the Society for Disability Studies.

Tobias Hecht, Ph.D. received his PhD in social anthropology from Cambridge. He is the author of *At Home in the Street: Street Children of Northeast Brazil* (Cambridge UP), which won the Margaret Mead Award, and *After Life: An Ethnographic Novel* (Duke UP). He has received research awards from the H.F. Guggenheim Foundation, NSF, NEH and other institutions. He won second prize in the Hucha de Oro, which attracts more than 5,000 entries each year, for a short story.

Devva Kasnitz, Ph.D. trained as a cultural geographer at Clark University and then as a medical anthropologist at The University of Michigan, with postdoctoral work at Northwestern University and at the University of California, San Francisco in health policy and disability. She has worked in the area of disability studies for the last 34 years while still maintaining an interest in ethnicity and immigration. She was on the founding boards of: the Society for Disability Studies, the Anthropology and Disability Research Interest Group, and the Association of Programs for Rural Independent Living, and has mentored a generation of disability studies scholars in the US, Australia, and Guatemala. She has directed research at the World Institute on Disability and the Association of Higher Education and Disability. She is currently Adjunct Professor at the City University of New York. She has received research funding from NIH, NIMH, NIDRR, the American Anthropological Association, The Felton Bequest, and Sprint Foundation. She was a 2000 NIDRR Switzer Fellow and is the 2014 recipient of the Society for Disability Studies, Senior Scholar Award. She was the Director of a California independent living center and currently represents disabled citizens on the state Telecommunications Access for the Deaf and Disabled Administrative Committee, California. Her current work focuses on speech impairment and the politics of social participation and on disability services in higher education. With Pamela Block, a book on speech impairment is forthcoming. She lives in Northern California behind the redwood curtain surrounded by her family and by spinning wheels, looms, and baskets full of yarn and fiber waiting to become cloth.

Petra Kuppers, Ph.D. is a disability culture activist, a community performance artist, and Professor of English, Women's Studies, Art and Design and Theatre at the University of Michigan, Ann Arbor. She also teaches in Goddard College's Low Residency MFA in Interdisciplinary Arts. She leads The Olimpias, a performance research collective (www.olimpias.org). Her books include *Disability and Contemporary Performance: Bodies on Edge* (Routledge, 2003), *The Scar of Visibility: Medical Performance and Contemporary Art* (Minnesota, 2007) and *Community Performance: An Introduction* (Routledge, 2007). Edited work includes *Somatic Engagement* (2011), and *Community Performance: A Reader* (2007). Her *Disability Culture and Community Performance: Find a Strange and Twisted Shape* (Palgrave, 2011, paperback 2013) explores The Olimpias' arts-based research methods, and won the Biennial Sally Banes Prize by the American Society for Theatre Research. She is also the author of a textbook, *Studying Disability Arts and Culture: An Introduction* (Palgrave, 2014).

Jessica Lehman is proud to serve as Executive Director at San Francisco Senior and Disability Action, an organization committed to mobilizing seniors and people with disabilities to fight for justice on health care, housing, transportation and other issues. She previously worked as a community organizer at ACORN and then at an independent living center, where she founded the Disability Action Network, a grassroots group of people with disabilities building a voice for their community. As a person with a disability who employs home attendants, Jessica supports domestic worker rights as a founding member and leader of Hand in Hand: the Domestic Employers Network. She leads monthly Organizer's Forum calls, as part of the National Disability Leadership Alliance, to share ideas and experiences related to organizing the disability community. Jessica coaches and plays on a power soccer team in Hayward and loves to cook in her home in Oakland, California.

Rachel Liebert, Originally from Aotearoa New Zealand, I am a PhD Candidate in Critical Psychology and an Adjunct Professor in Interdisciplinary and Disability Studies at the City University of New York. Previous research projects have interrogated SSRI-induced violence and the rise in 'bipolar disorder' diagnoses, and my dissertation uses ethnography to trace the circulation of 'paranoia' within the neoliberal security state. This work has been published in Social Science & Medicine, Women's Studies Quarterly, The Journal of Theoretical and Philosophical Psychology, and Affilia, among others, as well as mobilized for creative, collaborative activism against the privatization and policing of our psyches, bodies, and desires through the 'mental health', 'sexual health', 'criminal justice', and 'public education' industries. At this time I am also co-editing a Special Feature for Feminism & Psychology on/by/with 'young feminists' and conducting participatory action research with young people living in public housing in Brooklyn. Overall I am committed to participatory, performative, and non-imperialist epistemologies – interested ultimately in how to nourish spaces for dissent, imagination, and connection.

Susan Magasi, Ph.D. is Assistant Professor, Department of Occupational Therapy. Dr. Magasi earned her PhD in Disability Studies at the University of Illinois at Chicago. Upon completion of her post-doctoral fellowships in outcomes and health services research at the Rehabilitation Institute of Chicago and Northwestern University's Feinberg School of Medicine, Dr. Magasi joined David Cella's Center for Outcomes Research and Education before accepting a faculty position in the Department of Medical Social Science at Northwestern University. Dr. Magasi served as a co-investigator on several major NIH-funded instrument development initiatives including the NIH Toolbox Assessment for Neurological and Behavioral and the NIH PROMIS Initiative. Dr. Magasi is a qualitative methodologist on numerous federal, foundation and industry-sponsored research grants. A frequent guest lecturer in qualitative methods, Dr. Magasi has presented her qualitative work nationally and internationally. She is the co-editor of the forthcoming special issue "Current Thinking in Qualitative Research: Evidence-based practice, moral philosophies, and political struggle" in the journal *OTJR: Occupation, Participation, and Health*. Dr. Magasi is deeply committed to the identification and elimination of health and healthcare disparities experienced by people with disabilities. Based on a deep-seated belief that people who experience health and participation inequities are best situated to identify both the source of their own inequities and potential solutions, she favors the use of mixed methods research within a community-based participatory research model.

Neil Marcus is an icon in US disability culture. In the 1980s and 1990s, he performed his stage show *Storm Reading* over 300 times all over the US, the UK and Canada. Parts of it were on Maria Shrivers Sunday Today Show. Neil has also written and performed other plays in the SF Bay Area, and is a frequent guest in Butoh and Contact Improv Festivals. His philosophy, art, performance and teachings speak to the idea that we cannot afford to judge or put limits on one another (including ourselves) because we as inter-related beings are limitless. His plays and dances have been staged all over the world since the 1980's. His poetry has found its way to many people, on the back of fridge magnets, policy statements for NGOs, university reading lists, and in many people's private stash of important things to know about life. His poem Disabled Country has been a keystone of the disability arts movement. Neil is still recognized in the street for his role in an episode of ER. Neil engages in his own ongoing street theater show, singing, clowning and performing in the everyday. His book *Special Effects* was published in 2011 by Publication Studio. *Cripple Poetics: A Love Story*, in collaboration with Petra Kuppers, was published in 2008 by Homofactus press.

Anahi Guedes de Mello, is a Ph.D. student in anthropology at the Graduate Program in Social Anthropology, at the Federal University of Santa Catarina (UFSC), in Florianopolis, Brazil. She is a Researcher of the Nucleus of Gender Identity and Subjectivities (NIGs), at the UFSC's Department of Anthropology, and of the Nucleus of Disability Studies (NED), at the UFSC's Department of Psychology. She has been developing research around the following themes: gender and disability, crip theory, sexualities, violence against women with disabilities, accessibility in communication, assistive technology and inclusive education—always focusing on the Brazilian reality.

Mansha Mirza, Ph.D., OTR/L, MSHSOR, Assistant Professor in the Department of Occupational Therapy at the University of Illinois at Chicago. She has an interdisciplinary background in occupational therapy, health services research, and disability studies. Dr. Mirza's research and academic interests focus on delivery of disability and health related services in resource-limited situations of humanitarian relief, experiences of refugees with disabilities in resettlement and in refugee camps, and health disparities among refugees and immigrants settled in the US. Dr. Mirza has been awarded multiple grants to fund her research in this area. She has presented at several national conferences and has numerous publications to her credit including 14 peer-reviewed journal articles and three book chapters.

Leroy F. Moore Jr. is a Black writer, poet, hip-hop\music lover, community activist and feminist with a physical disability. He has been sharing his perspective on identity, race & disability for the last 13 years or so. His work began in London, England where he discovered a Black Disabled Movement which help led to the creation of his lecture series: *On the Outskirts: Race & Disability*. Leroy is Co-founder of the Sins Invalid performance project and its Community Relations Director. Leroy is also a contributing writer and performer for many Sins Invalid shows. He is also the creator of Krip-Hop Nation (Hip-Hop artists with disabilities and other disabled musicians from around the world) and produced Krip-Hop Mixtape Series. With Binki wio of Germany and Lady MJ of the UK, he started what is now known as Mees With Disabilities, an international movement. Leroy formed one of the first organizations for people of color with disabilities in the San Francisco Bay area that lasted 5 years. He is founding member and current

Chair of the Black Disability Studies Working Group with the National Black Disability Coalition. Leroy was Co Host of a radio show in San Francisco at KPOO 89.5 FM, Berkeley at KPFA 94.1 FM. He has studied, worked and lectured in the field of race and disability concerning blues, hip-hop, and social justice issues in the United States, United Kingdom, Canada and South Africa. Leroy is one of the leading voices around police brutality and wrongful incarceration of people with disabilities and has studied, worked and lectured in the field of race and disability concerning blues, hip-hop, and social justice issues in the US, UK, Canada and the Netherlands. Leroy is currently writing a Krip-Hop book with Professor Terry Rowden and working on his poetry/lyrics book, *The Black Kripple Delivers Poetry & Lyrics*. Leroy has won many awards for his advocacy from the San Francisco Mayor's Disability Council under Willie L. Brown to the Local Hero Award in 2002 from Public Television Station, KQED in San Francisco. Leroy has interviewed hip-hop\soul\blues\jazz artists with disabilities; the Blind Boys of Alabama, Jazz elder Jimmy Scott, Hip-Hop star, Wonder Mike of the Sugar Hill Gang, DJ Quad of LA, Paraplegic MC of Chicago, Rob DA Noize Temple of New York to name a few. Leroy has a poetry CD, entitled *Black Disabled Man with a Big Mouth & A High I.Q.* and has put out his second poetry CD entitled *The Black Kripple Delivers Krip Love Mixtape*. Leroy is a longtime columnist, one of the first columns on race & disability that started in the early 90's at Poor Magazine in San Francisco www.poormagazine.org, Illin-N-Chillin. kriphopnation@gmail.com blackkrip@gmail.com Facebook/kriphopnation, https://twitter.com/kriphopnation

Denise M. Nepveux, Ph.D. is an Assistant Professor of Occupational Therapy at Utica College. She received her Ph.D. in disability studies from University of Illinois at Chicago and a postdoctoral fellowship from Syracuse University. Since 2011, she has engaged in elder community organizing with the Ida Benderson Seniors Action Group of Syracuse, NY. As a 2002 Fulbright Scholar, Denise documented life stories of women in Ghana's disability movement. She continues to study activism, cultural production, development and policy on disability in Africa. She has also published participatory research on sexual health knowledge, identity and access of LGBT youth self-advocates in Ontario. A believer in melding scholarship, arts and community work, she creates populist musical theater with the Dream Freedom Revival of Central New York.

Akemi Nishida is a Ph.D. candidate in Critical Social Personality Psychology at The Graduate Center of The City University of New York. She is also a faculty member of the Disability Studies, MA. program at the CUNY School of Professional Studies. Her dissertation critically examines relationship building between poor disabled people receiving long-term care via Medicaid and their care providers, and how this relationship (or solidarity) building is impacted by the neoliberal public care system and various social injustices. In her narrative Nishida advocates for a role of interdependence as a means to resist neoliberalism and actualize a just society. Particularly, she practices and writes about ways to nurture interdependent relationships among those who embody different capacities, needs, and social standpoints. Such topics are also explored in her previous research concerning political development of disability rights and justice activists, coming of age experiences for disabled young women, and resistance against neoliberal academia. She has received research funding from the American Association of University Women, YAI National Institute for People with Disabilities, and the CUNY Graduate Center. Nishida is a current member of The Disability Justice Collective, and a former organizer for the People of Color Caucus for the Society for Disability Studies. Working alongside of her fellow NYC disability activists, Nishida started Krips Occupy Wall Street (later dubbed the Disability Caucus) concurrent with the rise of Occupy Wall Street. Her research, teaching, and community organizing value artful, accessible, liberating, and collective methodologies. She strives to learn about, create, and practice caring collectives with a diverse groups and in various spheres.

Adriano Henrique Nuernberg, Ph.D. is a researcher and professor in the area of disability studies and educational psychology. His work seeks to promote the social model perspective, and to explain the importance of removing barriers to social participation of people with disabilities. At the university level he has developed several studies aimed at promoting equal access to knowledge for students with disabilities. As a teacher, he guides research and extension work that results in the better inclusion of children and youth with disabilities. He was recognized with three national awards for his work related to disability and human rights perspectives. He has published several articles that advocate equality for people with disabilities in education and health. Dr. Nuernberg is currently interested in the field of Disability Studies in Education as a powerful field to support his work related about inclusive education.

Marta Peres, Ph.D. is a teacher (UFRJ/Universidade Federal do Rio de Janeiro), PhD in Sociology (University of Brasilia/UnB, 2005), post-PhD in Anthropology (IFCS/UFRJ, 2006) and she is participating now in another post-PhD program at the University of São Paulo (USP), in Diversitas – studies of diversity, intolerance and conflict. She works in different disciplines offered to undergraduate Dance courses. She graduated in Contemporary Dance (Angel Vianna, 1990) and in Physical Therapy (IBMR, 1995), has a master's degree in Health Sciences (UnB, 2000). She worked as a dance teacher at Rehabilitation Sarah Hospital with patients and inpatients with different kind of disabilities (1996/2000). She coordinates Paratodos, a teaching/research/extension Project in dance & health, which involves people being treated in mental health services, people with physical and visual disabilities. She directed the dance/theater play "The Quantic of the Bodies" (Brasilia/2004) of "Wheels Company," a group with wheelchair users and non-disabled dancers, "68 to Vera" (Rio/2008), was one of the choreographers of scenic cantata "Carmina Burana" (Rio/2009) and collaborated with the Norwegian group "Non-Stop Theater," linked to social work Graduation and participants with disabilities, the University of Namsos, Norway (2011). She participated and presented papers at Spinal Cord Injury Congress in Beijing (China, 2003), at the "Festival of the Moving Body" (Stony Brook University, Long Island, New York, 2012), and Hemi Convergence (LA, 2013) with Healing Arts Collective.

Nick Pollard, Ph.D. is a senior lecturer in Occupational Therapy at Sheffield Hallam University (since 2003) and previously worked in psychiatric settings. He and his colleagues in the profession have been concerned with developing a socially committed stance within occupational therapy. He has co-edited a number of key books which critically explore aspects of occupational therapy practices and their political context: *Occupational Therapy Without Borders* (2005, second volume 2010), *A Political Practice of Occupational Therapy* (2008), and the *Politics of Occupation-Centered Practice* (2012). This writing contributed to his 2014 PhD thesis, by publication. Nick has also authored papers on community based rehabilitation, meaningfulness and occupation, and writing activities and community publication. He co-edited an expanded second edition of Morley and Worpole's *The Republic of Letters* (2009), about the UK community publishing movement. Between 2010 and 2014 he was a director and chairperson of Pecket Learning Community, a peer-tuition led basic adult education college archiving project. Between 1990 and 2007 he was a director and magazine editor for the Federation of Worker Writers and Community Publishers.

Eva L. Rodriguez, Ph.D., OTR/L is the Program Chairperson of the Occupational Therapy Program at Stony Brook University in Stony Brook, NY since 2010 and has been a faculty member at that program since 1996. Eva holds a Doctorate of Philosophy in Post-Secondary and Adult Education from Capella University, a Masters of Sciences in Post-Secondary and Adult Education, also from Capella University, a Master's of Arts from Leslie University on Pediatric Dysphagia, and a Bachelor's of Sciences in Occupational Therapy from City University of New York at York College. Eva holds certifications in the models of practice of Sensory Integration and also in Neurodevelopmental Treatment. She is also a mother and an occupational therapist (since 1984) that has learned to advocate for changes in the school system because her son has taught her a different viewpoint. Eva has worked in the school systems for 24 years as an occupational therapist and continues to have a strong interest in research of self-determination and self-advocacy in youth with disabilities. She has done research and has co published articles addressing these areas in youth with Pediatric Multiple Sclerosis. Eva wrote a grant for the Bethel Hobbs Farm in Centereach, NY, a volunteer run farm, to provide accessibility for all volunteers within the community. The faculty and students at the Stony Brook University Occupational Therapy Program then build the accessible garden. She is currently working with Nassau BOCES and the Community Engagement and Development Program of School of Health Technology and Management at Stony Brook, to identify factors that limit students with disabilities in attending large 4 year colleges. Eva is also currently attending training sessions to be a Certified Driver Rehabilitation Specialist.

Katherine D. Seelman, Ph.D. is Associate dean of Disability Programs and Professor of Rehabilitation Science and Technology at the School of Health and Rehabilitation Sciences, University of Pittsburgh. She holds secondary appointments in the School of Public Health and the Center for Bioethics, and an adjunct position at Xian Jiatong University, China. Formerly serving as Co-Research Director she is now Senior Policy Adviser for the National Science Foundation-supported Quality of Life Technology Engineering Research Center which is housed in the Robotics Institute at Carnegie Mellon University. Seelman has a lifetime interest in science, technology, public policy and disability. President Obama appointed her to the National Council on Disability in May 2014. She was one of two from the US serving on the World Health Organization's 9-member international editorial committee to guide the development of the first *World Report on Disability* and presented a chapter of the Report, for which she was a principal author for information technology, in 2011 at the United Nations. During the Clinton Administration, she served for 7 years as the Director of the National Institute on Disability and Rehabilitation Research in Washington, D.C. She was the recipient of the University of Pittsburgh Chancellor's Distinguished Service Award in 2007. Dr. Seelman, who is hard-of-hearing, serves as adviser to the University's Students for Disability Advocacy and is co-chair of the City of Pittsburgh-Allegheny County Task Force on Disability. She is widely published and the recipient of many awards.

José Otavio Pompeu e Silva, Ph.D., OTRL has a degree in Occupational Therapy from the Federal University of São Carlos (1999), Master of Arts from the State University of Campinas (2006) and Doctorate of Arts from the State University of Campinas (2011). He conducted postdoctoral studies at the PACC/UFRJ (2012). He has specialized in management of Distance Education at Lante/UFF. He is currently an assistant professor at the Federal University of Rio de Janeiro in Tércio Pacitti Institute of Computer Applications and Research (NCE/UFRJ), where develops research in neuroscientific and computational interfaces. He has experience in the area of digital culture, accessibility, rehabilitation, art and mental health.

Jean Stewart, a writer and activist, became disabled in '78 as a result of pesticide exposure. This launched a life of disability and environmental activism and mid-wifed her acclaimed novel, The Body's Memory (St. Martin's Press). Her stories, poems, and essays have been widely anthologized. Jean Stewart has been a music school director, concert/festival producer, research botanist, blueberry raker, music journalist, special ed teacher, university instructor in women's lit, radio producer, and community organizer. She founded and directed an independent living center in upstate New York; founded and directed the Disabled Prisoners' Justice Fund; and immersed herself in Deaf culture and American Sign Language. Stewart traveled to Cuba for an international disability rights conference; to India for the World Social Forum, where she co-organized a disability rights panel; to Brazil (World Social Forum); and to Mexico, where she spent time with Oaxacan disability rights activists. She actively participates in movements to end war and occupation (including Israel's occupation of Palestine), eliminate the death penalty, support the rights of non-human animals, stop the devastation humans seem determined to wreak on the planet, secure economic justice for all (ie an end to capitalism), and enact single payer health care. One of the proud 99 %, she continues raising hell as a member of CUIDO, Communities United in Defense of Olmstead, a grassroots, in-your-face disability rights group based in Berkeley, CA.

Rick Stoddart is passionate about being regarded as a man in his own right, a thinker, as capable of doing meaningful work and remaining in charge of his own affairs, without regard to the relatively minor matter that he has cerebral palsy.

Sunaura Taylor, MFA is an artist, writer and activist. Taylor's artworks have been exhibited at venues across the country, including the CUE Art Foundation, the Smithsonian Institution and the Berkeley Art Museum. She is the recipient of numerous awards including a Joan Mitchell Foundation MFA Grant and an Animals and Culture Grant. Her written work has been printed in various edited collections as well as in publications such as the Monthly Review, Yes! Magazine, American Quarterly and Qui Parle. Taylor worked with philosopher Judith Butler on Astra Taylor's film *Examined Life* (Zeitgeist 2008). Taylor holds an MFA in art practice from the University of California, Berkeley. Her book Beasts of Burden, which explores the intersections of animal ethics and disability studies, is forthcoming from the Feminist Press. She is currently a PhD student in American Studies in the Department of Social and Cultural Analysis at NYU.

Emmitt H. Thrower was born in Dallas Arkansas and raised in NYC. He is a retired NYC Police Officer and is the founder and President of the not for profit "Wabi Sabi Productions Inc." His mission is to use performance and entertainment to organize and address community issues especially around youth. He has vast experience performing on stage as an actor as well as directing, producing and writing numerous stage plays. He is an experienced Videographer and Editor and is producing several documentary films including one on police brutality against people with disabilities entitled *Where is Hope?*. He is the recipient of the "Katrina Award," the "Independent Spirit Award" in culture, as well as being an AUDELCO award nominated actor. Emmitt has been the Chair of the "Otto Awards" for political theater in NYC since its inception in 1998. He is a member of Actors Equity. And best of all he is married and the proud father of three grown sons. (See: et34888@aol.com, www.oldlionsstillroar.com, www. wabisabiproductions.com/, www.whereishope.webs.com)

Tiny aka Lisa Gray-Garcia is a poverty scholar, revolutionary journalist, teacher, Po' Poet and welfareQUEEN, Mixed Race, Boriken-Taino, Roma mama of Tiburcio, daughter of Dee, and the co–founder of POOR Magazine/Prensa POBRE/PoorNewsNetwork. She founded Escuela de la gente/PeopleSkool- a poor and indigenous people-led skool and the Race, Poverty Media Justice Institute which trains people with race, class or formal education privilege how to implement Revolutionary Giving as well as the Po Poets Project, welfareQUEENs & the

Theatre of the POOR to name a few. She is also the author of Criminal of Poverty: Growing Up Homeless in America, co-editor of A Decolonizers Guide to A Humble Revolution, Born & Raised in Frisco (a series of Anti-gentrification narratives) The DGZ—De-Gentrification Zones—a poor people-led plan to anti-gentrification and currently working on her second book—*Poverty SkolaShip #101: A PeoplesTeXt*. In 2011 she co-launched The Homefulness Project—a landless peoples, self-determined land liberation movement in the Ohlone territory known as Deep East Oakland (Ohlone Land), CalifaZtlan, Turtle Island. In 2014 she launched a curriculum and series of workshops centered around a concept she calls Community Reparations and Revolutionary Giving to support other poor and indigenous people-led movements. (See: www.tinygraygarcia.com, www.racepovertymediajustice.org)

David Turnbull is a freelance writer, occupational philosopher, teacher of ethics, disability advocate and environmental activist. His interests include writing philosophically about human occupation (see http://nodangerousthoughts.com/), the ongoing intellectual development of older people through involvement in the University of the Third Age, teaching ethics to therapy and medical students, advocating for people with disability against perceived injustice, and being involved in efforts to protect endangered species and habitats in the environment where he lives.

Melanie Yergeau, Ph.D. is an autistic activist and an Assistant Professor of English at the University of Michigan. She has published in *College English*, *Disability Studies Quarterly*, *Computers and Composition Online*, and *Kairos: A Journal of Rhetoric, Technology, and Pedagogy*. Additionally, Melanie is an editor for Computers and Composition Digital Press, an imprint of Utah State University Press. She is a co-author of the *SAGE Reference Series on Disability: Arts and Humanities* and co-editor of the disability and rhetoric special issue of DSQ. Melanie has served on the boards of the Autistic Self-Advocacy Network (ASAN) and the Autism National Committee. She is currently at work on a book project titled *Authoring Autism*.

Index

© Springer Science+Business Media Dordrecht 2016
P. Block et al. (eds.), *Occupying Disability: Critical Approaches to Community, Justice, and Decolonizing Disability*, DOI 10.1007/978-94-017-9984-3